FIRST AID

SURGERY clerkship

THE STUDENT TO STUDENT GUIDE

SERIES EDITORS:

LATHA G. STEAD, MD
Assistant Professor of Emergency Medicine
Mayo Medical School
Rochester, Minnesota

S. MATTHEW STEAD, MD, PhD
Fellow in Pediatric Neurology
Mayo Graduate School of Medicine
Rochester, Minnesota

MATTHEW S. KAUFMAN, MD
Resident in Internal Medicine
Long Island Jewish Medical Center
New Hyde Park, New York

TITLE EDITORS:

NISHANT ANAND
Mayo Medical School
Class of 2004

TARA SOTSKY KENT, MD
Resident in General Surgery
Montefiore Medical Center
Albert Einstein College of Medicine
Bronx, New York

McGraw-Hill
Medical Publishing Division

New York   Chicago   San Francisco   Lisbon   London   Madrid
Mexico City   Milan   New Delhi   San Juan   Seoul
Singapore   Sydney   Toronto

First Aid for the® Surgery Clerkship

Copyright © 2003 by The **McGraw-Hill** Companies, Inc. All rights reserved. Printed in the United States of America. Except as permitted under the United States Copyright Act of 1976, no part of this publication may be reproduced or distributed in any form or by any means, or stored in a data base or retrieval system, without the prior written permission of the publisher.

4 5 6 7 8 9   CUS/CUS   0 9 8 7 6 5

ISBN 0-07-136422-6

Notice

Medicine is an ever-changing science. As new research and clinical experience broaden our knowledge, changes in treatment and drug therapy are required. The authors and the publisher of this work have checked with sources believed to be reliable in their efforts to provide information that is complete and generally in accord with the standards accepted at the time of publication. However, in view of the possibility of human error or changes in medical sciences, neither the authors nor the publisher nor any other party who has been involved in the preparation or publication of this work warrants that the information contained herein is in every respect accurate or complete, and they disclaim all responsibility for any errors or omissions or for the results obtained from use of the information contained in this work. Readers are encouraged to confirm the information contained herein with other sources. For example and in particular, readers are advised to check the product information sheet included in the package of each drug they plan to administer to be certain that the information contained in this work is accurate and that changes have not been made in the recommended dose or in the contraindications for administration. This recommendation is of particular importance in connection with new or infrequently used drugs.

This book was set in Goudy by Rainbow Graphics.
The editor was Catherine A. Johnson.
The production supervisor was Catherine Saggese.
Project management was provided by Rainbow Graphics.
The index was prepared by Angie Wiley Indexing Services
Von Hoffmann was the printer and binder.
This book is printed on acid-free paper.

Cataloging-in-Publication Data is on file for this title at the Library of Congress.

Contributing Authors

GAL AHARONOV, MD
Resident in General Surgery
University of Southern California
Los Angeles, California
Ear, Nose, and Throat

ALEJANDRO BAEZ, MD
Resident in Emergency Medicine
Mayo Graduate School of Medicine
Rochester, Minnesota
Hernia and Abdominal Wall Problems

KENNETH CHENG, MD
Resident in Anesthesia
Montefiore Medical Center
Bronx, New York
Anesthesia; The Pancreas

JASON HATFIELD, MD
Resident in Emergency Medicine
Jacobi-Montefiore EM Program
Bronx, New York
Fluids, Electrolytes, and Nutrition; Pediatric Surgery

MICHELLE HIGLEY, MD
Resident in Anesthesia
The Appendix; The Spleen

LAURIE KIRSTEIN, MD
Resident in General Surgery
Montefiore Medical Center
Bronx, New York
The Hepatobiliary System

JORDAN MOSKOFF, MD
Resident in Emergency Medicine
Jacobi-Montefiore EM Program
Bronx, New York
Critical Care

VIPUL PATEL, MD
Resident in Orthopedic Surgery
New York University
New York, New York
Orthopedics

TODD PATRICK, MD
Resident in Neurosurgery
Mayo Graduate School of Medicine
Rochester, Minnesota
Neurosurgery

LEON SANCHEZ, MD
Instructor in Emergency Medicine
Beth Israel Deaconess Hospital
Boston, Massachusetts
Trauma

VERNON SMITH. MD
Resident in Emergency Medicine
Mayo Graduate School of Medicine
Rochester, Minnesota
Cardiothoracic Surgery

ROGER TILLOTSON, MD
Resident in Emergency Medicine
State University of New York at Brooklyn
Brooklyn, New York
The Esophagus; Wounds

JESSICA WANG, MD
Attending in Emergency Medicine
Jacobi Medical Center
Bronx, New York
The Genitourinary System

MUHAMMAD WASEEM, MD, FAAP
Assistant Professor of Emergency Medicine
Weill Medical College, Cornell University
New York, New York
Pediatric Surgery

Contents

Introduction

This clinical study aid was designed in the tradition of the *First Aid* series of books. It is formatted in the same way as the other books in the series. You will find that rather than simply preparing you for success on the clerkship exam, this resource will also help guide you in the clinical diagnosis and treatment of many of the problems seen by surgeons.

The content of the book is based on the objectives for medical students laid out by the Association for Surgical Education (ASE). Each of the chapters contain the major topics central to the practice of general surgery and have been specifically designed for the third-year medical student learning level. The book is divided into general surgery, which contains topics that comprise the core of the rotation, and subspecialty surgery, which may be of interest but is generally considered not as high yield for the clerkship. Knowledge of a subspecialty topic may be useful if observing a related surgery, or if requesting a letter from a surgeon in this field.

The content of the text is organized in the format similar to other texts in the *First Aid* series. Topics are listed by bold headings, and the "meat" of the topic provides essential information. The outside margins contain mnemonics, diagrams, summary or warning statements and tips. Tips are categorized into Exam Tip , Ward Tip , and OR Tip .

Acknowledgments

We would like to thank the following individuals for their help with this manuscript:

MEDICAL STUDENT REVIEWER
Erik P. Hess
University of Alabama at Birmingham
Class of 2002

FACULTY REVIEWERS
Arun Chervu, MD, FACS
Vascular Surgeon, Private Practice
Vascular Surgical Associates, PC
Marietta, Georgia

Daniel Cullinane, MD, FACS
Consultant, Dept. of Trauma, Critical and General Surgery
ATLS Course Director
Mayo Clinic
Rochester, Minnesota

Stephanie Donnelly, MD
Fellow, Dept. of Trauma, Critical and General Surgery
Mayo Clinic
Rochester, Minnesota

David Farley, MD, FACS
Consultant, Dept. of Trauma, Critical and General Surgery
General Surgery Residency Program Director
Mayo Clinic
Rochester, Minnesota

Michael S. Malian, MD, FACS
General Surgeon, Private Practice
Minneapolis, Minnesota

Gregory J. Schears, MD
Assistant Professor of Anesthesiology and Pediatrics
Mayo Clinic
Rochester, Minnesota

Deepak Talreja, MD
Fellow, Dept. of Cardiology
Mayo Clinic
Rochester, Minnesota

We also wish to thank Drs. Luis Haro and Annie Sadosty for contributing vascular and cervical spine images from their personal library, and Ms. Julie Montgomery for her help in securing permissions.

How to Succeed in the Surgery Clerkship

The surgery clerkship is unique among all the medical school rotations. Even if you are dead sure you do not want to be a surgeon, it can be a very fun and rewarding experience if you approach it prepared. There are three key components to the rotation: (1) what to do in the OR, (2) what to do on the wards, and (3) how to study for the exam.

IN THE OPERATING ROOM . . .

One of the most fun things on the surgery rotation is the opportunity to scrub in on surgical cases. The number and types of cases you will scrub in on depends on the number of residents and students on that service and how busy the service is that month. At some places, being able to go to the OR is considered a privilege rather than a routine part of the rotation. A few tips:

- **Eat before you begin the case.** Some cases can go on for longer than planned and it isn't cool to leave early because you are hungry (read unprepared!) or, worse, to pass out from exhaustion. As a student, your function in the OR will most likely be to hold retraction. This can be tedious, but it is important to pay attention and do a good job. Not pulling in the right direction obscures the view for your attending, and pulling too hard can destroy tissue. Many students get light-headed standing in one position for an extended period of time, especially when they are not used to it. Make sure you shift your weight and bend your knees once in a while so you don't faint. If you feel you are going to faint, then say something—ask one of the surgical techs to take over or state discreetly that you need relief. Do not hold on to the bitter end, pass out, and take the surgical field with you (believe it or not, this has actually happened; we print this advice from real experience).
- **Find out about the case as much as possible beforehand.** Usually, the OR schedule is posted the night before, so you should be able to tell. Read up on the procedure as well as the pathophysiology of the underlying condition. Know the important anatomic landmarks.
- **Find out who you are working with.** If you can, do a quick bibliography search on the surgeon you will be working with. It can never hurt to know which papers (s)he has written, and this may help to spark conversation and distinguish you among the many other students they will have met.
- **Assess the mood in the OR.** The amount of conversation in the OR directed to you varies by attending. Some are very into teaching and will engage you during most of the surgery. Many others act as if you aren't even there. Some will interact if you make the first move; others nuke all efforts at interaction. You'll have to figure it out based on the situation. Generally, if your questions and comments reflect that you have read about the procedure and disease, things will go well.
- **Keep a log of all surgeries** you have attended, scrubbed on, or assisted with (see Figure 1-1). If you are planning to go into general surgery or a surgical subspecialty, it can be useful during residency interviews for conveying how much exposure/experience you have had. This is particularly true if your school's strength is clinical experience. The log can also be useful if you are requesting a letter from the chairman of surgery whom you have never worked with. It gives her/him an idea of what you have been doing with your rotation. Many rotations will set a minimum number of surgeries you are to attend. Try to attend as many as possible, and document them. This serves both to increase your exposure, and confirm your interest.

	Operation	S/O	Attending	Date	MR #	Comments
1	Cholecystectomy	S	Dr. Wolfe	5/28/2003	123456	Got to close, placed 28 nonabsorbable sutures
2	Appendectomy	S	Dr. Tau	5/30/2003	246800	Used laparoscope
3	Cataract surgery	O	Dr. Mia	6/1/2003	135791	

S, scrubbed in; O, observed; MR, patient's medical record number.

FIGURE 1-1. Example of an operative case log.

ON THE WARDS . . .

Be on Time

Most surgical ward teams begin rounding between 6 and 7 A.M. If you are expected to "pre-round," you should give yourself at least 10 minutes per patient that you are following to see the patient and learn about the events that occurred overnight. Like all working professionals, you will face occasional obstacles to punctuality, but make sure this is occasional. When you first start a rotation, try to show up at least 15 minutes early until you get the routine figured out.

Dress in a Professional Manner

Even if the resident wears scrubs and the attending wears stiletto heels, you must dress in a professional, conservative manner. Wear a *short* white coat over your clothes unless discouraged.

> **Men** should wear long pants, with cuffs covering the ankle, a long collared shirt, and a tie. No jeans, no sneakers, no short-sleeved shirts.
> **Women** should wear long pants or knee-length skirt, blouse or dressy sweater. No jeans, no sneakers, no heels greater than 1½ inches, no open-toed shoes.
> **Both men and women** may wear scrubs occasionally, especially during overnight call or in the operating room. Do not make this your uniform.

Act in a Pleasant Manner

The surgical rotation is often difficult, stressful, and tiring. Smooth out your experience by being nice to be around. Smile a lot and learn everyone's name. If you do not understand or disagree with a treatment plan or diagnosis, do not "challenge." Instead, say "I'm sorry, I don't quite understand, could you please explain . . ." Be empathetic toward patients.

Be Aware of the Hierarchy

The way in which this will affect you will vary from hospital to hospital and team to team, but it is always present to some degree. In general, address your questions regarding ward functioning to interns or residents. Address your medical questions to attendings; make an effort to be somewhat informed on your subject prior to asking attendings medical questions.

Address Patients and Staff in a Respectful Way

Address patients as Sir, Ma'am, or Mr., Mrs., or Miss. Do not address patients as "honey," "sweetie," and the like. Although you may feel that these names are friendly, patients will think you have forgotten their name, that you are being inappropriately familiar, or both. Address all physicians as "doctor" unless told otherwise.

Take Responsibility for Your Patients

Know everything there is to know about your patients, their history, test results, details about their medical problem, and prognosis. Keep your intern or resident informed of new developments that he or she might not be aware of, and ask for any updates you might not be aware of. Assist the team in developing a plan and speaking to radiology, consultants, and family. Never give bad news to patients or family members without the assistance of your supervising resident or attending.

Respect Patients' Rights

1. All patients have the right to have their personal medical information kept private. This means do not discuss the patient's information with family members without that patient's consent, and do not discuss any patient in hallways, elevators, or cafeterias.
2. All patients have the right to refuse treatment. This means they can refuse treatment by a specific individual (you, the medical student) or of a specific type (no nasogastric tube). Patients can even refuse life-saving treatment. The only exceptions to this rule are if the patient is deemed to not have the capacity to make decisions or understand situations (in which case a health care proxy should be sought) or if the patient is suicidal or homicidal.
3. All patients should be informed of the right to seek advanced directives on admission. Often, this is done by the admissions staff, in a booklet. If your patient is chronically ill or has a life-threatening illness, address the subject of advanced directives with the assistance of your attending.

Volunteer

Be self-propelled, self-motivated. Volunteer to help with a procedure or a difficult task. Volunteer to give a 20-minute talk on a topic of your choice. Volunteer to take additional patients. Volunteer to stay late.

Be a Team Player

Help other medical students with their tasks; teach them information you have learned. Support your supervising intern or resident whenever possible. Never steal the spotlight, steal a procedure, or make a fellow medical student look bad.

Be Honest

If you don't understand, don't know, or didn't do it, make sure you always say that. Never say or document information that is false (a common example: "bowel sounds normal" when you did not listen).

Keep Patient Information Handy

Use a clipboard, notebook, or index cards to keep patient information, including a miniature history and physical, lab, and test results at hand.

Present Patient Information in an Organized Manner

Here is a template for the "bullet" presentation:

> This is a [age] year old [gender] with a history of [major history such as HTN, DM, coronary artery disease, CA, etc.] who presented on [date] with [major symptoms, such as cough, fever and chills], and was found to have [working diagnosis]. [Tests done] showed [results]. Yesterday the patient [state important changes, new plan, new tests, new medications]. This morning the patient feels [state the patient's words], and the physical exam is significant for [state major findings]. Plan is [state plan].

The newly admitted patient generally deserves a longer presentation following the complete history and physical format.

Some patients have extensive histories. The whole history can and probably should be present in the admission note, but in ward presentation it is often too much to absorb. In these cases it will be very much appreciated by your team if you can generate a **good summary** that maintains an accurate picture of the patient. This usually takes some thought, but it's worth it.

Presenting the Chest Radiograph (CXR)

A sample CXR presentation may sound like:

> This is the CXR of Mr. Jones. The film is an AP view with good inspiratory effort. There is an isolated fracture of the 8th rib on the right. There is no tracheal deviation or mediastinal shift. There is no pneumo- or hemothorax. The cardiac silhouette appears to be of normal size. The diaphragm and heart borders on both sides are clear; no infiltrates are noted. There is a central venous catheter present, the tip of which is in the superior vena cava.

The key elements of presenting a CXR are summarized in Figure 1-2.

- First, confirm that the CXR belongs to your patient
- If possible, compare to a previous film

Then, present in a systematic manner:
1. *Technique*
   Rotation, anteroposterior (AP) or posteroanterior (PA), penetration, inspiratory effort.

2. *Bony structures*
   Look for rib, clavicle, scapula, and sternum fractures.

3. *Airway*
   Look for tracheal deviation, pneumothorax, pneumomediastinum.

FIGURE 1-2. How to present a chest radiograph (CXR).

4. *Pleural space*
Look for fluid collections, which can represent hemothorax, chylothorax, pleural effusion.

5. *Lung parenchyma*
Look for infiltrates and consolidations: These can represent pneumonia, pulmonary contusions, hematoma, or aspiration. The location of an infiltrate can provide a clue to the location of a pneumonia:

- Obscured right (R) costophrenic angle = right lower lobe
- Obscured left (L) costophrenic angle = left lower lobe
- Obscured R heart border = right middle lobe
- Obscured L heart border = left upper lobe

6. *Mediastinum*
- Look at size of mediastinum—a widened one (> 8 cm) goes with aortic rupture.
- Look for enlarged cardiac silhouette (> ½ thoracic width at base of heart), which may represent congestive heart failure (CHF), cardiomyopathy, hemopericardium, or pneumopericardium.

7. *Diaphragm*
- Look for free air under the diaphragm (suggests perforation).
- Look for stomach, bowel, or NGT tube above diaphragm (suggests diaphragmatic rupture).

8. *Tubes and lines*
- Identify all tubes and lines.
- An endotracheal tube should be 2 cm above the carina. A common mistake is right mainstem bronchus intubation.
- A chest tube (including the most proximal hole) should be in the pleural space (not in the lung parenchyma).
- An NGT tube should be in the stomach, and uncoiled.
- The tip of a central venous catheter (central line) should be in the superior vena cava (not in the right atrium).
- The tip of a Swan–Ganz catheter should be in the pulmonary artery.
- The tip of a transvenous pacemaker should be in the right atrium.

FIGURE 1-2. (Continued)

Types of Notes

In addition to the admission H&P and the daily progress note, there are a few other types of notes you will write on the surgery clerkship. These include the preoperative, operative, postoperative, and procedure notes. Samples of theses are depicted in Figures 1-3 through 1-6.

Under sterile conditions following anesthesia with 5 cc of 2% lidocaine with epinephrine and negative wound exploration for foreign body, the laceration was closed with 3-0 Ethilon sutures. Wound edges were well approximated and no complications occurred. Wound was dressed with sterile gauze and triple antibiotic ointment.

FIGURE 1-3. Sample procedure note (for wound repair).

Pre-op diagnosis:	Abdominal pain
Procedure:	Exploratory laparotomy
Pre-op tests:	List results of labs (CBC, electrolytes, PT, aPTT, urinalysis), ECG, CXR
	(Most adult patients require coagulation studies; patients over 40 usually need ECG and CXR—these are institution specific.)
Blood:	How many units of what type were crossmatched and available; or, "none" if no blood needed
Orders:	e.q., colon prep, NPO after midnight, preoperative antibiotics

FIGURE 1-4. Sample preoperative note.

Pre-op diagnosis:	Abdominal pain
Post-op Dx:	Small bowel obstruction
Procedure:	Segmental small bowel resection with end-to-end anastomosis
Surgeon:	Dr. Attending
Assistant:	Your Name Here
Anesthesia:	GETA (general endotracheal anesthesia)
	EBL (estimated blood loss): 100 cc
	Fluid replacement: 2000 cc crystalloid, 2 units FFP
	UO = 250 cc
Findings:	10 cm of infarcted small bowel
	Dermoid tumor, left ovary
Complications:	None

Wound was clean/clean contaminated/contaminated/dirty. (pick one)

Closure: 0-0 prolene for fascia, 3-0 vicryl SQ staples for skin.

Procedure tolerated well, patient remained hemodynamically stable throughout. Instrument, sponge, and needle counts were correct. Patient was extubated in the OR and transferred to the recovery room in stable condition.

FIGURE 1-5. Sample operative note.

Postoperative day:	1
Procedure:	Colon resection with diverting colostomy
Vitals:	
Intake and output:	For intake include all oral and parenteral fluids and TPN
	For output include everything from all drains, tubes, and Foley
Physical examination:	Note particularly lung and abdominal exam, and comment on wound site.
Labs:	
Assessment:	
Plan:	

FIGURE 1-6. Sample postoperative note.

YOUR ROTATION GRADE

Many students worry about their grade in this rotation. There is the perception that not getting honors in surgery pretty much closes the door to obtaining a residency spot in general or subspecialty surgery (ophthalmology, otorhinolaryngology, neurosurgery, plastic surgery, urology). While this is not necessarily true, the medicine and surgery clerkships are considered to be among the most important in medical school, so doing well in these is handy for all students. Usually, the clerkship grade is broken down into three or four components.

- *Inpatient evaluation.* This includes evaluation of your ward time by residents and attendings and is based on your performance on the ward. Usually, this makes up about half your grade and can be largely subjective.
- *Ambulatory evaluation.* This includes your performance in clinic, including clinic notes and any procedures performed in the outpatient setting.
- *Written examination.* Most schools use the NBME or "Shelf" examination. Some schools have their own homemade version, very similar to the NBME's. The test is multiple choice. This portion of the grade is anywhere from 20% to 40%, so performance on this multiple-choice test is vital to achieving honors in the clerkship. More on this below.
- *Objective Structured Clinical Examination (OSCE).* Some schools now include an OSCE as part of their clerkship evaluation. This is basically an exam that involves a standardized patient and allows assessment of a student's bedside manner and physical examination skills. This may comprise up to one fourth of a student's grade. It is a tool that will probably become more and more popular over the next few years.

HOW TO STUDY

Make a List of Core Material to Learn

This list should reflect common symptoms, illnesses, and areas in which you have particular interest, or in which you feel particularly weak. Do not try to learn every possible topic. The Association for Surgical Education (*www.surgicaleducation.com*) has put forth a manual of surgical objectives for the medical student surgery clerkship, on which this book is based. The ASE emphasizes:

Symptoms and Lab Tests
- Abdominal masses
- Abdominal pain
- Altered mental status
- Breast mass
- Jaundice
- Lung nodule
- Scrotal pain and swelling
- Thyroid mass
- Fluid, electrolyte, and acid–base disorders
- Multi-injured trauma patient

Common Surgeries
- Appendectomy
- Coronary artery bypass grafting (CABG)
- Cholecystectomy
- Exploratory laparotomy
- Breast surgery
- Herniorraphy
- Peptic ulcer disease (PUD) surgery
- Bariatric surgery

We also recommend:
- Preoperative care
- Postoperative care
- Wound infection
- Shock

The core of the general surgery rotation consists of the following chapters:

2. The Surgical Patient
3. Wounds
4. Fluids, Electrolytes, and Nutrition
5. Critical Care
6. Trauma
7. Thermal Injury
8. The Breast
9. Endocrine System
10. Acute Abdomen
11. The Esophagus
12. The Stomach
13. Small Bowel
14. Large Bowel
15. The Appendix
16. The Hepatobiliary System
17. The Pancreas
18. The Spleen
19. Hernia and Abdominal Wall Problems
24. Cardiothoracic Surgery
25. Vascular Surgery

The other chapters are somewhat less important, as they focus on subspecialty surgery. The subspecialty chapters are comprehensive and less "high yield" than the abdominal chapters, but they are an excellent primer for anyone considering going into subspecialty surgery. We kept the detail in these chapters due to feedback from several students who wanted a concise but comprehensive overview of surgical subspecialties.

You will notice that the chapters will discuss pathophysiology and in general a lot of things that seem like they belong in a medicine book. The reason for this is that **the NBME clerkship exam covers the medicine behind surgical disease.** The exam does not ask specifics of operative technique. So, in a way, you are studying for three distinct purposes. The knowledge you need on the wards is the day-to-day management know-how. The knowledge you want in the OR involves surgical knowledge of anatomy and operative technique (see OR TIPs). The knowledge you want on the end of rotation examination is the epidemiology, risk factors, pathophysiology, diagnosis, and treatment of major diseases seen on a general surgery service.

As You See Patients, Note Their Major Symptoms and Diagnosis for Review

Your reading on the symptom-based topics above should be done with a specific patient in mind. For example, if a patient comes to the office with a thyroid mass, read about Graves' disease, Hashimoto's, thyroid cancer, and the technique of needle aspiration in the review book that night.

Select Your Study Material

We recommend:
- This review book, *First Aid for the Surgery Clerkship*
- A major surgery textbook such as *Schwartz's Principles of General Surgery* (costs about $140)
- A full-text online journal database, such as *www.mdconsult.com* (subscription is $99/year for students)
- A small pocket reference book to look up lab values, clinical pathways, and the like, such as *Maxwell Quick Medical Reference* (ISBN 0964519119, costs $7)
- A small book to look up drugs, such as *Pocket Pharmacopoeia* (Tarascon publishers, $8)

Prepare a Talk on a Topic

You may be asked to give a small talk once or twice during your rotation. If not, you should volunteer! Feel free to choose a topic that is on your list; however, realize that this may be considered dull by the people who hear the lecture. The ideal topic is slightly uncommon but not rare, for example: bariatric surgery. To prepare a talk on a topic, read about it in a major textbook or a review article not more than 2 years old, and then search online or in the library for recent developments or changes in treatment.

Procedures

During the course of the surgery clerkship, there is a set of procedures you are expected to learn or at least observe. The common ones are:
- Intravenous line placement
- Nasogastric tube placement
- Venipuncture (blood draw)
- Foley (urinary) catheter placement
- Wound closure with sutures/staples
- Suture/staple removal
- Surgical knots (hand and instrument ties)
- Dressing changes (wet to dry, saline, Vaseline gauze)
- Incision and drainage of abscesses
- Technique of needle aspiration (observe)
- Ankle–brachial index (ABI) measurement
- Evaluation of pulses with Doppler
- Skin biopsy (punch and excisional)
- Removal of surgical drains
- Transillumination of scrotum

If you have read about your core illnesses and core symptoms, you will know a great deal about the medicine of surgery. To study for the clerkship exam, we recommend:

2 to 3 weeks before exam: Read this entire review book, taking notes.
10 days before exam: Read the notes you took during the rotation on your core content list, and the corresponding review book sections.
5 days before exam: Read this entire review book, concentrating on lists and mnemonics.
2 days before exam: Exercise, eat well, skim the book, and go to bed early.
1 day before exam: Exercise, eat well, review your notes and the mnemonics, and go to bed on time. Do not have any caffeine after 2 P.M.

Other helpful studying strategies include:

Study with Friends

Group studying can be very helpful. Other people may point out areas that you have not studied enough, and may help you focus on the goal. If you tend to get distracted by other people in the room, limit this to less than half of your study time.

Study in a Bright Room

Find the room in your house or in your library that has the best, brightest light. This will help prevent you from falling asleep. If you don't have a bright light, get a halogen desk lamp or a light that simulates sunlight (not a tanning lamp).

Eat Light, Balanced Meals

Make sure your meals are balanced, with lean protein, fruits and vegetables, and fiber. A high-sugar, high-carbohydrate meal will give you an initial burst of energy for 1 to 2 hours, but then you'll drop.

Take Practice Exams

The point of practice exams is not so much the content that is contained in the questions, but the training of sitting still for 3 hours and trying to pick the best answer for each and every question.

Tips for Answering Questions

All questions are intended to have one best answer. When answering questions, follow these guidelines:

Read the answers first. For all questions longer than two sentences, reading the answers first can help you sift through the question for the key information.

11

Look for the words EXCEPT, MOST, LEAST, NOT, BEST, WORST, TRUE, FALSE, CORRECT, INCORRECT, ALWAYS, and NEVER. If you find one of these words, circle or underline it for later comparison with the answer.

Evaluate each answer as being either true or false. Example:

Which of the following is *least* likely to be associated with pulmonary embolism?

      A. Tachycardia **T**

      B. Tachypnea **T**

      C. Chest pain ? **F not always**

      D. Deep venous thrombosis ? **T not always**

      E. Back pain **F ? aortic dissection**

By comparing the question, noting LEAST, to the answers, "E" is the best answer.

Finally, as the boy scouts say, "BE PREPARED."

High-Yield Facts

The Surgical Patient

PREOPERATIVE EVALUATION

Assess Risks

- Thorough history and physical exam
- Optimization of any medical problems, i.e., cardiac or pulmonary diseases

Anesthetic History

Note any prior anesthetics and associated complications.

Medications

Know all medications patient is taking.

As a general rule:
- Continue preoperative antihypertensive medications except for diuretics and possibly angiotensin-converting enzyme (ACE) inhibitors.
- Hold aspirin for 10 days.
- Generally hold insulin on day of surgery.
- Consider holding nonsteroidal anti-inflammatory drugs (NSAIDs) and selective COX-2 inhibitors also.

Allergies

Antibiotics are the most common drug allergy.

Social History

Smoking, alcohol, drugs.

The ASA Physical Status Classification System (1999)

System used by American Society of Anesthesiologists to classify patient's preoperative physical status, but does not necessarily predict anesthetic risk. Classification is based on patient's physical exam and medical history, not on the surgery planned.

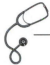

Ask yourself: What does the patient need in order to undergo the operation with the lowest risk possible?

Aspirin and NSAIDs can inhibit platelet activity and exacerbate bleeding.

Smoking increases pulmonary complications under general anesthesia (ideally should stop smoking 8 weeks prior to anesthesia).

P1: A normal, healthy patient
P2: A patient with mild systemic disease
P3: A patient with severe systemic disease
P4: A patient with severe systemic disease that is a constant threat to life
P5: A moribund patient who is not expected to survive without the operation
P6: A declared brain-dead patient whose organs are being removed for donor purposes
E: Indicates emergency surgery designation used in addition to above P codes

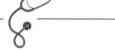
Evaluate Organ Systems

- Consent for the procedure
- Full set of labs, including complete blood count (CBC), chemistries with liver function tests, coags
- Type and hold in blood bank, possibly crossed for several units depending on the case
- Electrocardiogram (ECG)
- Chest x-ray
- Urinalysis (UA)

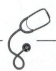
Evaluate Airway

Mallampati Classfication (Figure 2-1) predicts difficulty of intubation. Test is performed with the patient in the sitting position, the head held in a neutral position, the mouth wide open, and the tongue protruding to the maximum.

- *Class I:* Visualization of soft palate, fauces, uvula, anterior and posterior tonsillar pillars
- *Class II:* Visualization of soft palate, fauces, uvula
- *Class III:* Visualization of soft palate, base of uvula
- *Class IV:* Nonvisualization of soft palate

Talk to Patient and/or Family

- Explanation of upcoming operation, its risks, benefits, and alternatives
- Verification of patient's and family's understanding of procedure

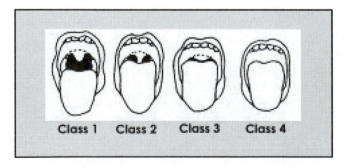

FIGURE 2-1. Mallampati Classification of ease of intubation.

Facts

- Approximately 33% of patients undergoing surgery have coronary artery disease (CAD) or risk factors for it.
- 1 to 2% of patients > 40 years old have perioperative cardiac complications.

Obtain Historical Information

- Previous myocardial infarction (MI)
- Angina
- Cardiac meds
- Hypertension (HTN)
- Vascular disease
- Arrhythmias

Examine Patient

- Assess rate and rhythm.
- Determine origin of any murmurs.
- Note crackles, peripheral edema, or any sign of congestive heart failure (CHF).

Complete Needed Further Workup

- For a patient > 35 years old, with no cardiac history: Obtain ECG (if normal, no further workup required).
- For a patient of any age with cardiac history, or for an older patient: Obtain ECG.
  - Consider stress test and echocardiogram.

Describe Individual Risk

Goldman's risk assessment for noncardiac surgery (see Figure 2-2).
- Relative risk of infarction/cardiac death (%):
  - No previous MI   0.1–0.6
  - MI more than 6 months previous   4
  - Transmural MI within 3 months   37
  - Prior bypass (CABG)   1.2/–
- Risk levels:
  1. **High risk:** History or ECG evidence of infarction, angina, angio-documented significant CAD, prior CABG
  2. **Intermediate risk:** Evidence of noncoronary atherosclerosis
  3. **Low risk:** No clinical atherosclerosis, but high risk factor profile
  4. **Negligible risk:** Low risk factor profile

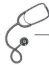

Patients with aortic stenosis are at increased risk for ischemia, MI, and sudden death.

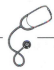

Stress test is positive if ST depressions > .2mV are present or if there is an inadequate response of heart rate to stress or hypotension.

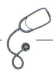

Echo is concerning when there is evidence of aortic stenosis (AS) or if the ejection fraction (EF) is < 35%.

Negligible and low-risk patients require only history and physical (H&P) and ECG. Higher-risk patients may require further workup as described above.

HIGH-YIELD FACTS

The Surgical Patient

Points		Probability of life-threatening complications
S3 gallop or JVD on exam	11	
MI within 6 months	10	**Add points to get risk**
> 5 PVCs/minute	7	0–5 = class I = 1%
Rhythm other than sinus rhythm (SR) or SR with APCs on last ECG	7	6–12 = class II = 5%
Age > 70	5	13–25 = class III = 11%
Emergent operation	4	> 25 = class IV = 22%
Intrathoracic, intraperitoneal, or aortic surgery	3	
Significant aortic stenosis	3	
Poor general medical condition	3	

FIGURE 2-2. Goldman's risk assessment for noncardiac surgery.

(Reproduced, with permission, from Goldman L, Caldera DL, Nussbaum SR, et al. Multifactorial index of cardiac risk in noncardiac surgical procedures. *New Eng J Med* 297:1977, 845.)

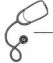

Echocardiography:
- Sensitivity 90–100%
- Specificity 50–80%
- Fixed defects, or defects that persist with time, indicate infarcted or scarred tissue.
- Reversible defects are more concerning: Normal and fixed defects have similar negative predictive values for cardiac events.

Tests

Stress Test (Thallium)

- Conducted with dipyridamole or adenosine (chemical vasodilators).
- Thallium's uptake by myocardium is proportional to coronary blood flow. When blood flow is limited by narrowed vessels, initial scans show a defect, but delayed scans do not. This is called a *reversible* defect, and indicates viable myocardium with decreased perfusion.
- Possible steps to optimization:
  - Wait more than 6 months after an MI, when possible.
  - Unstable angina may require preoperative revascularization.
  - If rapid atrial fibrillation is present, achieve rate control, consider cardioversion or anticoagulation.
  - Medical optimization of CHF patients.

Echocardiography

- Assesses valvular function, ventricular function, and wall motion.
- Look at wall motion abnormalities induced by stress (exercise or drugs).

Exercise Stress Test

- Involves continuous ECG monitoring for an episode of exercise
- Positive stress test: Sustained ST depressions, associated with less than ideal increase in heart rate or blood pressure, angina, or arrhythmia

SPECIFIC CARDIAC PROBLEMS

Congestive Heart Failure (CHF)

- Preop evidence of CHF = 16% risk of perioperative pulmonary edema.
- No preop evidence of CHF, but history of it = 6% risk perioperative pulmonary edema.
- New CHF (mortality is 15–20%) is usually secondary to fluid overload, end of positive pressure ventilation, myocardial depression (from anesthetic agents), or postoperative hypertension.
- Risk of pneumonia also increased.

Ischemic Heart Disease

- If CAD, surgical mortality is increased threefold.
- Overall, 0.13% patients have perioperative MIs.
- If patient required CABG prior to gastrointestinal (GI) surgery, wait 30 days in between operations.
- Mortality of perioperative MI is approximately 25% (usually occurs within 3 days of surgery, is often asymptomatic, and is associated with intraoperative hypertension, hypotension, or tachycardia).

Valvular Disease

- Only aortic disease has been found to affect mortality (when area of orifice < 1cm² or transverse pressure gradient > 50 mm Hg).
- Valvular AS: Surgical mortality 13%.
- Assess valve function with echocardiogram.
- Patient may need valve replacement first (prior to other planned surgery).
- *Endocarditis prophylaxis* for patients with mitral valve prolapse (MVP) or prosthetic valves: One option as follows:
  - 30 minutes before incision: ampicillin and gentamicin (or vancomycin and gentamicin if penicillin allergic)
  - 6 hours after incision: amoxicillin or second dose of ampicillin and gentamicin

Aortic stenosis:
- Harsh murmur at right second intercostal space that radiates to carotids
- Presents with angina, dyspnea on exertion, syncope

Hypertension

- Poorly controlled HTN is indicated by diastolic blood pressure (dBP) > 110 or systolic blood pressure (sBP) > 160: Associated with blood pressure lability, dysrhythmia, ischemia, MI, neurologic complications, intraoperative hypotension, postoperative hypertension, and renal failure.
- Antihypertensive meds should be continued up to time of surgery.
- Diuretics should be avoided the morning of surgery.

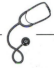

Risk of endocarditis:
- Moderate risk: Hypertrophic cardiomyopathy, MVP
- High risk: Prosthetic valve, congenital abnormality such as tetralogy of Fallot

Arrhythmia

- Patients in nonsinus rhythm have operative mortality of 18%.
- Risk is higher if arrhythmia is supraventricular tachycardia (SVT), atrial fibrillation, or atrial flutter.

PULMONARY RISK ASSESSMENT

Risk Factors for Pulmonary Complications

- Known pulmonary disease
- Abnormal pulmonary function tests (PFTs) (FEV < 11, max breathing capacity < 50% predicted)
- Smoking
- Age > 60
- Obesity
- Upper abdominal or thoracic surgery
- Long OR time

Up to 35% of postoperative deaths are due to pulmonary complications.

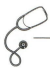
Goals to Reduce Risks

- Decrease or cease smoking (benefit if at least 8 weeks preoperatively).
- Increase/optimize bronchodilator therapy.

Preoperative Steps

- Usual history, physical exam.
- CXR if over age 40.
- If patient has risk factors for pulmonary complications, or will be undergoing upper abdominal surgery, obtain preoperative spirometry and ABG.
- FEV_1 (forced expiratory volume in 1 second)
- MBC (maximal breathing capacity)

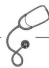

Major abdominal surgery decreases vital capacity by 50% and functional residual capacity by 30%.

- $FEV_1 < 70\%$ predicted indicates increased risk.
- If $VO_2 > 20$, patient is not likely to have pulmonary complications.

SPECIFIC PULMONARY PROBLEMS

Asthma

- Assess frequency and severity of attacks.
- Increased risk of bronchospasm during intubation and extubation.
- Continue bronchodilator therapy on day of surgery.
- If operation must occur during acute exacerbation, give twice usual PO dose of steroids, or 1 mg/kg methylprednisone preop and then q6h.

Chronic Obstructive Pulmonary Disease (COPD)

- Bronchitis and emphysema
- Arterial blood gas (ABG): $PCO_2 > 50$ indicates increased risk for postoperative respiratory failure.

Deep Vein Thrombosis/Pulmonary Embolism (DVT/PE)

- High-risk procedures:
  - Long duration of surgery
  - Orthopedic
  - Pelvic
  - Abdominal cancer surgery
- High-risk patient:
  - History of DVT/PE
  - Coagulopathic
  - On estrogen
  - Immobile/paralyzed
  - Obese
  - Age > 40
- Prophylaxis is warranted for moderate- and high-risk patients.
  - Perioperative subcutaneous (SQ) heparin reduces the risk of DVT by two thirds and PE by 50% (can be given 2 hours prior to induction of anesthesia).
  - Sequential compression devices (SCDs) work via stimulation of endothelial cell fibrinolytic activity.

Calf DVT is more common than proximal DVT (per risk group, risk of calf DVT is about 4 to 10 times greater).

Risk of PE in high-risk patients is 1–5%, and in low-risk patients is < .01%.

Postoperative Pulmonary Problems

Adult Respiratory Distress Syndrome (ARDS)
- Patient unable to maintain adequate oxygenation/ventilation/tissue delivery.
- Causes: Pneumonia, decompensation in COPD, trauma/flail chest.
- Defining concepts:
  - Acute lung injury
  - Bilateral infiltrates (white out); normal tissue interspersed with diseased tissue
  - $PaO_2/FiO_2 < 200$
  - PCWP < 19; no CHF
- Management
  - Positive end-expiratory pressure (PEEP)/PEEP trial
  - Pressure limited ventilation
  - Permissive hypercapnia
  - Prone position

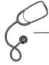

SQ heparin causes thrombocytopenia in 6% (caution when platelets < 100,000). An alternative is low-molecular-weight heparin.

Pulmonary Edema
- Fluid enters alveolus, especially likely in ARDS, pancreatitis, sepsis.
- Causes/contributing factors: Fluid overload, MI, sepsis, valvular dysfunction, liver failure.
- Presentation: Dyspnea, tachypnea, wheezing, rales, bronchospasm.
- Management: Oxygen, upright position, furosemide, Swan–Ganz catheter (may be useful in some situations).

Because of the method by which they work, one SCD should work as well as two if one leg is injured.

Fat Embolism
- Marrow fat enters bloodstream and goes to lung
- Basics
  - Eighty to 100% of these patients are trauma/accident victims.
  - Occurs in 26% of patients with one fracture.
  - Occurs in 44% of patients with multiple fractures.
- Management
  - Immobilize (splint) fracture
  - Consider corticosteroids
- Outcome: Death is uncommon.

Atelectasis
- Collapse of alveoli
- Secondary to changes from normal physiology, with anesthesia, diaphragmatic dysfunction, patient position, and postoperative pain.
- Secretions accumulate leading to bacterial overgrowth and increased risk for pneumonia.
- *Incentive spirometry* maintains lung inflation.
- Expectorant, N-acteyl cysteine (Mucomist®), and bronchdilators may also be useful at times.

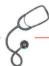

Atelectasis and/or pneumonia affect 20–40% of all postoperative patients.

Pneumonia
- Signs and symptoms:
  - Fever
  - Cough
  - Dyspnea
  - Pleuritic chest pain
  - Purulent sputum
  - Bronchial breath sounds, dullness, rales

The mortality of elderly patients with postoperative pneumonia is 50%.

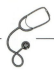

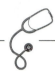

Aspiration

- Patient will have wheezing, hypoxia, bronchorrhea, cyanosis.
- Chemical pneumonitis often leads to bacterial pneumonia.
- Management:
  - Suction
  - Lavage
  - Endotracheal tube when indicated
  - Pulmonary toilet

Ways to Decrease Complications

1. Incentive spirometry
2. Chest physical therapy
3. Postural drainage where needed
4. Humidified oxygen

DIABETES MELLITUS AND OTHER ENDOCRINE DISEASE RISK ASSESSMENT

Operative Mortality

Similar to nondiabetic patients when matched by age, sex, and incidence of cardiovascular disease.

Preoperative Evaluation

- End organ assessment is crucial:
  - Patients with nephropathy will tolerate hypovolemia poorly and will be susceptible to nephrotoxicity of any contrast used.
  - Patients with autonomic neuropathy will be more likely to have gastroparesis, and so will be more susceptible to aspiration during intubation.

Preoperative Steps

- Glucose control is essential to minimize risk of infection.
- Usual medications:
  - Oral hypoglycemics: Discontinue the night before surgery except chlorpropamide (stop 2 to 3 days prior).
  - Insulin: Give one half the usual A.M. dose the morning of surgery.
- These patients may benefit from an early OR time and will need careful instruction with respect to their usual medications.

Thyroid

- Aim for euthyroid state.
- Thyrotoxicity increases risk for cardiovascular dysfunction, CHF, shock.

Parathyroid

- Watch for hypo/hypercalcemia.
- *Chvostek's sign:* Look for facial twitch when tapping CN VII; indicates hypocalcemia.
- *Trousseau's sign:* Carpopedal spasm with tourniquet; also indicates hypocalcemia.

Adrenal

- Addison's disease:
  - Patients unable to respond to stress of operation.
  - Require stress-dose steroids.

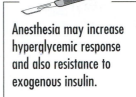

Anesthesia may increase hyperglycemic response and also resistance to exogenous insulin.

HEPATIC RISK ASSESSMENT

Child's Classification of Operative Risk for Patients with Cirrhosis

See Table 2-1.

Cautions

- Watch for prolonged elevations in drug levels in patients with preoperative liver dysfunction.
- Acute hepatitis is relative contraindication with 10% increase in morbidity/mortality if viral origin.
- Recommend abstinence from alcohol; alcohol's hypermetabolic state causes increased need for amino acids (by 2×).
- Attempt to control ascites prior to elective surgery, with fluid restriction, diuretics, and nutritional therapy.

- $NH_3 > 150$: Mortality 80%
- PT > 2: Mortality 40–60%

TABLE 2-1. Child's classification of operative risk.

	A	B	C
Ascites	None	Controlled	Uncontrolled
Total bilirubin	< 2	2–3	> 3
Encephalopathy	None	Minimal	Advanced
Nutrition	Excellent	Good	Poor
Albumin	> 3.5	3–3.5	< 3
Operative mortality	2%	10%	50%

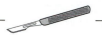

Increased BUN and creatinine indicate a loss of at least 75% of renal reserve.

Preoperative Evaluation

- Check blood urea nitrogen (BUN) and creatinine.
- Estimate preoperative creatinine clearance:
  $[(140 - age) * wt]/72 * creatinine$.
- Maintain intravascular volume.
- Ensure electrolytes are repleted; correct acidosis.
- Dialysis patients should be dialyzed within 24 hours of surgery to best control creatinine and electrolytes.

The risk of bleeding increases in patients with BUN > 100.

Intraoperative Problems

- Risk factors for development of acute renal failure:
  - Renal ischemia
  - Exposure to nephrotoxins (including contrast dye)
  - Sepsis
  - CHF

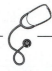

The most common complication in dialysis patients is *hyperkalemia* (in nearly 1/3 of patients).

Dialysis

- Overall mortality for dialysis-dependent patients: 5% (even when dialyzed within 24 hours of surgery).
  - Acute renal failure that develops in perioperative period requiring dialysis is associated with a mortality of approximately 50–80%.
- Morbidity: Shunt thrombosis, pneumonia, wound infection, hemorrhage.

Postoperative Complications

- Hyperkalemia:
  - Treat with IV calcium, D_{50}, insulin, bicarbonate, albuterol, and kayexalate (when possible).
- Anuria/oliguria:
  - Causes: Retention, inadequate resuscitation, ATN, renal failure
  - Urinary retention:
    - Major abdominal surgery: 4–5%
    - Anorectal surgery > 50%
    - Stress, pain, spinal anesthesia, and anorectal reflex increase β-adrenergic stimulation, preventing release of urine.
    - Patients have urgency, discomfort, fullness on palpation of bladder.
    - Treatment: Straight catheterization twice 6 hours apart; if patient fails to void then, place indwelling Foley catheter.
    - May try prazosin or phenoxybenzamine.

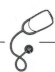

To determine source of a renal problem:
- $FENa > 1$ = intrinsic damage
- Specific gravity = 1.010 in ATN
- $U_{Na} < 10$ in prenal

Return of Bowel Function

Small intestine then *stomach* then *colon*.
hours   24 hrs?   ~3-4 days

Ileus

- Incidence after GI surgery: 5%.
- In general, await return of bowel function before advancing diet.

Clostridium difficile Colitis

- Variable presentation from mild diarrhea and discomfort to severe pain, tenderness, fever, elevated white blood count (WBC).
- Associated with: Age, prior residence in nursing home, renal failure, immunocompromised state, antibiotic use (especially cefoxitin), small or large bowel obstruction, GI surgery, NGT for > 48 hours.
- Treatment: PO metronidazole or as second line, vancomycin.

Preoperative Labs

- Check complete blood count (CBC).
- Blood should be typed and crossed for at least 2 units for most operations.
- Discuss possible need for transfusion, as some patients may have religious beliefs that preclude transfusion.

Anemia

- Determine cause.
- Postpone elective operations when possible; patients who will not tolerate anemia well include those with chronic hypoxia, ischemic heart disease, or cerebral ischemia.
- Sickle cell patients have increased risk of vaso-occlusive crises with operations. (This increased risk does not generally include patients with sickle cell trait.)
  - Minimize risk by maintaining euvolemia.

Thrombocytopenia

See Figure 2-3.

Urination requires release of β-adrenergic receptors in smooth muscles of bladder neck and urethra, parasympathetic stimulation of bladder contraction.

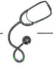

To estimate when bowel function will return, allow one postoperative day per decade for major abdominal surgery.

HIGH-YIELD FACTS

The Surgical Patient

Platelets	Likelihood of bleed perioperatively
> 150,000	Normal
100,000–150,000	Unlikely
50,000–100,000	Unlikely with adequate hemostasis
20,000–50,000	Possible excessive surgical bleeding
10,000–20,000	Spontaneous mucosal and cutaneous bleeding
< 10,000	Major spontaneous mucosal bleed, including GI tract

FIGURE 2-3. Risk of postoperative bleeding by platelet count.

Coagulopathy

- Check prothrombin time (PT) and partial thromboplastin time (PTT) preoperatively.
- Note that elevated values should be expected in patients with liver disease.
- Patients on aspirin should discontinue it at least one week prior.
- Factor abnormalities should be addressed (for example with hemophilia).

- Risk of bleeding is further increased at any platelet level if patient is septic or has a functional platelet deficit.
- One unit of platelets raises platelet count by 5,000 to 10,000.

CONSIDERATIONS OF BASELINE STATUS

Nutrition

Assessment
- Ideal body weight (IBW) = 106 lb + 6/inch over 5 ft (male) or 100 lb + 5/inch over 5 ft (female)
- Body mass index (BMI) = kg/m^2

Effect on Nutritional State/Needs With
- *Brief fasting:* Increased circulation of glucose, TAG, amino acids, fatty acids.
- *Prolonged fasting:* Decrease by 25% in resting energy expenditure with conservation of protein stores.
- *Starvation:* Decreased body fat, cell mass. Increased extracellular fluid.
- *Surgery or critical illness:* Increased demand for gluconeogenesis, increased muscle protein catabolism.
- *Elective surgery:* Minimal effect.

PT will decrease by 2 sec/day when warfarin is witheld.

Activities of Daily Living (ADL)

Consider whether patient will tolerate any necessary rehabilitation and effect of operation and immobile time on eventual functional status.

Mental Status

- Consider who makes decisions for the patient.
- Determine ahead of time in case any further decisions need to be made while patient is unable to do so.

- Ideal BMI = 19 – 25.
- Increased risk if < 80% or > 120% of IBW, or recent change of > 10% body weight.
- Consider baseline state of patient: Well-nourished with acute illness versus chronically ill, alcoholic, obese.

NPO

- To decrease the risk of aspiration with intubation, patients should refrain from solids 6 to 8 hours prior, and from liquids 2 to 3 hours prior to surgery.
- In bowel surgery, when patients require bowel preps, the duration of NPO may be preceded by a day of clear liquids only with the prep to clear the bowel of stool and facilitate the operation.

To simplify instructions, we tell patients to be NPO after midnight the night prior to elective surgery.

Bowel Preparation

- Purpose: To clear bowel of stool, thereby reducing bacterial count and risk of contamination with fecal spillage.
- Types:
  - Mechanical prep: Facilitates operation.
  - Oral antibiotics (neomycin, erythromycin base): Nadir bacterial count at commencement of operation if doses given at 1 P.M., 2 P.M., 11 P.M., the day prior (for a first case).

Remember that the bowel prep is a source of iatrogenic fluid loss. Elderly or chronically ill patients may not tolerate this loss without IV fluid replacement.

Usual Medications

- **Aspirin:** Avoid 7 days preoperatively to allow platelets to regenerate.
- **Warfarin (Coumadin):**
  - 3 options: Avoid 3 days prior to operation and resume POD #2; admit preoperatively and change to heparin which can be held only a couple of hours ahead; change to low-molecular-weight heparin (SQ).
- **Antihypertensives:** Continue, especially β-blockers; hold diuretics the morning of surgery.
- **Antithyroid medications:** Hold on morning of surgery.
- **Thyroid replacement:** Give on morning of surgery.
- **Oral hypoglycemics:** Avoid on day of surgery.
- **Insulin:** Give half usual dose on morning of surgery.

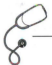

$t_{1/2}$ thyroxine = 7 days so it can be held for several postoperative days without much effect.

By Type of Surgery

1. In general: Cefazolin
2. Colorectal surgery, appendectomy: Cefoxitin or cefotetan
3. Urologic procedures: Ciprofloxacin
4. Head and neck: Cefazolin or clindamycin and gentamicin

Antibiotic prophylaxis: Single dose 30 minutes prior to skin incision, and again 6 hours later if operation is ongoing.

HIGH-YIELD FACTS

The Surgical Patient

Wounds

INTRODUCTION

By definition, the end result of any surgical case is one type of wound or another. Surgeons define a successful surgical case as one in which the patient survives, the pathology is removed and/or corrected, and the patient's wound heals. To accomplish this, it is important to understand the processes involved in wound repair, and ways in which these processes can lead to complications.

STEPS OF WOUND HEALING

- Coagulation
- Inflammation
- Collagen synthesis
- Angiogenesis
- Epithelialization
- Contraction

Coagulation

- Begins essentially instantaneously following wound formation.
- Coagulation and complement cascades are activated, and platelets create a hemostatic plug.
- Release of various inflammatory mediators from activated platelets sets the stage for the steps that follow.
- Impaired by anticoagulants, antiplatelet agents, and coagulation factor deficiency.

Inflammation

- Occurs as the wound is inundated with macrophages and polymorphonuclear leukocytes in response to various inflammatory mediators.
- Bacteria, cellular debris, dirt, and other foreign materials are also cleared from the wound site.
- Impaired by: Steroids and other immunosuppressants, congenital or acquired immune-deficient states.

Collagen Synthesis

- Occurs by fibroblasts in the vicinity of the wound, in response to various growth factor peptides
- Impaired by vitamin deficiency (especially C) and protein–calorie malnutrition

Angiogenesis (Granulation)

- Occurs in response to peptide growth factors such as vascular endothelial growth factor (VEGF).
- Presence of these new vascular networks is what gives granulation tissue its characteristic beefy-red appearance.

Epithelialization

- Occurs with the migration of epithelial cells over the wound defect.
- Integrity of the basement membrane is restored as type IV collagen and other matrix components are deposited.
- Foreign bodies, such as suture material, and necrotic tissue remain separated from the wound by the migrating epithelial cells.
- Once this step has occurred, the wound is essentially waterproofed.

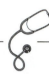

Contraction

- Process by which the surrounding uninjured skin is pulled over the wound defect, and the size of the scar is reduced.
- Made possible by the action of myofibroblasts, which possess a contraction mechanism similar to that seen in muscle cells.
- A long process that takes many months before it is complete.
- *Do not confuse wound contraction with scar contracture, as the latter occurs after wound repair has ceased. Scar contracture can lead to undesirable effects since architecture of the surrounding tissue may become distorted.*

SURGICAL WOUND CLASSIFICATION

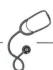

Clean

For a wound to be considered "clean," the following must be true:
- Wound created in a sterile and nontraumatic fashion, in an area that is free of preexisting inflammation.
- The respiratory, alimentary, genital, or urinary tract was not entered
- All persons involved in the case maintained strict aseptic technique.

Clean-Contaminated

- The respiratory, alimentary, genital, or urinary tract was entered, but there was no significant spillage of its contents (e.g., feces), and there was no established local infection.
- There was only a minor break in aseptic technique.

Contaminated

- There was gross spillage from the gastrointestinal tract.
- The genitourinary and biliary tracts were entered in the presence of local infection (e.g., cholangitis).
- The wound was the result of recent trauma.
- There was a major break in aseptic technique.

Dirty/Infected

- The wound was the result of remote trauma and contains devitalized tissue.
- There is established infection or perforated viscera prior to the procedure.

TYPES OF WOUND HEALING

Primary (First) Intention

- Type of healing seen following closure of clean surgical wounds, or traumatic lacerations in which there is minimal devitalized tissue, and minimal contamination.
- Edges of the incisional defect are approximated with the use of sutures or staples.
- Since the defect is very small, reepithelialization occurs rapidly, and overall healing time is short.
- Wounds closed primarily may have their dressing changed after 24 to 48 hours. By this time, epithelialization should be complete, and a less bulky dressing can be applied.
- Wound strength reaches its maximum at about 3 months and is generally 70–80% that of normal skin.

Generally, clean traumatic lacerations are closed with sutures or staples (primary intention) if less than 6 to 8 hours old.

Second Intention

- Type of healing seen following closure of wounds that are not approximated with sutures.
- Reason for not using sutures may be (1) that the wound edges cannot be apposed because the defect is very large (e.g., donor site of skin graft); or (2) that the surgeon chooses not to close the wound primarily because of the high risk of infection.
- Wounds healing by second intention should be packed loosely with moist gauze and covered with a sterile dressing. The wound should be assessed daily for the development of granulation tissue and the presence of infection.

Third (Delayed Primary) Intention

- Type of healing seen following closure of wounds in which there is obvious gross contamination at the incisional site (i.e., the wound is classified as contaminated or dirty).
- An example of where delayed primary closure is often used is s/p removal of a ruptured appendix in which there was leakage of pus into

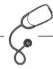

Sutures are utilized in primary and delayed primary intention healing only.

the peritoneal cavity. In such cases, the parietal peritoneum and fascial layers are closed, and antibiotics are administered. The skin and subcutaneous tissue are not sutured until 3 to 5 days later after bacterial contamination has decreased.

FACTORS AFFECTING WOUND HEALING

Sutures are tied to approximate, not strangulate, a healing wound!!!

- Wound infection (see next section)
- Tissue perfusion
- Oxygen
- Malnutrition
- Vitamin and trace element deficiency (vitamin C, vitamin A, zinc, copper)
- Smoking
- Foreign body
- Chronic disease

WOUND INFECTIONS

Infections that involve both deep and superficial tissues are classified as deep incisional SSIs.

Classification

Surgical site infections (SSIs) generally occur within 30 postoperative days. Depending on their location, they may be classified as superficial incisional, deep incisional, or organ/space infections.

> **Superficial incisional SSIs** exist when there is involvement by infection of the skin and subcutaneous tissue in the vicinity of the incision.
> **Deep incisional SSIs** exist when there is involvement by infection of deeper soft tissues that were divided by the incision such as fascia or muscle.
> **Organ/space SSIs** exist when there is infection of any anatomical structure remote from the incisional site but was manipulated during the procedure.

Early surgical site infections that occur in the first 24 hours postoperatively are most commonly due to *Streptococcus* or *Clostridium*. These bacteria grow very fast because they excrete enzymes that digest local tissue and impair host defenses. Infections due to other bacteria generally become apparent later (4 to 5 days postoperatively) because they lack such virulence factors.

Pathophysiology

Many of the factors that impair wound healing will also increase the risk of wound infections.

Depend on:
- Factors relating to microorganism:
  - The magic number is 10^5 (dose of contaminating microorganisms required to result in an increased risk of wound infection)
- Factors relating to the patient—increased risk with:
  - Infection that is *remote* from the surgical site
  - Diabetes
  - Smokers
  - Immunosuppressive agents, such as corticosteroids

- Severe protein–calorie malnutrition
- AIDS, disseminated malignancy, and any other immunocompromised state
- Factors relating to surgical technique:
  - Preoperative considerations:
    - Patient skin preparation, scrubbing, and the administration of antimicrobial prophylaxis
  - Intraoperative considerations:
    - Strict attention to aseptic technique.
    - OR should be well ventilated and maintained under positive pressure to prevent the entrance of pathogens from the corridor.
    - Avoid excessive use of electrocautery and tying sutures too tightly.
  - Postoperative considerations:
    - Proper wound management and discharge instructions are key.
    - Wound management will differ depending on whether the wound is closed by primary, secondary, or delayed primary intention (see above).

NORMAL FLORA

- Most common source of a wound infection is the host's normal flora.
- See Table 3-1.

COMMON SURGICAL PATHOGENS

- The organism responsible for causing a surgical site infection is best identified by culturing the involved region.
- The most likely causative organism can be predicted based on the site of the operation:
  - **Staphylococcus aureus and coagulase-negative staphylococci** are commonly isolated from wounds that follow thoracic (cardiac and noncardiac), neurological, breast, ophthalmic, vascular, and orthopedic surgery.

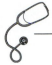

Hair in the vicinity of the incision should be shaved immediately before the procedure, preferably with electric clippers.

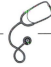

In the healthy individual, the lower respiratory tract and the upper urinary tract are essentially sterile.

TABLE 3-1. Normal flora by body part.

Body part	Normal flora
Skin	*Staphylococcus epidermidis, Staphylococcus aureus*, diphtheroids, streptococci, *Pseudomonas aeruginosa*, anaerobes, *Candida*
Upper respiratory tract	*Streptococcus viridans, Streptococcus pyogenes, Streptococcus pneumoniae, Neisseria, Staphylococcus epidermidis, Haemophilus influenzae*
Esophagus and stomach	Lactobacilli
Small bowel	Streptococci, Enterobacteria, *Bacteroides* spp., and very low density of lactobacilli
Large bowel	*Bacteroides*, Enterobacteria (e.g., *E. coli, Klebsiella* spp., *Salmonella*), *Staphylococcus aureus, Clostridium* spp.
Lower urinary tract	*Staphylococcus epidermidis*, streptococci, diphtheroids, gram-negative rods
Vagina	Lactobacilli

- **Gram-negative bacilli and anaerobes** are commonly isolated from wound infections that develop following appendectomy, colorectal, biliary tract, OB/GYN, and urological cases.
- **Streptococci and oropharyngeal anaerobes** are commonly isolated from wounds that follow head and neck procedures in which the mucosa of the oral cavity is involved.

Signs and Symptoms of Wound Infections

- Classic signs:
  - Calor (heat, warmth)
  - Rubor (redness)
  - Tumor (swelling)
  - Dolor (pain)
- More severe infections may produce systemic symptoms such as fever, chills, and rigors.
- Unusual for a wound infection to cause fever before postoperative day 3.
- Other causes of postoperative fever include urinary tract infection (UTI) (owing to prolonged placement of a Foley catheter), deep venous thrombosis (DVT)/thrombophlebitis, and certain medications.

DIAGNOSTIC APPROACH

- Physical exam should be directed at the surgical wound, looking for signs of infection such as induration, warmth, erythema, or frank purulent discharge.
- Any discharge present should be sent for microbiological culture.
- The febrile patient should be evaluated with an appropriate fever workup: CBC, blood and urine cultures, urinalysis, and chest x-ray should be sent.
- If an intra-abdominal abscess is suspected, a computed tomography (CT) scan may be useful.
- Lumbar puncture may be required for the patient with fever and altered mental status, especially in a patient that is status post craniotomy for a neurosurgical procedure.

TREATMENT

- Wound abscesses (superficial SSIs) require incision and drainage followed by thorough irrigation.
- Deeper SSIs may require surgical debridement.
- Systemic antibiotic therapy is required for deep SSIs; they may or may not be required for superficial SSIs, depending on the severity of the infection.
- Peritoneal abscesses (organ/space SSI) may be treated by CT-guided percutaneous drainage; those that cannot be drained percutaneously may require open drainage.

The benefits of surgical antimicrobial prophylaxis are maximized if the chosen antibiotic:

- Provides appropriate coverage against the most probable contaminating organisms
- Is present in optimal concentrations in serum and tissues at the time of incision
- Is maintained in therapeutic levels throughout the operation

General Principles

- First- and second-generation cephalosporins: For gram-positive cocci
- Third-generation cephalosporins: For gram-negative rods
- Metronidazole or clindamycin: For anaerobes
- Aminoglycosides: For gram-negative rods
- Vancomycin: For methicillin-resistant *Staphylococcus aureus*

OTHER WOUND COMPLICATIONS

Hematoma = blood

DEFINITION

Collection of blood that may form in the vicinity of a surgical wound.

CAUSES

Incomplete hemostasis, which may be caused by:

- Inadequate intraoperative hemostasis
- The administration of anticoagulants or antiplatelet agents (e.g., aspirin)
- Presence of a coagulation disorder (e.g., factor VIII deficiency, von Willebrand's disease)

SIGNS AND SYMPTOMS

- Localized fluctuant swelling
- Discoloration at the wound site
- Signs of hypovolemia such as tachycardia and hypotension with very large hematomas

TREATMENT

- Small hematomas may be left alone and allowed to reabsorb spontaneously, while larger hematomas may require aspiration.

COMPLICATIONS

- Pain
- Increased risk of wound infection (because the pooled blood is an excellent growth medium for microorganisms)

Seroma = fluid not blood

DEFINITION

Collection of fluid in the vicinity of a wound that is not blood or pus.

CAUSES

Creation of a potential space combined with disruption of local draining lymphatic channels (e.g., mastectomy).

TREATMENT

- Placement of a closed drainage system primarily will help prevent seroma formation.
- Seromas are treated by aspiration of the fluid followed by drain placement.

COMPLICATIONS

Like hematomas, a seroma increases the risk of infection due to the presence of nutrients in which microorganisms can grow.

Wound Failure

DEFINITIONS

- Occurs when there has been complete or partial disruption of one or more layers of the incisional site
- Termed **dehiscence** if it occurs early in the postoperative course before all stages of wound healing have occurred
- Termed incisional hernia when it occurs months or years after the surgical procedure

CAUSES

Poor operative techniques that may lead to wound failure include the following:

- *Suture material with inadequate tensile strength.* Since absorbable sutures lose their tensile strength rather quickly, nonabsorbable sutures should be used to close the fascia.
- *Inadequate number of sutures.* Sutures should be placed no greater than 1 cm apart; if placed greater than 1 cm apart, herniation of viscera may occur between sutures.
- *Too small bite size.* Sutures should be placed no less than 1 cm from the wound edge; if placed closer to the wound edge, the fascia may tear.

Patient factors may be divided into:

1. Systemic illnesses that impair wound healing, such as malnutrition, corticosteroid therapy, sepsis, uremia, liver failure, or poorly controlled diabetes; and
2. Physical factors that place stress on the incisional site, such as coughing/retching, obesity, and the presence of ascites.

TREATMENT

- Immediate treatment of wound dehiscence involves minimizing contamination of the operative site by the placement of sterile packing. The patient must then be brought back to the OR to reclose the incision.
- Incisional hernia must be treated promptly, especially if the patient is symptomatic (e.g., abdominal pain, nausea, vomiting). This is because strangulation of the bowel may occur, resulting in necrosis and increased morbidity. Incisional hernias are repaired by repairing the fascial defect, with or without the use of a synthetic mesh to reinforce the defect.

Complications of Scar Formation

Skin: Keloid in susceptible individuals (e.g., African-Americans, Hispanics), scar carcinoma

GI tract: Small bowel obstruction secondary to adhesions or stricture formation

Liver: Intrahepatic or extrahepatic cholestasis secondary to stricture formation

Musculoskeletal: Pain or limited range of motion (ROM) secondary to osteoarthritis or ankylosis

Heart: Pericardial tamponade secondary to rupture of ventricular aneurysm, congestive heart failure (CHF) secondary to ruptured chordae tendinea and resulting incompetent valve

Nerve: Paresis/paralysis/paresthesia/anesthesia secondary to failure of nerve conduction

Fluids, Electrolytes, and Nutrition

ANATOMY OF BODY FLUIDS

See Figure 4-1.

Total Body Water

- 50–70% of total body weight
- Made up of two compartments—ICF and ECF
- Greater in lean individuals because fat contains little water
- Greatest percentage in newborns, then decreases with age

Intracellular Fluid (ICF)

- Mostly in skeletal muscle mass (thus slightly lower in females than males)

Extracellular Fluid (ECF)

- Made up of plasma and interstitial (extravascular) fluid.
- This is where most fluid equilibration occurs.

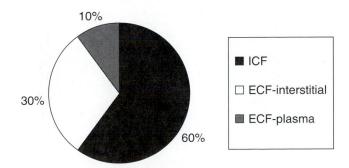

FIGURE 4-1. Composition of body fluids.

Plasma osmolality (Posm) = 2[Na] + glucose/18 + blood urea nitrogen (BUN)/2.8

Water Movement Between ICF and ECF

- **Osmolality.** The amount of water in a compartment is determined by the number of osmotically active particles in that compartment. Osmotic equilibrium is maintained because of permeability of cell membranes and endothelium.
- **Nonisotonic fluid shifts.** When the osmolality of either ICF or ECF changes, water moves along the osmotic gradient from the hypotonic compartment to the hypertonic compartment until a new osmotic equilibrium is reached. At this point, each compartment has a new volume and osmolality.
- **Isotonic fluid shifts.** Iso-osmotic fluid gains and losses are distributed only within the ECF because without a change in osmolality, water will not shift between compartments.

Even without intake, you must excrete 800 mL/day in urine waste products.

Water Movement Within ECF

- Starling forces—some fluid movement between the plasma and interstitial fluid is governed by the balance between plasma hydrostatic pressure and interstitial oncotic pressure on one side and plasma oncotic pressure and tissue hydrostatic pressure on the other.

See Table 4-1.

Insensible loss increases with fever and hyperventilation.

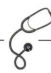

May lose 1,500 mL/day with an unhumidified tracheostomy and hyperventilation.

TABLE 4-1. Water, Na, K balance in normal patient.

	Water (mL/day)	Na (mEq/day)	K (mEq/day)
Intake			
Liquid	800–1,500	50–150	50–80
Solid	500–1,000		
Output—Sensible			
Urine	800–1,500	10–150	50–80
Sweat	0–100	10–60	0–10
Output—Insensible			
Lungs	250–450	0	0
Skin	250–450	0	0

See Figure 4-2.
- Distal tubules—reabsorption of Na in exchange for K and H secretion.
  - Affected by adrenocorticotropic hormone (ACTH) and aldosterone.
- Aldosterone directly stimulates K secretion and Na reabsorption from the distal tubule.

Volume Deficit (Dehydration)

Most common fluid disorder.

CAUSES

- Loss of gastrointestinal (GI) fluid—vomiting, nasogastric (NG) suction, diarrhea, fistular drainage
- Fluid sequestered in injuries or infection (third spacing):
  - Intra-abdominal and retroperitoneal infection
  - Peritonitis
  - Intestinal obstruction
- Burns
- Fever
- Osmotic diuresis
- Postoperative
- Inadequate input during procedure

SIGNS AND SYMPTOMS

See Table 4-2.
- (CNS) and cardiovascular (CV) signs occur early with acute loss.
- CV signs are secondary to a decrease in plasma volume.
- Tissue signs may be absent until the deficit has existed for 24 hours.
- Tissue signs may be difficult to assess in the elderly patient or patient with recent weight loss.

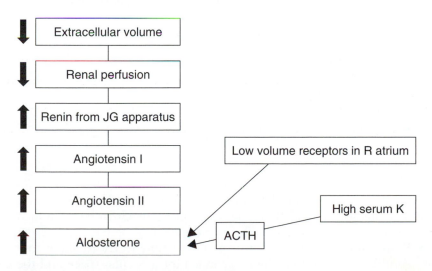

FIGURE 4-2. Renal mechanism of fluid and electrolyte balance.

TABLE 4-2. Dehydration: Signs and symptoms.

	Volume Deficit	
	Moderate	**Severe**
CNS	■ Sleepiness ■ Apathy ■ Slow responses ■ Anorexia ■ Cessation of usual activity	■ Decreased tendon reflexes ■ Anesthesia of distal extremities ■ Stupor ■ Coma
GI	■ Progressive decrease in food consumption	■ Nausea, vomiting ■ Refusal to eat ■ Ileus and distention
CV	■ Orthostatic hypotension ■ Tachycardia ■ Collapsed veins ■ Collapsing pulse	■ Cutaneous lividity ■ Hypotension ■ Distant heart sounds ■ Cold extremities ■ Absent peripheral pulses
Tissue signs	■ Soft, small tongue with longitudinal wrinkling ■ Decreased skin turgor	■ Atonic muscles ■ Sunken eyes
Metabolism	Mild temperature decrease: 97°–99° F	Marked temperature decrease: 95°–98° F

- Body temperature varies with environment—cool room may mask fever.
  - After partial correction of volume deficit, the temperature will generally rise to the appropriate level.
- Severe volume depletion depresses all body systems and interferes with the clinical evaluation of the patient.
- Volume depleted patient with severe sepsis from peritonitis may be afebrile and have normal white blood count (WBC), complain of little pain, and have unremarkable findings on abdominal exam. This may change dramatically when the ECF is restored.
- History items important for evaluating fluid deficits include:
  - Weight change, intake (quantity and composition), output, general medical status
- Degree of dehydration dependent on acute loss of body weight and is assessed clinically:
  - Mild—3% for adults, 5% for kids
  - Moderate—6% for adults, 10% for kids
  - Severe—9% for adults, 15% for kids

TREATMENT

- Goal is to replace this deficit in most patients over the next 24 hours.
- The amount of fluid the patient is missing needs to be combined with the expected maintenance fluid for the next 24 hours.
- Rehydration is done over this period of time to try to allow continual equilibration between the reexpanded intravascular space and the contracted ECF and ICF.

- The initial intervention is to give a fairly large aliquot of fluid as a volume expander. 20 mL/kg of normal saline (NS) or Ringer's lactate (LR) is given over the first hour. During the remaining 8 hours, the expected maintenance fluid is given plus about one half of the remaining calculated loss. Over the remaining 16 hours, the other one half of the remaining calculated loss is given along with the assumed maintenance fluid.

COLLOID VS. CRYSTALLOID

- Dehydration and hypovolemia are treated with volume expansion.
- Volume expansion can be accomplished with crystalloid (NaCl, Ringer's lactate, D_5W, etc.) or colloid (albumin, blood products).

Crystalloid
- In most cases, the initial therapy is to give 2 L or 20 mg/kg bolus through two large-bore (> 16 gauge in adults) IVs.
- Goal is to expand the intravascular space.
- Use isosmotic solutions.
- Since there is equilibration between ICF and ECF, only two thirds of any volume of isotonic crystalloid will stay intravascularly.

Colloid
- Used to stimulate the liver to release albumin (up to 50 g or 40% of the normal intravascular pool) within 3 hours of the hypovolemia.
- Stay mainly within intravascular space *if* the capillary membranes are intact.
- Possible increased incidence of pulmonary embolism (PE) and respiratory failure (controversial).
- Expensive
- Indications:
  - If hypovolemia persists after 2 L of crystalloid.
  - Patients with excess Na and water, but are hypovolemic—such as ascites, CHF, postcardiac bypass patients.
  - Patients unable to synthesize enough albumin or other proteins to exert enough oncotic pressure—such as liver disease, transplant recipients, resections, malnutrition.
  - Severe hemorrhage or coagulopathy—packed red blood cells (PRBCs) and fresh frozen plasma (FFP) may increase hematocrit to help correct coagulopathy.

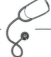

When replacing fluids, remember that:
- Large volumes may lead to peripheral and/or pulmonary edema.
- Large amounts of dextrose may cause hyperglycemia.
- Large amounts of NS may cause hyperchloremic metabolic acidosis.
- Ringer's lactate given when patient is hypovolemic and in metabolic alkalosis (i.e., from NG tube, vomiting) may worsen the alkalosis when the lactate is metabolized.

VOLUME EXCESS

Isotonic

CAUSES

Isotonic
- Iatrogenic—intravascular overload of IV fluids with electrolytes
- Increased ECF without equilibration with ICF—especially postoperative or trauma when the hormonal responses to stress are to decrease Na and water excretion by kidney
- Often secondary to renal insufficiency, cirrhosis, or CHF

Third spacing is the shift of ECF from the plasma compartment to elsewhere, such as the interstitial or transcellular spaces.

Hypotonic

- Inappropriate NaCl-poor solution as a replacement for GI losses (most common)
- Third spacing
- Increased antidiuretic hormone (ADH) with surgical stress, inappropriate ADH (SIADH)

Hypertonic

- Most common cause: excessive Na load without adequate water intake:
  - Water moves out of the cells because of increased ECF osmolarity.
  - Causes an increase in intravascular and interstitial fluid.
  - Worse when renal tubular excretion of water and/or Na is poor.
- Can also be caused by rapid infusion of nonelectrolyte osmotically active solutes such as glucose and mannitol.

SIGNS AND SYMPTOMS

See Table 4-3.

TREATMENT

- Restriction of Na and fluids for isotonic hypervolemia
- Free water replacement for hypertonic hypervolemia (will correct hypertonicity, which should lead to diuresis of excess fluid)

TABLE 4-3. Signs and symptoms of volume excess.

	Volume Excess	
	Moderate	**Severe**
CNS	None	None
GI	*At operation:* Edema of stomach, colon, lesser and greater omenta, and small bowel mesentery	
CV	Increased: Pulse pressure Venous pressure ■ Cardiac output ■ Pulmonic 2nd sound ■ Distention of peripheral veins ■ Loud heart sounds ■ Functional murmurs ■ Bounding pulse ■ Gallop	■ Pulmonary edema
Tissue signs	■ Pitting edema ■ Basilar rales	■ Anasarca ■ Moist rales ■ Vomiting ■ Diarrhea
Metabolism	None	None

- Saline for hypotonic hypervolemia (again, will correct hypotonicity, which should then correct the hypervolemia)
- Diuresis with furosemide 10 to 50 mg:
  - Be sure to replace K as needed.
  - Be careful not to overdiurese—must maintain kidney and brain perfusion as well as appropriate cardiac output.
- Cardiotonic drugs, O_2, artificial ventilation for cardiac failure and respiratory insufficiency as needed

ONGOING FLUID LOSS

- Besides normal maintenance loss, there may be other ongoing losses.
- You cannot simply collect all the patient's urine, stool, and vomit and add up the total because some loss of fluid in urine and stool is assumed in the original maintenance assumptions.
- Rule of thumb: Replace one half of the "usual" ongoing losses along with the assumed maintenance and the rehydration replacement fluid.
- Electrolyte content of the ongoing loss can be either assumed based on serum electrolyte values or can be determined by direct electrolyte measurement of the fluid. (See Table 4-4.)

CAUSES

- Fever
  - Each °C above 37°C adds 2.0 to 2.5 mL/kg/day of insensible water loss.
- Loss of body fluids:
  - From vomit, NG suction, fistulas
- Third-space losses:
  - Adults—approximately 1 L of third-space fluid intra-abdominally for each quadrant of the abdomen that is traumatized, inflamed, or operated on.
- Kids—approximately one fourth of calculated maintenance fluid per 24 hour period is sequestered for each quadrant of the abdomen that is traumatized, inflamed, or operated on.
- Burns:
  - See Thermal Injury chapter for estimating volume losses and replacement.
- Osmotic diuresis:
  - Secondary to urea, mannitol, or glucose.
  - Urine electrolytes should be checked to determine the appropriate replacement fluid, if one is necessary.

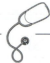

Estimating daily caloric expenditure:
- Up to 10 kg: 100 kcal/kg/day
- 11–20 kg: 1,000 kcal + 50 kcal/kg/day for each kg above 10 kg
- > 20 kg 1,500 kcal + 20 kcal/kg/day for each kg above 20 kg

100 mL of water is lost per 100 kcal energy expended.

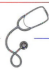

Calculating fluids/hr:
- Up to 10 kg: 100 mL/kg/day = 4 mL/kg/hr
- 11–20 kg: 1,000 mL + 50 mL/kg/day for each kg above 10 kg = 40 mL/hr + 2 mL/kg/hr for each kg above 10 kg
- > 20 kg: 1,500 mL + 20 mL/kg/day for each kg above 20 kg = 60 mL/hr + 1 mL/kg/hr for each kg above 20 kg

The average (70 kg) adult patient needs about 2.5 L/day (1,000 + 500 + (20 × 50) = 2,500) or 100 mL/hr (2,500/24 = 104) *unless other factors warrant a higher rate.*

Calculating free water deficit (FWD):
- FWD = normal body water (NBW) – current body water (CBW)
- NBW = 0.6 × body weight in kg
- CBW = (NBW) [normal serum Na/measured serum Na]

TABLE 4-4. Composition of GI secretions.

	Volume (L/day)	Electrolytes (mEq/L)			
		Na$^+$	K$^+$	Cl$^-$	HCO$_3^-$
Saliva	1.0–1.5	30	20	35	15
Gastric juice, pH < 4	2.5	60	10	90	—
Gastric juice, pH > 4	2.0	100	10	100	—
Bile	1.5	145	5	110	40
Duodenum	—	140	5	80	50
Pancreas	0.7–1.0	140	5	75	90
Ileum	3.5	130	10	110	30
Cecum	—	80	20	50	20
Colon	—	60	30	40	20
Sweat	0–3.0	50	5	55	—
New ileostomy	0.5–2.0	130	20	110	30
Adapted ileostomy	0.4	50	5	30	25
Colostomy	0.3	50	10	40	20

ASSESSING HYDRATION STATUS

Vital Signs

- Early signs of hypovolemia: Tachycardia, decreased pulse pressure, orthostatic blood pressure (BP).
- BP is not persistently lowered until 20–30% of circulating volume is lost.

Physical Exam in Hypervolemia

- Jugular venous distention (JVD)
- Rales
- S$_3$
- Edema

Physical Exam in Hypovolemia

- Flat neck veins
- Poor tissue turgor
- Dry mucous membranes
- Cool extremities

Input, Output, Weight

Daily weight is one of the best methods for assessing volume status.

Urine Output (UO)

- Normal urine output: 0.5 cc/kg/hr for adults, 1 cc/kg/hr for kids
- Low UO: Hypovolemia, renal failure, low flow states
- High UO: Hypervolemia, diabetes insipidus, osmotic diuresis, postobstructive diuresis

Lab

- Check daily serum electrolytes on intensive care unit (ICU) patients
- BUN/creatinine (Cr) > 20 and FeNa < 1% indicates hypovolemia.
- BUN/Cr < 15 indicates adequate hydration.

SODIUM BALANCE

Hyponatremia

< 130 mEq/L.

Hyponatremia with Hypotonicity

Hypovolemia
- May be from diuretics or vomiting
- Often with K deficit

Hypervolemia
- May be from CHF, cirrhosis, or nephrotic syndrome
- Increased thirst and vasopressin
- Edematous state

Euvolemia
- SIADH:
  - Most common cause of normovolemic hyponatremia
  - Increased vasopressin release from posterior pituitary or ectopic source causes decreased renal free water excretion
  - Signs and symptoms:
    - Hypo-osmotic hyponatremia
    - Inappropriately concentrated urine (urine osmolality > 100 mOsm/kg)
    - Euvolemia
    - Normal renal, adrenal, and thyroid function
  - Causes—neuropsychiatric disorders, malignancies (especially lung), and head trauma
- Glucocorticoid deficiency (Addison's disease)—cortisol deficiency causes hypersecretion of vasopressin
- Hypothyroidism—causes decreased CO and glomerular filtration rate (GFR), which leads to increased vasopressin secretion
- Primary polydipsia—usually seen in psychiatric patients who compulsively drink massive volumes of water

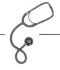

Chronic hyponatremia may be asymptomatic until < 120 mEq/L.

Fluids, Electrolytes, and Nutrition

Hyponatremia with hypertonicity: Things go UP!
- ICP
- Reflexes
- Muscle activity

You're so full of water that your kidneys clamp down and your head pops off like a toy sprinkler.

Hyponatremia with High Plasma Osmolality

CAUSES

Rapid infusion of glucose or mannitol will cause increased osmotic pressure that shifts fluid from the ICF to the ECF.

SIGNS AND SYMPTOMS

- Increased intracranial pressure—may induce hypertension (HTN)
- Hyperactive reflexes
- Muscle twitching
- Oliguric then anuric renal failure
- Salivation, lacrimation, watery diarrhea

TREATMENT

- Correct underlying disorder.
- Raise plasma Na (lower ICF volume)—restrict water intake.
- ECF volume contraction—Na repletion with saline isotonic to the patient, in order to avoid rapid changes in ICF volume.

Hypernatremia

DEFINITION

> 145 mEq/L.

SYMPTOMS

- Restlessness, weakness, delirium
- Hypotension and tachycardia
- Decreased saliva and tears
- Red, swollen tongue
- Fever
- Oliguria

TREATMENT

Stop ongoing water loss. Correction of hypovolemia, if present. Replace water deficit with D5W. Correct ½ of water deficit in first 24 hours; remaining water deficit over next 1 to 2 days.

POTASSIUM BALANCE

- 98% of K is in ICF.
- Released into ECF in response to severe injury, surgical stress, or acidosis.

Hypokalemia

DEFINITION

< 3.5 mEq/L.

CAUSES

- Excessive renal secretion:
  - Renal tubular excretion of K increases when large quantities of Na are available for excretion.
  - The more Na available for reabsorption, the more K is exchanged for Na in the lumen.
  - Thus, K requirements for prolonged or massive isotonic fluid volume replacement are increased.
- Movement of K into cells.
- Prolonged administration of K-free parenteral fluids
- Total parenteral hyperalimentation with inadequate K replacement.
- Loss in GI secretions.
- Diuretics

SIGNS AND SYMPTOMS

- Weakness → flaccid paralysis
- Decreased reflexes
- Paralytic ileus
- Electrocardiogram (ECG) (see Figure 4-3):
  - Flattened T waves, ST depression, U wave
  - Arrhythmias, signs of low voltage

TREATMENT

- No more than 40 mEq should be added to a liter of IV fluid.
- Rate should not exceed 40 mEq/hr.
- Don't give to oliguric patient.

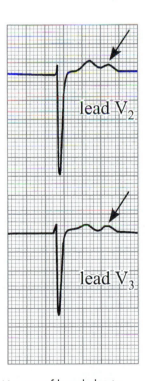

FIGURE 4-3. ECG demonstrating U wave of hypokalemia.

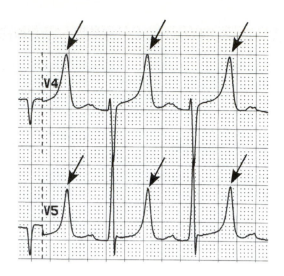

FIGURE 4-4. Peaked T waves in hyperkalemia.

Hyperkalemia

DEFINITION

> 5 mEq/L.

CAUSES

Rarely found when renal function is normal.

SIGNS AND SYMPTOMS

- ECG:
  - *Early:* Peaked T waves, wide QRS, ST depression
  - *Late:* Disappearance of T waves, heart block, **sine wave,** cardiac arrest
- GI: nausea, vomiting, intermittent intestinal colic, diarrhea

See Figures 4-4 and 4-5.

TREATMENT

- Kayexalate—cation exchange resin.

- 10% calcium gluconate 1 g IV—monitor ECG
  - Temporarily suppresses myocardial effects, but does not move potassium
- Albuterol
- 45 mEq $NaHCO_3$ in 1 L $D_{10}W$ with 20 units of regular insulin:
  - Promotes cellular reuptake of K—transient relief of hyperkalemia
- Dialysis (last resort)

Lower extracellular K^+ (acute treatment)—albuterol, $NaHCO_3$, insulin; lower total body K^+—Kayexalate, dialysis.

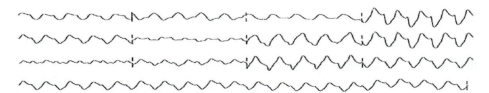

FIGURE 4-5. Sine waves in hyperkalemia.

- 1,000 to 1,200 mg normal—most is in the bone in the form of phosphate and carbonate
- Normal daily intake—1 to 3 g
- Most excreted via stool (~200 mg via urine)
- Normal serum level—8.5 to 10.5 mg/dL:
    - Half of this is nonionized and bound to plasma protein. **Correcting for low albumin 0.8 (normal albumin–observed albumin) + observed calcium**
    - An additional nonionized fraction (5%) is bound to other substances in the ECF.
    - Ratio of ionized to nonionized Ca is related to pH (see Figure 4-6):
        - Acidosis causes increase in ionized fraction.
        - Alkalosis causes decrease in ionized fraction.
    - Ionized calcium most accurate measure of calcium

Hypocalcemia

DEFINITION

< 8 mg/dL.

CAUSES

- Acute pancreatitis
- Massive soft-tissue infections (necrotizing fasciitis)
- Acute/chronic renal failure
- Pancreatic/small bowel fistulas
- Hypoparathyroidism (common after parathyroid or thyroid surgery)
- Hypoproteinemia (often asymptomatic)
- Severe depletion of Mg
- Severe alkalosis may elicit symptoms in patient with normal serum levels because there is a decrease in the ionized fraction of total serum Ca.

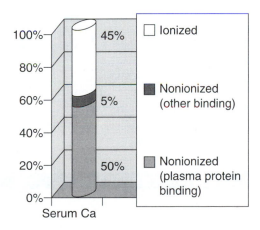

FIGURE 4-6. Concentration of ionized and nonionized calcium in serum.

- Numbness and tingling of fingers, toes, and around mouth
- Increased reflexes
- Chvostek's sign: tapping over the facial nerve in front of the tragus of the ear causes ipsilateral twitching
- Trousseau's sign: carpopedal spasm following inflation of sphymo-manometer cuff to above sBP for several minutes
- Muscle and abdominal cramps
- Convulsions
- ECG—prolonged QT interval

TREATMENT

- IV Ca gluconate or Ca chloride.
- Monitor QT interval on ECG.

Hypercalcemia

DEFINITION

> 15 mg/dL.

CAUSES

- Hyperparathyroidism
- Cancer (especially breast, multiple myeloma)
- Drugs (e.g., thiazides)

SIGNS AND SYMPTOMS

- Fatigue, weakness, anorexia, weight loss, nausea, vomiting
- Somnambulism, stupor, coma
- Severe headache, pain in the back and extremities, thirst, polydipsia, polyuria
- Death

TREATMENT

- Vigorous volume repletion with salt solution—dilutes Ca and increases urinary Ca excretion:
  - May be augmented with furosemide.
- Definitive treatment of acute hypercalcemic crisis in patients with hyperparathyroidism is immediate surgery.
- Treat underlying cause.

INDICATIONS FOR NUTRITIONAL SUPPORT

Enteral
- Gut works
- Oral intake not possible—altered mental state, ventilator, oral/pharyngeal/esophageal disorders
- Oral intake not sufficient for metabolic requirements—anorexia, sepsis, severe trauma/burns
- Presence of malnutrition and wasting

Parenteral (TPN)

- Enteral feeding not possible—GI obstruction, ileus
- Enteral intake not sufficient for metabolic requirements—chronic diarrhea/emesis, malabsorption, fistulas, chemotherapy, irradiation therapy
- Risk of aspiration
- Adjunctive support necessary for managing disease—pancreatitis, hepatic failure, renal failure, chylothorax
- Presence of malnutrition and wasting

Malnutrition and Wasting

KWASHIORKOR (PROTEIN MALNUTRITION)

- Adequate fat reserves with significant protein deficits
- Slight or no weight loss
- Low visceral proteins (albumin, prealbumin, transferrin)
- Edema often present
- Seen in acutely stressed patients

MARASMUS (PROTEIN–CALORIE MALNUTRITION)

- Weight loss with fat and muscle wasting
- Visceral proteins normal or slightly low
- Seen in chronic malnutrition

NUTRIENT REQUIREMENTS

Calorie Requirements

- **Harris–Benedict equation**—used to estimate basal energy expenditure.
- **Fick equation**—used to estimate BEE in patients with Swan–Ganz catheters:

$$BEE = (SaO_2 - SvO_2) \times CO \times Hb \times 95.18$$

- General estimation of BEE:
  Males: BEE = **25 kcal/kg/day**
  Females: BEE = **22 kcal/kg/day**
  - Multiply this by the desired goal:
    - Nonstressed patient: BEE × 1.2
    - Postsurgery: BEE × 1.3 to 1.5
    - Trauma/sepsis/burns: BEE × 1.6 to 2.0
    - Fever: 12% increase per °C

ENTERAL NUTRITION

Continuous

Suggested for initiation of feedings and for those who are at risk for aspiration, have high residuals, have diarrhea, or are being fed via duodenum/jejunum.

Intermittent

- Schedule:
    - Intermittent feeds around the clock.
    - Intermittent/continuous feed during day/night hours only.
    - Offer meals and administer feed only when intake is inadequate.
- Order:
    - Total volume of feed/day.
    - Rate and frequency of feed.
    - Type and volume of flush solution.
    - Specify pump or gravity drip.

Complications

- Diarrhea:
    - Exclude other causes: Antibiotics, Mg, sorbitol, infections (send stool for *Clostridium difficile* assay).
    - Dilute hypertonic formulas and lower rate of infusion.
    - Switch formulas.
    - Use loperamide only as a last resort.
- Aspiration:
    - Add drops of methylene blue to feeding and check respiratory secretions for color.
    - Check respiratory secretions with glucose strips.
    - Keep head of bed elevated.
    - Consider surgical jejunostomy.
- Obstruction of feeding tube:
    - Improper flushing—flush with warm water before and after medications.
    - Thick formulas—dilute formula.
    - Inappropriate use of medications—avoid sucralfate and psyllium.
- High gastric residual volumes:
    - Increase risk of aspiration
    - Mechanical problems:
        - Gastric outlet obstruction
        - Small bowel obstruction
    - Functional problems:
        - Gastroparesis
        - Ileus
        - Meds that slow GI motility—opiates and anticholinergics
    - Diagnosis—obstructive series, endoscopy, contrast radiography
    - Treatment:
        - Promotility agents (metoclopramide 10 mg PO or IV qid; cisapride 10 to 20 mg PO qid).
        - Switch to low-fat formula (fat slows gastric emptying).
- Esophagitis:
    - Common in patients with NG tubes.
    - Use H_2 blockers or proton pump inhibitors.

ACID–BASE DISORDERS

Assess the acid–base disorder step by step (Figure 4-7):
- Is the primary disorder an acidosis (pH < 7.40) or alkalosis (pH > 7.40)?
- Is the disorder respiratory (pH and P_{CO_2} move in opposite directions)?

Causes of elevated anion gap metabolic acidosis:

MUDPILES

Methanol, metabolism (inborn errors)

Uremia

Diabetic ketoacidosis

Paraldehyde

Iron, isoniazid

Lactic acidosis

Ethylene glycol

Salicylates, strychnine

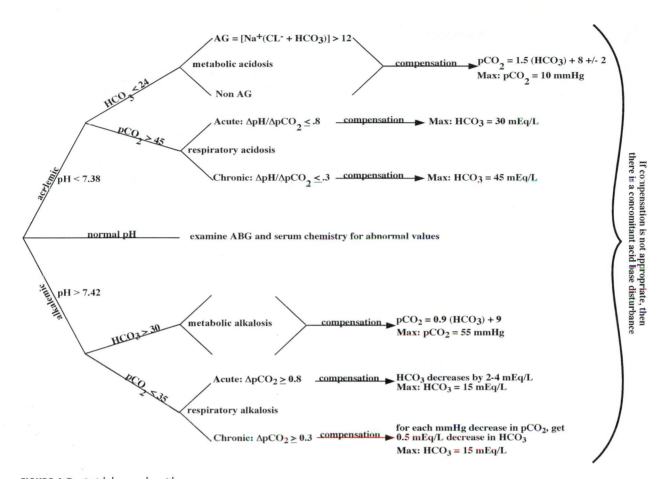

FIGURE 4-7. Acid–base algorithm.
(Reproduced, with permission, from Stead L. *BRS Emergency Medicine*. Philadelphia, PA: Lippincott Williams & Wilkins, 2000.)

- Is the disorder metabolic (pH and P_{CO_2} move in same direction)?
- Is the disorder a simple or mixed disorder?

Use the following general rules of thumb for acute disorders:
- Metabolic acidosis: P_{CO_2} drops ~1.5 (drop in HCO_3)
- Metabolic alkalosis: P_{CO_2} rises ~1.0 (rise in HCO_3)
- Respiratory acidosis: HCO_3 rises ~0.1 (rise in P_{CO_2})
- Respiratory alkalosis: HCO_3 drops ~0.3 (drop in P_{CO_2})

Compensation beyond above parameters suggests mixed disorder.

METABOLIC ACIDOSIS

Two varieties: Anion gap and nonanion gap

Calculating the Anion Gap
$AG = Na - [Cl + HCO_3]$
Normal $AG = 10$

Causes of normal anion gap metabolic acidosis:
HARD UP
Hyperparathyroidism
Adrenal insufficiency, anhydrase (carbonic anhydrase) inhibitors
Renal tubular acidosis
Diarrhea

Ureteroenteric fistula
Pancreatic fistulas

METABOLIC ALKALOSIS

Two mechanisms:
- Loss of H$^+$:
  - Renal: Mineralocorticoid excess, diuretics, potassium-losing nephropathy
  - GI: Vomiting, gastric drainage, villous adenoma of colon
- Gain HCO$_3$: Milk–alkali syndrome, exogenous NaHCO$_3$

RESPIRATORY ACIDOSIS

Hypercapnia secondary to one of two mechanisms:
- Hypoventilation (brain stem injury, neuromuscular disease, ventilator malfunction)
- Ventilation–perfusion (V/Q) mismatch (COPD, pneumonia, pulmonary embolism, foreign body, pulmonary edema)

RESPIRATORY ALKALOSIS

- Hyperventilation secondary to anxiety, increased intracranial pressure (ICP), salicylates, fever, hypoxemia, systemic disease (sepsis), pain, pregnancy, CHF, pneumonia, asthma, liver disease
- Alkalosis causes decrease in serum K and ionized Ca, resulting in paresthesias, carpopedal spasm, and tetany.

Critical Care

DEFINITION

Inadequate perfusion and oxygen delivery to tissues

PHYSIOLOGY OF SHOCK AND TYPES OF SHOCK

Tissue perfusion is determined by:
1. Cardiac output (CO) (and CO = Stroke volume × Heart rate)
2. Systemic vascular resistance (SVR)

The deterioration of one of these factors can cause shock. Shocks are classified into different types according to which of these factors is abnormal. The three major types of shock are **hypovolemic, distributive,** and **cardiogenic.**

If the skin is warm, it is distributive shock. If the skin is cold and clammy, it is hypovolemic or cardiogenic shock.

Hypovolemic Shock

DEFINITION

Decreased tissue perfusion secondary to rapid volume/blood loss, i.e., preload. **CO is consequently decreased.** The causes include bleeding, vomiting/diarrhea, and third spacing (e.g., from burns or pancreatitis).

SIGNS AND SYMPTOMS

Early on, patients will have orthostatic hypotension, tachycardia, and cool skin. As the condition progresses, they are hypotensive, have decreased pulse pressure, become confused, and have cold, clammy skin due to "clamping down" of peripheral vessels.

CLASSIFICATION OF SEVERITY OF HYPOVOLEMIC SHOCK

Class I: Loss of < 20% of circulating blood volume. Manifestations include slight tachycardia. No change in BP or urine output.
Class II: Loss of 20 to 40% of blood volume. Manifestations include tachycardia, tachypnea, capillary refill time > 2 seconds, orthostatis, and decreased pulse pressure. Agitation or confusion may be present.
Class III: Loss of > 40% of circulating blood volume. All of the above plus lethargy and decreased urine output.

Of the vital organs, the first "casualty" of hypovolemic or cardiogenic shock (both "cold shocks") is the kidneys, as blood is shunted away from the constricted renal arteries. Therefore, it is crucial to monitor for renal failure. An adequate urine output is a crucial sign that the treatment is adequate.

Adequate (at minimum)
urine output is 0.5
cc/kg/hr.

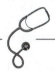

Gram-negative bacteria are
notorious for causing septic
shock.

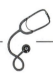

Poor prognostic signs in
septic shock:
- DIC
- Multiple organ failure

Even when SIRS criteria are
met, infection is present <
50% of the time.

Treatment

- Fluids first!! Isotonic fluids are the best volume repleters; hence, use normal saline or lactated Ringer's.
- Replacement of blood, if hemorrhage is cause
- Treat underlying cause (i.e., surgical correction if patient has ongoing hemorrhage).

Distributive Shock

DEFINITION

A family of shock states that are caused by systemic vasodilation (i.e., severe decrease in SVR). They include septic shock, neurogenic shock, and anaphylactic shock. These patients will have warm skin from vasodilation.

SEPTIC SHOCK

Infection that causes vessels to dilate and leak, causing hypotension refractory to fluid recuscitation.

Lab/Physical Findings

- Fever, tachypnea
- Metabolic acidosis, hyperglycemia
- Positive blood cultures (often negative, however, particularly if drawn after antibiotics are started)

Treatment

- Fluids!!
- Antibiotics (**start early** and empirically treat until blood cultures come back—do not wait for blood cultures)
- If blood pressure unresponsive to fluids, the following pressors are classically used: norepinephrine (Levophed) or dopamine (high dose)

The Continuum: SIRS, Sepsis, Severe Sepsis, and Septic Shock

Septic shock is the most severe manifestation of infection in a continuum. Milder manifestations of infection are classified as SIRS, sepsis, and severe sepsis.

- **SIRS (systemic inflammatory response syndrome):** To meet the SIRS criteria, you need two of the following:
  - Temp > 38°C or < 36°C
  - Pulse > 90/min
  - Respiratory rate > 20/min
  - $PaCO_2$ < 32 mm Hg
  - WBC > 12,000 or < 4,000
  - > 10% bands
- **Sepsis:** Sepsis is SIRS + a known source of infection.
- **Severe sepsis:** Severe sepsis is sepsis + organ dysfunction (e.g., renal failure, altered mental status, ARDS, etc.). Hypotension is present, but it responds to fluid resuscitation.
- **Septic shock:** Septic shock is sepsis that is refractory to fluid resuscitation.

ANAPHYLACTIC SHOCK

Systemic type I hypersensitivity reaction causing chemically mediated angioedema and increased vascular permeability, resulting in hypotension and/or airway compromise.

Physical Findings

- Urticaria
- Swelling
- Angioedema of lips and throat
- Wheezing

Treatment

- Intubation if airway compromise
- Epinephrine
- Antihistamines (diphenhydramine)
- Steroids

NEUROGENIC SHOCK

CNS injury causing disruption of the sympathetic system, resulting in unopposed vagal outflow and vasodilation. It is characterized by hypotension and bradycardia (no sympathetic response of vasoconstriction and tachycardia).

Treatment

- Fluids
- If needed, the pressor dopamine or dobutamine is classically used.
- Atropine and/or pacemaker for bradycardia

Cardiogenic Shock

Pump failure, resulting in decreased CO. This can be caused by myocardial infarction, arrhythmias, valvular defects, or extracardiac obstruction (tamponade, pulmonary embolism, tension pneumothorax). Wedge pressure and systemic vascular resistance are elevated.

FINDINGS

Patients will have cold, clammy skin from clamping down of peripheral vessels. Additionally, they will have jugular venous distention (JVD), dyspnea, and bilateral crackles on lung exam. Chest x-ray will show bilateral pulmonary congestion.

TREATMENT

Left heart failure or biventricular failure:
- Diuretics
- Nitrates (decrease preload)
- Classically, the following pressors can be used:
    - Dopamine (medium dose)
    - Dobutamine
    - Amrinone
- Intra-aortic balloon pump can be used to decrease the work of the heart.

Isolated right heart failure: Give fluids (maintains preload).

See Table 5-1.

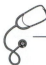

Causes of anaphylaxis: Drugs (penicillin), radiocontrast, insect bites (honeybee, fire ant, wasps), and food (shellfish, peanut butter).

Remember, type I hypersensitivity reactions are immunoglobulin E (IgE) mediated and require prior exposure.

Look for neurogenic shock following history of spinal trauma or spinal anesthesia.

Cardiogenic shock, like hypovolemic shock, often results in renal insult from peripheral vasoconstriction. It is crucial to monitor urine output.

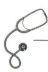

The Swan–Ganz catheter has *never* been proven to improve morbity or mortality in any study.

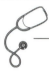

Risks of the Swan–Ganz:
- Infection
- Arrhythmia (the guidewire can irritate the endocardium and trigger this)

How is the wedge pressure obtained? The "wedge" pressure is obtained by inflating the distal end of the Swan–Ganz and "floating" this "balloon" down pulmonary artery until it "wedges." The pressure measured equals the pulmonary capillary pressure, and this, theoretically, represents the left atrial pressure, and ultimately the left ventricular end-diastolic pressure (LVEDP).

What is the significance of the wedge pressure? It reflects the left ventricular pressure, which will be increased with left ventricular failure.

TABLE 5-1. Types of shock and their hemodynamic profiles.

	Wedge (PCWP)	Cardiac Output	Systemic Vascular Resistance (SVR)
Hypovolemic shock	↓	↓	↑
Cardiogenic shock	↑	↓	↑
Distributive shock	↓ or normal	↑	↓

SWAN–GANZ CATHETER

The Swan–Ganz catheter is often used with intensive care unit (ICU) and shock patients in order to obtain information relevant to fluid and volume status. It is threaded through the vena cava (superior or inferior) → right atrium → right ventricle → pulmonary artery.

The following are some of the measurements obtainable through the Swan–Ganz that will allow a better understanding of the different types of shock.

- **Pulmonary capillary wedge pressure (PCWP)** (normal 6 to 12 mm Hg). This reflects the pressures of the left ventricle (end-diastolic pressure). It can be thought of as preload.
  Clinical context: If the pump fails, pressures in the left ventricle increase and you will have an increased wedge.
- **Cardiac output (CO)** (normal 4 to 8 mm Hg). Remember, CO = Stroke volume × Heart rate. The Swan–Ganz allows CO to be measured via the **thermodilutional technique:** The temperature change is measured at the distal end of catheter when cold fluid is injected from proximal port. The difference in temperature reflects the cardiac output. CO can also be thought of as pump function.
  Clinical context: If you have an MI and lose wall motion, your stroke volume will be decreased and, therefore, so will your CO. Likewise, if you hemorrhage and have no preload, your stroke volume will decrease as well.
- **Systemic vascular resistance (SVR)** (usually divided by body surface area to give systemic vascular resistance index [SVRI]) (normal 1,500 to 2,400). SVR reflects the vascular resistance across the systemic circulation (it can be thought of as afterload as well).
  Clinical context: Distributive shock causes vessels to dilate and leak, causing SVR to decrease. Cardiogenic and hypovolemic shock results in vasoconstriction, causing SVR to increase.

A group of vasoactive drugs that are the final line of defense in treating shock

EFFECTS AND SIDE EFFECTS

Generally, pressors are used to increase CO or SVR. All of them have important side effects that can limit their use.

These side effects are easily predicted based on the drug's action. For example, in addition to stimulating β_1 receptors, dobutamine stimulates β_2 (which causes vasodilation). The β_2 stimulation causes the side effect of hypotension.

Furthermore, remember that virtually any direct stimulation of the heart (β_1) can cause the side effect of arrhythmias.

Dobutamine

> **Action:** Strong stimulation β_1 receptors (ionotropic/chronotropic effects on the heart) with a mild stimulation of β_2 (vasodilation)
> **Result:** ↑ CO, ↓ SVR
> **Typical use:** Cardiogenic shock

Isoproterenol

Similar to dobutamine.

> **Action:** Strong stimulation of β_1 receptors (ionotropic/chronotropic effects on the heart) and β_2 (vasodilation)
> **Result:** ↑ CO, ↓ SVR
> **Typical use:** Cardiogenic shock with bradycardia

Milrinone

Milrinone is technically not a pressor, but it is an important drug used in the ICU.

> **Action:** Phosphodiesterase inhibitor, which results in increased cyclic AMP. This has positive ionotropic effects on the heart and also vasodilates.
> **Result:** ↑ CO, ↓ SVR
> **Typical use:** Heart failure/cardiogenic shock

Dopamine

Dopamine has different action depending on the dose.

> **Low Dose (1 to 3 µg/kg/min): "Renal Dose"**
> **Action:** Stimulation of dopamine receptors (dilates renal vasculature) and mild β_1 stimulation
> **Typical use:** Renal insufficiency

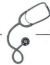

The concept of low-dose dopamine being a "renal dose" and helping perfuse the kidney has been debunked. It dilates the vasculature, but no evidence shows that it is renal protective or improves renal failure.

Intermediate Dose (5 to 10 µg/kg/min): "Cardiac Dose"
Action: Stimulation of dopamine receptors, moderate stimulation of β_1 receptors (heart ionotropy/chronotropy), and mild stimulation of α_1 receptors (vasoconstriction)
Result: ↑CO
Typical use: Cardiogenic shock

High Dose (10 to 20 µg/kg/min)
Action: Stimulates dopamine receptors, β_1 receptors (heart ionotropy/chronotropy), and strong stimulation of α_1 receptors (vasoconstriction)
Result: ↑↑SVR
Typical use: Cardiogenic or septic shock

Norepinephrine

Action: Strong stimulation of α_1 receptors (vasoconstriction), moderate stimulation of β_1 receptors (heart ionotropy/chronotropy)
Result: ↑↑SVR, ↑CO
Typical use: Septic shock

Epinephrine

Action: Strong stimulation of β_1 receptors (heart ionotropy/chronotropy), strong stimulation of α_1 receptors (vasoconstriction), moderate stimulation of β_2 receptors (dilates bronchial tree)
Result: ↑↑SVR, ±/− ↑CO, bronchodilation
Typical use: Anaphylaxis, septic shock, cardiopulmonary arrest

Phenylephrine

Action: Strong stimulation of α_1 receptors (vasoconstriction)
Result: ↑↑SVR
Typical use: Septic shock, neurogenic shock, anesthesia-induced hypotension

Sodium Nitroprusside

This is not a pressor, but it is an important vasoactive drug.

Action: Venodilation and arterial dilation
Result: Decrease preload and afterload
Typical use: Low cardiac output with high BP

Note: Nitroglycerin has less arterial dilation, except in the coronary arteries, which it effectively dilates. It is used for anginal pain in low doses and to reduce BP in high doses.

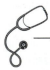

What are the indications for intubation? Intubation is a clinical decision, based on clinical circumstance as well as physiologic derangements. It is not based on any absolute numbers.

MECHANICAL VENTILATION

The decision to put someone on a ventilator is clinical; there are no finite lab values that tell you exactly when to intubate. A blood gas, for example, may contribute evidence that leads you in that direction, but intubation and mechanical ventilation is not done based on numbers alone.

The goals of mechanical ventilation are to:
1. Improve gas exchange
2. Decrease the work of breathing

There are different ways to provide ventilatory support via mechanical ventilation, and the main options are discussed below.

Pressure Support

An initial "boost of pressure" triggered by the patient's initiation of a breath. This boost helps the patient to overcome the resistance of the endotracheal tube. This mode can be used alone, as the only ventilator setting, or in conjunction with the IMV mode (see below). Pressure support is typically set at 8 to 20.

Pressure support is an important weaning mode.

Assist-Control Mechanical Ventilation (AC)

A set tidal volume is given a set number of times per minute. If the patient initiates a breath himself, the vent responds by giving the preset tidal volume.

Intermittent Mandatory Ventilation (IMV)

When the patient initiates a breath, the vent responds by giving pressure support (a boost of pressure to overcome initial resistance—see above), but the amount of tidal volume will be determined by the patient's inspiratory effort. As a backup, if the patient does not initiate breaths, a set tidal volume is automatically given a certain number of times per minute (like AC mode).

IMV theoretically allows the patient to "exercise" his respiratory muscles and therefore condition him for weaning off the vent. This concept has *never* been proven.

Continuous Positive Airway Pressure (CPAP)

Continuous positive pressure, with no variation with the breathing cycle. The patient must breathe on his own.

Positive End-Expiratory Pressure (PEEP)

Positive pressure is provided at the end of a breath to maintain alveoli open. PEEP is typically set at 5 to 20.

Setting the Ventilator

Several parameters have to be set for the vent. You need to define the mode (e.g., AC, IMV), respiratory rate, tidal volume, and the FIO_2.

> **Mode:** Choose AC, IMV, PS, or CPAP.
> **Respiratory rate** (for AC or IMV only): Usually 10 to 20
> **Tidal volume** (for AC or IMV only): Usually 400 to 600 cc (6.8 cc/kg)
> **FIO_2:** Always start at 100% and titrate down, maintaining the pulse ox > 90%.

PEEP is used primarily in congestive heart failure (CHF) or acute respiratory distress syndrome (ARDS). It maintains alveoli open, allowing more time for gas exchange. It is therefore used to increase the oxygen level. Problems with PEEP can be hypotension (decreases preload).

What are the causes of failure to wean off the vent?
1. Secretions
2. Drugs (usually, sedatives)
3. Alkalemia (remember, H^+ stimulates respiration)
4. Endotracheal tube is too small bore (patient will have to overcome a lot of resistance)
5. Diaphragm dysfunction

Try to titrate down the FIO_2 (< 50% is ideal) in order to avoid oxygen toxicity. Oxygen toxicity is thought to be caused by oxygen free radicals damaging the lung interstitium.

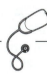

The chest x-ray does not reliably distinguish ARDS from CHF. A Swan–Ganz catheter can be useful in this matter.
- PCWP < 18 = ARDS
- PCWP > 18 = CHF

EXAMPLES

Typical AC mode setting:
AC 12, tidal volume 500 cc, $FIO_2 = 5$
Note: Can be used with or without PEEP, *no PS.*
Typical IMV mode setting:
IMV 12 (back-up rate), tidal volume 500 cc, PS = 8, $FIO_2 = 50\%$
Note: Can be used with or without PEEP.

Adjusting the Ventilator

MINUTE VENTILATION

Minute ventilation = Respiratory rate × Tidal volume. You can therefore adjust either the rate or the tidal volume to change the minute ventilation.

Know this simple rule: Increasing minute ventilation will decrease PCO_2 and increase pH. Decreasing minute ventilation will increase PCO_2 and decrease pH.

OXYGENATION

FIO_2 is the ventilator parameter that adjusts oxygenation.

ACUTE RESPIRATORY DISTRESS SYNDROME (ARDS)

Acute lung injury caused by inflammatory process in both lungs causing increased permeability of the capillaries and severe V/Q mismatch. These patients are tachypneic and hypoxic and have bilateral crackles on lung exam.

The diagnostic criteria are:
1. Bilateral, fluffy infiltrates on chest x-ray
2. Refractory hypoxemia
3. No evidence of heart failure (PCWP ≤ 18 mm Hg)

The diagnosis requires all three criteria.

CAUSES

There is a wide variety of causes of ARDS. The most common are:
- Sepsis (most common)
- Infectious pneumonia
- Blood products
- Aspiration
- Severe trauma, burns

MANAGEMENT

It is often necessary to intubate because of hypoxemia. Treat underlying cause. PEEP is often used to improve gas exchange and keep lungs open at relatively low lung volumes.

Trauma

ADVANCED TRAUMA LIFE SUPPORT (ATLS)

"Golden Hour" of Trauma

Period immediately following trauma in which rapid assessment, diagnosis, and stabilization must occur.

Prehospital Phase

Control of airway and external hemorrhage, immobilization, and rapid transport of patient to **NEAREST** appropriate facility.

Preparation

- Gown up, glove up, face shields on!
- Standard precautions!
- Set up: Airway equipment, monitor, O_2, Foley, IV and blood tubes (complete blood count [CBC], chemistry, prothrombin time/partial thromboplastin time [PT/PTT], type and cross, human chorionic gonadotropin [hCG], ± toxicologies), chest tube tray, etc.

Trauma History

Whenever possible take an **AMPLE** history
- Allergies
- Medications/Mechanism of injury
- Past medical history/Pregnant?
- Last meal
- Events surrounding the mechanism of injury

Primary Survey

Initial assessment and resuscitation of vital functions. Prioritization based on ABCs of trauma care.

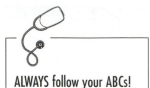

ALWAYS follow your ABCs!

Assume C-spine injury in trauma patients until proven otherwise.

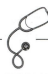

All trauma patients should receive supplemental O$_2$.

Draw blood samples at the time of intravenous catheter placement.

AVPU scale:
Alert
Verbal
Pain
Unresponsive

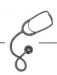

Don't forget to keep your patients **warm** (cover them up again as soon as possible).

ABCs

- Airway (with cervical spine precautions)
- Breathing and ventilation
- Circulation (and **Control of hemorrhage**)
- Disability (neurologic status)
- Exposure/Environment control
- Foley

Airway and C-spine

- Assess patency of airway.
- Use jaw thrust or chin lift initially to open airway.
- Clear foreign bodies.
- Insert oral or nasal airway when necessary. Obtunded/unconscious patients should be intubated. Surgical airway = cricothyroidotomy—used when unable to intubate airway.

Breathing and Ventilation

- Inspect, auscultate, and palpate the chest.
- Ensure adequate ventilation and identify and treat injuries that may immediately impair ventilation:
  - Tension pneumothorax
  - Flail chest and pulmonary contusion
  - Massive hemothorax
  - Open pneumothorax

Control of Hemorrhage

- Place two large-bore (14- or 16-gauge) IVs.
- Assess circulatory status (capillary refill, pulse, skin color) (see Shock section below).
- Control of life-threatening hemorrhage using direct pressure; do not "clamp" bleeding vessels with hemostats.

Disability

- Rapid neurologic exam
- Establish pupillary size and reactivity and level of consciousness using the AVPU or Glasgow Coma Scale.

Exposure/Environment/Extras

- Completely undress the patient, most often with the help of your trauma shears.
- Hook up monitors (cardiac, pulse oximetry, blood pressure [BP], etc.)

Foley Catheter

- Placement of a urinary catheter is considered part of the resuscitative phase that takes place during the primary survey.

- Important for monitoring urinary output, which is a reflection of renal perfusion and volume status.
- Adequate urinary output:
  - Adult: 0.5 cc/kg/hr
  - Child (> 1 year of age): 1.0 cc/kg/hr
  - Child (< 1 year of age): 2.0 cc/kg/hr
- Foley is contraindicated when urethral transection is suspected, such as in the case of a pelvic fracture. If transection suspected, perform retrograde urethrogram before Foley.

Signs of Urethral Transection
- Blood at the meatus
- A "high-riding" prostate
- Perineal or scrotal hematoma
- Be suspicious with any pelvic fracture.

Examine prostate and genitalia before placing a Foley.

Gastric Intubation

Placement of nasogastric (NG) or orogastric (OG) tube may reduce risk of aspiration by decompressing stomach, but does not assure full prevention.

Place OGT rather than NGT when fracture of cribriform plate is suspected.

RESUSCITATION

- Begins during the primary survey.
- Life-threatening injuries are tended to as they are identified.

Trauma resuscitation is a team sport with many different activities overlapping in both time and space.

Intravenous Catheters

The rate of maximal fluid administration is directly related to the internal diameter of the IV catheter (to the 4th power of the radius according to Poiseuille's law) and inversely related to the length of the tubing.

Intravenous Fluid

- Fluid therapy should be initiated with up to 2 L of an isotonic (either lactated Ringer's or normal saline) crystalloid (see below) solution.
- Pediatric patients should receive an IV bolus of 20 cc/kg.

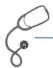

The antecubital fossae are a good place to find nice veins in which to place large-bore IVs.

Crystalloid vs. Colloid

- Crystalloids are sodium-based solutions that provide a transient increase in intravascular volume.
- Approximately one third of an isotonic solution will remain in the intravascular space. The remainder almost immediately distributes to the extravascular and interstitial spaces. This occurs because crystalloid solutions easily diffuse across membranes.
- Colloids have a harder time diffusing across membranes, thus remaining in the intravascular space for longer periods of time, thereby requiring smaller volumes for resuscitation. However, they are costly and carry the risks of transfusion reactions and viral transmission and have not been shown to improve outcomes.

Use **warmed** fluids whenever possible.

Body Water:
2/3 intracellular
1/3 extracellular:
    1/4 intravascular
    3/4 extravascular

- Crystalloids include saline and Ringer's lactate.
- Colloids include blood products such as red blood cells (RBCs) and albumin.

- Neither crystalloids nor colloid have been shown to be superior for volume resuscitation. Therefore, volume resuscitation begins with crystalloids (see below).

"3-to-1 Rule"

Used as a rough estimate for the total amount of crystalloid volume needed acutely to replace blood loss.

Shock

- Inadequate delivery of oxygen on the cellular level secondary to tissue hypoperfusion.
- In traumatic situations, shock is the result of hypovolemia until proven otherwise.

Hypovolemic Shock

Caused by the acute loss of blood in most cases. Blood volume estimate based on body weight in kilograms:
- Adults: 7% of weight
- Peds: 8–9% of weight

Example: 70-kg adult ($70 \times 7\% = 4.9$ liters of blood)

Classes of Hemorrhagic Shock

See Table 6-1.

TABLE 6-1. Types of hemorrhagic shock.

Class	Blood Loss (%)	Vol. Blood Loss (cc)	Heart Rate	Pulse Pressure	Systolic BP	Urine Output	Altered Mental Status?	Treatment
I	Up to 15	Up to 750	< 100	N	N	N	No	Crystalloids (3-to-1 rule). No blood products necessary.
II	15–30	750–1,500	↑	↓	↓	↓	No	Crystalloids initially, then monitor response. May or may not need blood products. Can wait for type-specific blood.
III	30–40	1,500–2,000	↑↑	↓↓	↓↓	↓↓	Yes	Crystalloids followed by type-specific blood products.
IV	>40	>2,000	↑↑↑	↓↓↓	↓↓↓	↓↓↓	Yes	2-L crystalloid bolus followed by uncrossed (O negative) blood. Death is imminent.

N, normal; ↑, increased; ↓, decreased.

Treatment of Hemorrhagic Shock

- Response to the initial fluid bolus (e.g., change in vital signs, urinary output, and/or level of consciousness) should direct further resuscitative efforts.
- Early blood transfusion and surgical intervention should be a consideration in patients who fail to respond to initial fluid resuscitation.

Hemorrhage is the most common cause of shock in the injured patient.

Nonhypovolemic Shock

- **Cardiogenic shock** during trauma may occur secondary to blunt myocardial injury, cardiac tamponade, tension pneumothorax, air embolus, or an acute myocardial infarction.
- **Neurogenic shock** may occur secondary to sympathetic denervation in patients who have suffered a spinal injury.
- **Septic shock** is due to infection and may be seen when there is a significant delay in patient arrival to the emergency department (ED) (> 24 hrs) or in patients with penetrating abdominal injuries, for example.

Radiologic and Diagnostic Studies

- X-rays of the chest, pelvis, and lateral cervical spine usually occur concurrently with early resuscitative efforts; however, this procedure should never interrupt the resuscitative process.
- Diagnostic peritoneal lavage (DPL) and focused abdominal sonogram for trauma (FAST) are also tools used for the rapid detection of intra-abdominal bleeding that often occurs early in the resuscitative process (see Abdominal Trauma).

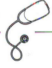

A "trauma series" consists of radiographs of the C-spine, chest, and pelvis.

Secondary Survey

- Begins once the primary survey is complete and resuscitative efforts are well under way.
- Head-to-toe evaluation of the trauma patient including a detailed history; frequent reassessment is key.
- Neurologic examination, procedures, radiologic examination, and laboratory testing take place at this time if not already accomplished.

"Fingers and tubes in every orifice."

Tetanus Prophylaxis

Immunize as needed.

HEAD TRAUMA

Anatomy and Physiology

Scalp
- The scalp consists of five layers.
- Highly vascular structure.
- May be the source of major blood loss.
- The loose attachment between the galea and the pericranium allows for large collections of blood forming a subgaleal hematoma.

Layers of the scalp:
Skin
Connective tissue
Aponeurosis (galea)
Loose areolar tissue
Pericranium

- Disruption of the galea should be corrected and may be done so with single-layer, interrupted 3.0 nonabsorbable sutures through the skin, subcutaneous tissue, and galea.
- Prophylactic antibiotics are not indicated in simple scalp lacerations.

Skull
- Rigid and inflexible (fixed volume)
- Composed of the cranial vault and base

Brain
- Makes up 80% of intracranial volume
- Partially compartmentalized by the reflections of dura (falx cerebri and tentorium cerebelli)

Cerebrospinal Fluid (CSF)
- Formed primarily by the choroid plexus at a rate of approximately 500 cc/day with 150 cc of CSF circulating at a given moment
- Cushions the brain

Cerebral Blood Flow
- Brain receives approximately 15% of cardiac output.
- Brain responsible for ~20% of total body O_2 consumption.

Cerebral Perfusion Pressure (CPP)
- CPP = MAP – ICP
- MAP = mean arterial blood pressure
- ICP = intracranial pressure
- Maintaining CPP in non-operative brain injury is the fundamental treatment.

Monro–Kellie Hypothesis

- The sum of the volume of the brain, blood, and CSF within the skull must remain constant. Therefore, an increase in one of the above must be offset by decreased volume of the others. If not, the ICP will increase.
- Increased ICP can thus result in cerebral herniation, or when ICP = systolic BP, cerebral blood flow ceases and brain death occurs.

Assessment

- History
- Identify mechanism and time of injury, loss of consciousness, concurrent use of drugs or alcohol, medications that may affect pupillary size (e.g., glaucoma medications), past medical history (especially previous head trauma and stroke with their residual effects, and previous eye surgery, which can affect pupillary size and response) and the presence of a "lucid interval."

Vital Signs

Cushing reflex:
- Brain's attempt to maintain the CPP
- Hypertension and bradycardia in the setting of increased ICP

CN III runs along the edge of the tentorium cerebelli.

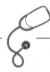

Concept of CPP is important in a hypertensive patient. Lowering the BP too fast will also decrease the CPP, creating a new problem.

Hypotension is usually not caused by isolated head injury. Look for other injuries in this setting.

- Search for signs of external trauma such as lacerations, hemotympponum, ecchymoses, and avulsions, as these may be clues to underlying injuries such as depressed or open skull fractures.
- Anisocoria (unequal pupils) are found in a small percentage (10%) of normal people; however, unequal pupils in the patient with head trauma are pathologic until proven otherwise.

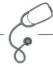

An enlarging pupil with a concurrent decrease in level of consciousness is strongly suggestive of uncal herniation.

Glasgow Coma Scale (GCS)

- The Glasgow Coma Scale may be used as a tool for classifying head injury (see Figure 6-1):

Severe head injury	GCS 8 or less
Moderate head injury	GCS 9 to 13
Mild head injury	GCS 14 or 15

Diagnostic Studies

- Assume C-spine injury in head injury patients and immobilize until cleared.
- Skull films have largely been replaced by computed tomography (CT) scan.
- Indications for head/brain CT:
  - Neurologic deficit
  - Persisting depression or worsening of mental status
  - Moderate to severe mechanism of injury
  - Depressed skull fracture or linear fracture overlying a dural venous sinus or meningeal artery groove (as demonstrated with skull x-rays)

Skin staples interfere with CT scanning and should therefore not be used until after CT scanning is complete.

Eyes	Open spontaneously	4
	Open to verbal command	3
	Open to pain	2
	No response	1
Best motor response	Obeys verbal command	6
	Localizes pain to painful stimulus	5
	Flexion–withdrawal	4
	Decorticate rigidity	3
	Decerebrate rigidity	2
	No response	1
Best verbal response	Oriented and converses	5
	Disoriented and converses	4
	Inappropriate words	3
	Incomprehensible sounds	2
	No response	1
TOTAL		**15**

FIGURE 6-1. Glasgow Coma Scale.

HIGH-YIELD FACTS

Trauma

Linear (Nondepressed)

Becomes clinically important if it occurs over the middle meningeal artery groove or major venous dural sinuses (formation of an epidural hematoma), air-filled sinuses, or if associated with underlying brain injury.

Stellate

Suggestive of a more severe mechanism of injury than linear skull fractures.

Depressed

- Carries a much greater risk of underlying brain injury and complications, such as meningitis and post-traumatic seizures.
- Treatment involves surgical elevation for depressions deeper than the thickness of the adjacent skull.

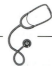

Ring test for CSF rhinorrhea (in the presence of epistaxis): Sample of blood from nose placed on filter paper to test for presence of CSF. If present, a large transparent ring will be seen encircling a clot of blood.

Basilar

- Often a clinical diagnosis and sign of a significant mechanism of injury.
- Signs include periorbital ecchymoses (Raccoon's eyes), retroauricular ecchymoses (Battle's sign), otorrhea, rhinorrhea, hemotympanum, and cranial nerve palsies.

Open

- A laceration overlying a skull fracture.
- Requires careful debridement and irrigation. Avoid blind digital probing of the wound.
- Obtain neurosurgical consultation.

Typical scenario: A 20-year-old female has brief loss of consciousness following head injury. She presents to the ED awake but is amnestic for the event and keeps asking the same questions again and again. *Think:* Concussion.

Cerebral Concussion

- Transient loss of consciousness that occurs immediately following blunt, nonpenetrating head trauma, caused by impairment of the reticular activating system.
- Recovery is often complete; however, residual effects such as headache may last for some time.

Diffuse Axonal Injury (DAI)

- Caused by microscopic shearing of nerve fibers, scattered microscopic abnormalities.
- Frequently requires intubation, hyperventilation, CPP monitoring, and admission to a neurosurgical intensive care unit (ICU).

- Patients are often comatose for prolonged periods of time.
- Mortality is approximately 33%.

FOCAL INTRACRANIAL LESIONS

Cerebral Contusion

- Occurs when the brain impacts the skull. May occur directly under the site of impact (coup) or on the contralateral side (contrecoup).
- Patients may have focal deficits; mental status ranges from confusion to coma.

Intracerebral Hemorrhage

Caused by traumatic tearing of intracerebral blood vessels. Difficult to differentiate from a contusion.

Epidural Hematoma

- Collection of blood between the dura and the skull.
- Majority associated with tearing of the middle meningeal artery from an overlying temporal bone fracture.
- Typically biconvex or lenticular in shape (see Figure 6-2).
- Patients may have the classic "lucid interval," where they "talk and die." Requires early neurosurgical involvement and hematoma evacuation.
- Good outcome if promptly treated.

Typical scenario: A 19-year-old male with a head injury has loss of consciousness followed by a brief lucid interval. He presents to the ED in a coma, with an ipsilateral fixed and dilated pupil and contralateral hemiparesis. *Think:* Epidural hematoma.

HIGH-YIELD FACTS

Trauma

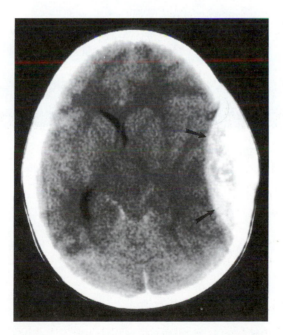

FIGURE 6-2. Epidural hematoma. Arrows indicate the characteristic lens-shaped lesion. (Reproduced, with permission, from Schwartz SI, Spencer SC, Galloway AC, et al. *Principles of Surgery,* 7th ed. New York: McGraw-Hill, 199: 1882.)

Subdural Hematoma

- Collection of blood below the dura and over the brain (see Figure 6-3). Results from tearing of the bridging veins, usually secondary to an acceleration–deceleration mechanism.
- Classified as acute (< 24 hours), subacute (24 hours–2 weeks), and chronic (> 2 weeks old).
- Acute and subacute subdurals require early neurosurgical involvement.
- Alcoholics and the elderly (patients likely to have brain atrophy), have increased susceptibility.

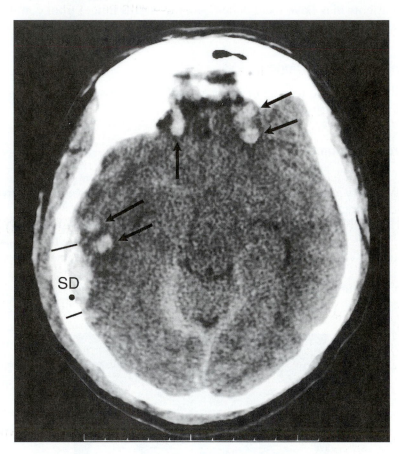

FIGURE 6-3. Subdural hematoma.

MANAGEMENT OF MILD TO MODERATE HEAD TRAUMA

- Safe disposition of the patient depends on multiple factors.
- Any patient with a persisting or worsening decrease in mental status, focal deficits, severe mechanism of injury, penetrating trauma, open or depressed skull fracture, or seizures, or who is unreliable or cannot be safely observed at home, should be admitted for observation.
- Patients with mild and sometimes moderate head trauma, brief or no loss of consciousness, no focal deficits, an intact mental status, a normal CT scan, and reliable family members who can adequately observe the patient at home can often be discharged with proper discharge instructions.
- Discharge instructions should include signs and symptoms for family members to watch for such as:
  - Persisting or worsening headache
  - Dizziness
  - Vomiting
  - Inequality of pupils
  - Confusion
- If any of the above signs are found, the patient should be brought to the ED immediately.

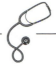

When in doubt, admit the patient for observation.

MANAGEMENT OF SEVERE HEAD TRAUMA

- Patients must be treated aggressively starting with the ABCs.
- Secure the airway via endotracheal intubation using topical anesthesia, intravenous lidocaine, and paralytics when necessary to prevent any further increase in the ICP.
- Maintain an adequate BP with isotonic fluids.
- Treatment of increased ICP:
  - Hyperventilation to an arterial P_{CO_2} of 28 to 32 will decrease the ICP by approximately 25% acutely (last resort only if herniation is imminent).
- Mannitol (1 g/kg in a 20% solution) is an osmotic diuretic and lowers ICP by drawing water out of the brain. Contraindicated in the hypotensive patient.
- Corticosteroids have not been shown to be useful in the patient with head trauma (used in penetrating spinal trauma).
- Consider prophylactic anticonvulsant therapy with phenytoin 18 mg/kg IV at no faster than 50 mg/min (usually at the discretion of the neurosurgeon).
- Acute seizures should be managed with diazepam or lorazepam and phenytoin.
- Early ICP measurement via ventriculostomy should begin in the ED and is also at the discretion of the neurosurgeon.
- Treat the pathology whenever possible (e.g., surgical drainage of a hematoma).

Measures to lower ICP:
HIVED
- **H**yperventilation
- **I**ntubation with pretreatment and sedation
- **V**entriculostomy (burr hole)
- **E**levate the head of the bed
- **D**iuretics (mannitol, furosemide)

General

Described in broad terms as penetrating vs. blunt injuries even though considerable overlap exists between the management of the two.

Anatomy

- The neck is divided into triangles (anterior and posterior) as well as zones (I, II, and III).

Anterior Triangle
- Bordered by the midline, posterior border of the sternocleidomastoid muscle (SCM), and the mandible

Posterior Triangle
- Bordered by the trapezius, posterior border of the SCM, and the clavicle. There is a paucity of vital structures in its upper zone (above the spinal accessory nerve). In the lower zone lie the subclavian vessels, brachial plexus, and the apices of the lungs.

Zones of the Neck
- Further division of the anterior triangle (see Figure 6-4):
  - Zone I lies below the cricoid cartilage.
  - Zone II lies between I and III.
  - Zone III lies above the angle of the mandible.
- These divisions help drive the diagnostic and therapeutic management decisions for penetrating neck injuries.

The majority of the vital structures of the neck lie within the anterior triangle.

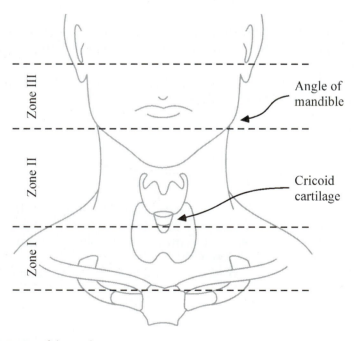

FIGURE 6-4. Zones of the neck.

Penetrating Injuries

Any injury to the neck in which the platysma is violated

Vascular Injuries
- Very common and often life threatening.
- Can lead to exsanguination, hematoma formation with compromise of the airway, and cerebral vascular accidents (e.g., from transection of the carotid artery or air embolus).

Nonvascular Injuries
- Injury to the larynx and trachea including fracture of the thyroid cartilage, dislocation of the tracheal cartilages and arytenoids, for example, leading to airway compromise and often a difficult intubation.
- Esophageal injury does occur, and as with penetrating neck injury is not often manifest initially (very high morbidity/mortality if missed).

Resuscitation

AIRWAY

- Special attention should be paid to airway management of the patient with neck trauma.
- Anatomy may be distorted and an apparently patent airway can rapidly evolve into a compromised, difficult airway.
- Initial attempts at securing the airway should be via endotracheal intubation; however, preparation for alternative methods of airway management, such as percutaneous transtracheal ventilation and surgical airway, should be readily available.

BREATHING

- Inability to ventilate the patient after an apparently successful intubation should prompt rapid reassessment of that airway.
- Creation and/or intubation of a "false lumen" in the patient with laryngotracheal or tracheal transection may be a fatal error if not identified immediately.
- Look for pneumohemothorax as the apices of the lungs lie in close proximity to the base of the neck.

CIRCULATION

- If the patient remains unstable after appropriate volume resuscitation, that patient should be taken rapidly to the OR for operative control of the bleeding.
- If injury to the subclavian vessels is suspected, IV access should be obtained in the opposite extremity, or more appropriately in the lower extremities.
- If a hemopneumothorax is suspected, and central venous access is necessary, a femoral line is the first option, followed by placement of the access on the side ipsilateral to the "dropped lung" (because the patient doesn't like it when both lungs are down!).

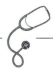

Fracture of the hyoid bone is suggestive of a significant mechanism of injury.

C-spine injuries are much more common with blunt neck injury.

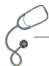

Avoid unnecessary manipulation of the neck as this may dislodge a clot.

Keep cervical in-line stabilization until C-spine fracture has been ruled out.

Tracheostomy is the procedure of choice in the patient with laryngotracheal separation.

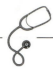

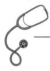

Secondary Survey

- After stabilization, the wound should be carefully examined.
- Obtain soft-tissue films of the neck for clues to the presence of a soft-tissue hematoma and subcutaneous emphysema, and a chest x-ray (CXR) for possible hemopneumothorax.
- Surgical exploration is indicated for:
  - Expanding hematoma
  - Subcutaneous emphysema
  - Tracheal deviation
  - Change in voice quality
  - Air bubbling through the wound
- Pulses should be palpated to identify deficits and thrills, and auscultated for bruits.
- A neurologic exam should be performed to identify brachial plexus and/or central nervous system (CNS) deficits as well as a Horner's syndrome.

Management

- Zone II injuries with instability or enlarging hematoma require exploration in the OR.
- Injuries to Zones I and III may be taken to OR or managed conservatively using a combination of angiography, bronchoscopy, esophagoscopy, gastrografin or barium studies, and CT scanning.

SPINAL TRAUMA

General

- Spinal trauma may involve injury to the spinal column, spinal cord, or both.
- Over 50% of spinal injuries occur in the C-spine, with the remainder being divided between the thoracic spine, the thoracolumbar junction, and the lumbosacral region.
- As long as the spine is appropriately immobilized, evaluation for spinal injury may be deferred until the patient is stabilized.

Anatomy

- There are 7 cervical, 12 thoracic, 5 lumbar, 5 sacral, and 4 coccygeal vertebrae.
- The cervical spine is the region most vulnerable to injury.
- The thoracic spine is relatively protected due to limited mobility from support of the rib cage (T1–T10); however, the spinal canal through which the spinal cord traverses is relatively narrow in this region. Therefore, when injuries to this region do occur, they usually have devastating results.
- The thoracolumbar junction (T11–L1) is a fairly vulnerable region as it is the area between the relatively inflexible thoracic region and the flexible lumbar region.

- The lumbosacral region (L2 and below) contains the region of the spinal canal below which the spinal cord proper ends and the cauda equina begins.

Pathology and Pathophysiology

Spinal injuries can generally be classified based on:
- Fracture/dislocation type (mechanism, stable vs. unstable)
- Level of neurological (sensory and motor) and bony involvement
- Severity (complete vs. incomplete spinal cord disability)

Neurogenic Shock

- A state of vasomotor instability resulting from impairment of the descending sympathetic pathways in the spinal cord, or simply a loss of sympathetic tone.
- Signs and symptoms include flaccid paralysis, hypotension, bradycardia, cutaneous vasodilation, and a normal to wide pulse pressure.

Spinal Shock

- State of flaccidity and loss of reflexes occurring immediately after spinal cord injury.
- Loss of visceral and peripheral autonomic control with uninhibited parasympathetic impulses.
- May last from seconds to weeks, and does not signify permanent spinal cord damage.
- Long-term prognosis cannot be postulated until spinal shock has resolved.

Spinal Cord Injuries

COMPLETE VS. INCOMPLETE

- Complete spinal cord injuries demonstrate no preservation of neurologic function distal to the level of injury. Therefore, any sensorimotor function below the level of injury constitutes an incomplete injury.
- Sacral sparing refers to perianal sensation, voluntary anal sphincter contraction, or voluntary toe flexion, and is a sign of an incomplete spinal cord injury (i.e., better prognosis).

Physical Exam

- Classification of spinal cord injuries as complete or incomplete requires a proper neurologic exam.
- The exam should include testing of the three readily assessable long spinal tracts (see Figure 6-5):
  - Corticospinal tract (CST)
    - Located in the posterolateral aspect of the spinal cord
    - Responsible for ipsilateral motor function
    - Tested via voluntary muscle contraction

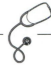

Mechanisms suspicious for spinal injury:
- Diving
- Fall from > 10 feet
- Injury above level of shoulders (C-spine)
- Electrocution
- High-speed motor vehicle crash (MVC)
- Rugby or football injury (tackling)

Deep tendon reflexes and sacral reflexes may be preserved in complete injuries.

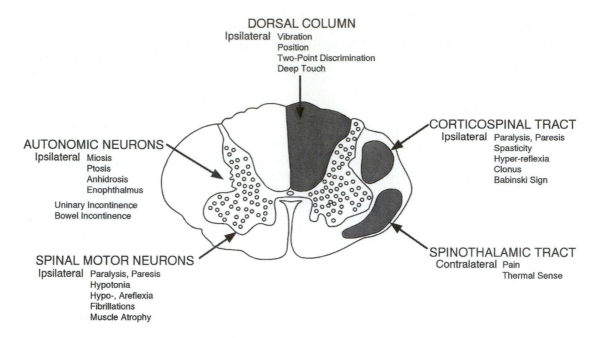

DORSAL COLUMN
Ipsilateral Vibration
Position
Two-Point Discrimination
Deep Touch

CORTICOSPINAL TRACT
Ipsilateral Paralysis, Paresis
Spasticity
Hyper-reflexia
Clonus
Babinski Sign

AUTONOMIC NEURONS
Ipsilateral Miosis
Ptosis
Anhidrosis
Enophthalmus

Uninary Incontinence
Bowel Incontinence

SPINAL MOTOR NEURONS
Ipsilateral Paralysis, Paresis
Hypotonia
Hypo-, Areflexia
Fibrillations
Muscle Atrophy

SPINOTHALAMIC TRACT
Contralateral Pain
Thermal Sense

FIGURE 6-5. Cross-section of the spinal cord and tracts. (Reproduced, with permission, from Afifi AA, Bergman RA. *Functional Neuroanatomy: Text and Atlas.* New York: McGraw-Hill, 1998: 92.)

- Spinothalamic tract (STT)
  - Located in the anteriolateral aspect of the spinal cord
  - Responsible for contralateral pain and temperature sensation and is tested as such
- Posterior columns
  - Located in the posterior aspect of the spinal cord
  - Responsible for ipsilateral position and vibratory sense and some light touch sensation
- Testing using a tuning fork and position sense of the fingers and toes

Spinal Cord Syndromes

ANTERIOR CORD SYNDROME

- Pattern seen with injury to the anterior portion of the spinal cord or with compression of the anterior spinal arteries (Artery of Adam Klewicz)
- Involves full or partial loss of bilateral pain and temperature sensation (STT) and paraplegia (CST) with preservation of posterior column function
- Often seen with flexion injuries
- Carries a poor prognosis

BROWN–SEQUARD SYNDROME

- Pattern seen with hemisection of the spinal cord usually secondary to a penetrating injury, but may also be seen with disc protrusion, hematoma, or tumor
- Consists of ipsilateral loss of motor function (CST) and posterior column function, with contralateral loss of pain and temperature sensation

Trauma

CENTRAL CORD SYNDROME

- Pattern seen with injury to the central area of the spinal cord often in patients with a preexisting narrowing of the spinal canal.
- Usually seen with hyperextension injuries, its cause is usually attributed to buckling of the ligamentum flavum into the cord and/or an ischemic etiology in the distribution of branches of the anterior spinal artery.
- Characterized by weakness greater in the upper extremities than the lower extremities, and distal worse than proximal.
- Has a better prognosis than the other partial cord syndromes with a characteristic pattern of recovery (lower extremity recovery progressing upward to upper extremity recovery, then the hands recover strength).

Typical scenario: A 70-year-old male presents to the ED after a whiplash injury. He is ambulating well but has an extremely weak handshake. *Think:* Central cord syndrome.

Treatment of Spinal Cord Syndromes

- Always start with the ABCs of trauma resuscitation.
- Maintain spinal immobilization throughout the resuscitation.
- Estimate level of neurologic dysfunction during the secondary survey.
- Obtain appropriate diagnostic studies.
- Establish early neurosurgical consultation.
- If penetrating spinal cord injury is diagnosed, begin high-dose methyl-prednisolone (must be given within 8 hours of injury and not for penetrating injury).
  - Loading dose of 30 mg/kg over 15 minutes during hour 1, followed by a continuous infusion of 5.4 mg/kg/hr over the next 23 hours.
- Consider traction devices in consultation with the neurosurgeon.
- Consider early referral to a regional spinal injury center.

C-SPINE FRACTURES AND DISLOCATIONS

General

As mentioned above, are usually classified on the basis of mechanism (flexion, extension, compression, rotation, or a combination of these), location, and/or stability.

IMAGING

- Three views of the cervical spine are obtained (lateral, anteroposterior [AP], and an odontoid view) for best accuracy.
- A lateral view alone will miss 10% of C-spine injuries.
- Adequate AP and lateral films will allow visualization of C1–T1.
- If C1–T1 still cannot be adequately visualized, CT scan is indicated.

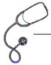

C-spine films are indicated for:

- Tenderness along C-spine
- Neurologic deficit
- Good mechanism of injury
- Presence of distracting injury
- Patients with altered sensorium

Reading a C-Spine Film

Alignment
- Evaluate the alignment of the four lordotic curves (see Figure 6-6):
  - Anterior margin of the vertebral bodies
  - Posterior margin of the vertebral bodies
  - Spinolaminar line
  - Tips of the vertebral body
    - In the adult, up to 3.5 mm of anterior subluxation is considered a normal finding.

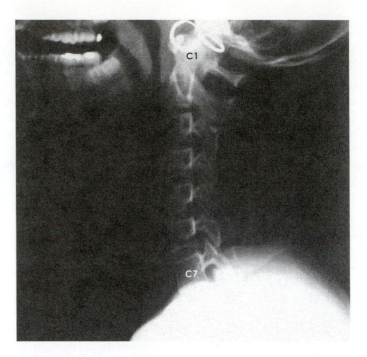

FIGURE 6-6. Lateral view of cervical spine.

- Most common level of fracture is C5.
- Most common level of subluxation is C5 on C6.

Bones
- Assess the base of the skull and each vertebral body, pedicle, facet, lamina, and spinous and transverse process for fracture/dislocation.

Cartilage
- Assess the intervertebral spaces and posterolateral facet joints for symmetry.

Soft Tissue
- Assess the prevertebral soft tissue: Wider than 5 mm suggests hematoma accompanying a fracture.
- Assess the predental space: Wider than 3 mm in adults and 4 to 5 mm in children is suggestive of a torn transverse ligament and fracture of C1.
- Assess the spaces between the spinous processes: Any increase in distance between the spinous processes is likely associated with a torn interspinous ligament and a spinal fracture.

ATLANTO-OCCIPITAL DISLOCATION
- Results from severe traumatic flexion.
- Survival to the hospital setting is rare.
- Traction is contraindicated.

JEFFERSON FRACTURE
- C1 (atlas) burst fracture.
- Most common C1 fracture.
- Consists of a fracture of both the anterior and posterior rings of C1.
- Results from axial loading such as when the patient falls directly on his or her head or something falls on the patient's head.
- Often associated with C2 fractures.

- Consider all C1 fractures unstable even though most are not associated with spinal cord injury.
- Seen as an increase in the predental space on lateral x-ray and displacement of the lateral masses on the odontoid view (see Figure 6-7).

C1 Rotary Subluxation

- Seen most often in children or in patients with rheumatoid arthritis.
- Seen as an asymmetry between the lateral masses and the dens on the odontoid view.
- Patients will present with the head in rotation and should not be forced to place the head in the neutral position.

Odontoid Fractures

See Figure 6-8.
- Type 1: Involves only the tip of the dens
- Type 2: Involves only the base of the dens
- Type 3: Fracture through the base and body of C2
- Generally unstable

Hangman's Fracture

See Figure 6-9.
- Fracture of both C2 pedicles ("posterior elements")
- Usually due to a hyperextension mechanism
- Unstable fracture; however, often not associated with spinal cord injury because the spinal canal is at its widest through C2

Some type 1 fractures may be stable when the transverse ligament remains intact.

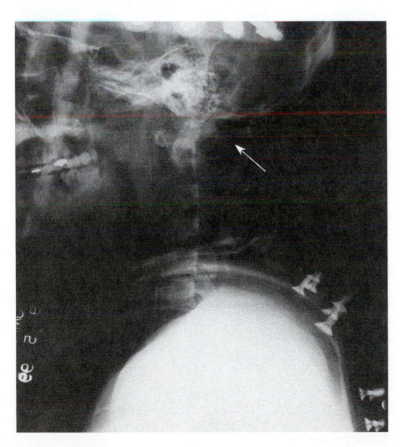

FIGURE 6-7. Jefferson fracture.

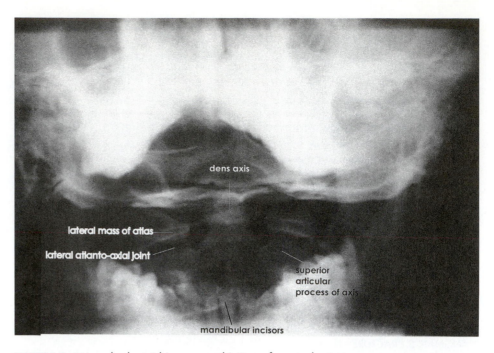

FIGURE 6-8. Normal odontoid (open mouth) view of cervical spine.

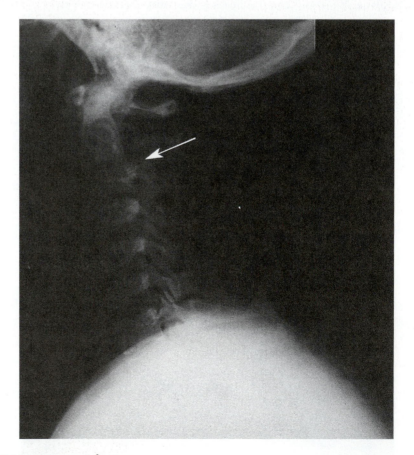

FIGURE 6-9. Hangman's fracture.

BURST FRACTURE OF C3–7

- An axial loading mechanism causing compression of a vertebral body with resultant protrusion of the anterior portion of the vertebral body anteriorly, and the posterior portion of the vertebral body posteriorly into the spinal canal, often causing a spinal cord injury (usually the anterior cord syndrome)
- Stable fracture when ligamentous structure remains intact

SIMPLE WEDGE FRACTURE

- A flexion injury causing compression on the anterior portion of the vertebral body
- Appears as a wedge-shaped concavity, with loss of vertebral height on the anterior portion of the vertebral body
- Usually stable when not associated with ligamentous damage

FLEXION TEARDROP FRACTURE

- A flexion injury causing a fracture of the anteroinferior portion of the vertebral body
- Appears as a teardrop-shaped fragment (see Figure 6-10)
- Unstable fracture because it is usually associated with tearing of the posterior ligament and often with neurologic damage

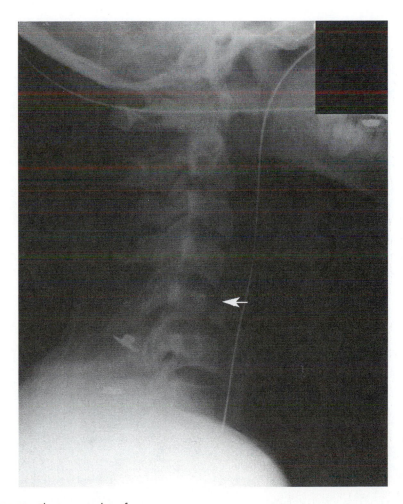

FIGURE 6-10. Flexion teardrop fracture.

EXTENSION TEARDROP FRACTURE

- Also appears as a teardrop-shaped fragment on the anteroinferior portion of the vertebral body.
- However, occurs as an extension injury with avulsion of the fragment, rather than a compression mechanism.
- The posterior ligaments are left intact, making this a stable fracture.
- However, differentiation between a flexion vs. extension teardrop fracture may be difficult and should be treated initially as if it were unstable.

CLAY SHOVELER'S FRACTURE

See Figure 6-11.
- Usually a flexion injury resulting in an avulsion of the tip of the spinous process (C7 > C6 > T1)
- May also result from a direct blow

UNILATERAL FACET DISLOCATION

- Occurs as a flexion–rotation injury
- Usually stable; however, is potentially unstable as it often involves injury to the posterior ligamentous structures
- Often identified on the AP view of the C-spine films when the spinous processes do not line up

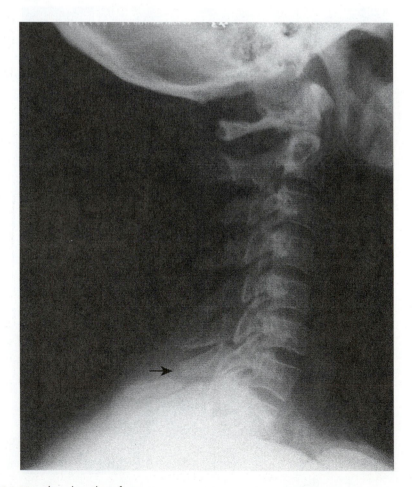

FIGURE 6-11. Clay shoveler's fracture.

BILATERAL FACET DISLOCATION

- Occurs as a flexion injury and is extremely unstable
- Associated with a high incidence of spinal cord injury
- Appears on lateral C-spine films as a subluxation of the dislocated vertebra of greater than one half the AP diameter of vertebral body below it

SUBLUXATION

- Occurs with disruption of the ligamentous structures without bony involvement.
- Potentially unstable.
- Findings on C-spine films may be subtle and flexion–extension views may be needed.

Thoracic Spine Fractures

- Most injuries occur at the junction between the relatively fixed upper thoracic spine and the mobile thoracolumbar region (T10–L5).
- When thoracic fractures do take place, the results are particularly more devastating.
- This occurs because the spinal canal through this region is relatively narrow and the blood supply to this region of spinal cord is in a watershed area (the greater radicular artery of Adamkiewicz enters the spinal canal at L1, but provides blood flow as high as T4).
- Most thoracic spine fractures are caused by hyperflexion leading to a wedge or compression fracture of the vertebral body.
- Most fractures/dislocations in this area are considered stable because of the surrounding normal bony thorax.
- However, as mentioned, neurologic impairment resulting from injuries in this area is often complete.

Thoracolumbar Junction and Lumbar Spine Fractures and Dislocations

COMPRESSION (WEDGE) FRACTURE

- Results from axial loading and flexion.
- Potentially unstable.
- Neurologic injury is uncommon.
- Treatment is symptomatic (patients usually experience pain and are at increased risk for the development of an ileus).

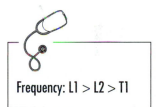

Frequency: L1 > L2 > T1

BURST FRACTURE

- Fracture of the vertebral end plates with forceful extrusion of the nucleus pulposus into the vertebral body causing comminution of the vertebral body.
- Results from axial loading.
- See loss of vertebral height on lateral spine film.

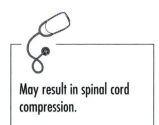

May result in spinal cord compression.

DISTRACTION OR SEAT-BELT INJURY

- Frequently referred to as a "Chance fracture."
- Horizontal fracture through the vertebral body, spinous processes, laminae, pedicles, and tearing of the posterior spinous ligament.
- Caused by an acceleration–deceleration injury of a mobile person moving forward into a fixed seat-belt.

FRACTURE–DISLOCATIONS

- Result from flexion with rotation
- Unstable and often associated with spinal cord damage

Sacral and Coccygeal Spine Fractures and Dislocations

- Fractures in this area are relatively uncommon.
- Sacral injuries often diagnosed via CT scan.
- Neurologic impairment is rare; however, damage to the sacral nerve roots results in bowel/bladder and sexual dysfunction as well as loss of sensory and motor function to the posterior lower extremities.

Coccygeal Spine Fractures and Dislocations

- Fractures of the coccyx are usually caused by direct trauma.
- Diagnosis is made on palpation of a "step-off" on rectal examination, and rectal bleeding must also be ruled out (severe fractures may lead to a rectal tear).
- Treatment of uncomplicated coccygeal fracture is symptomatic and includes pain management and a doughnut pillow.

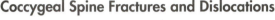

THORACIC TRAUMA

Pericardial Tamponade

- Life-threatening emergency usually seen with penetrating thoracic trauma, but may be seen with blunt thoracic trauma as well.
- Signs include tachycardia, muffled heart sounds, jugular venous distention (JVD), hypotension, and electrical alternans on electrocardiogram (ECG) (see Figure 6-12).
- Diagnosis may be confirmed with cardiac sonogram if immediately available (usually as part of FAST ultrasound).
- Requires immediate decompression via needle pericardiocentesis, pericardial window, or thoracotomy with manual decompression.

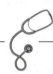
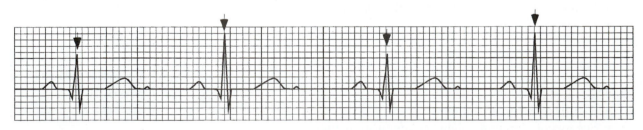

FIGURE 6-12. ECG demonstrating electrical alternans. Note alternating heights of the R in the QRS complexes.

HIGH-YIELD FACTS

Trauma

Cardiac Trauma

- Injury by chamber (cardiac injuries are frequently multichamber; thus, percentage > 100):
  - Right ventricle 40%
  - Left ventricle 40%
  - Right atrium 24%
  - Left atrium 3%
- Signs and symptoms: Beck's triad, pulsus paradoxus, elevated central venous pressure (CVP), hemodynamic instability, "good" mechanism

Diagnostic Tools
- Subxiphoid pericardial window:
  - Small window into pericardial sac through small midline incision.
  - Allows visual/manual inspection of heart.
  - If injury confirmed, incision can be extended for median sternotomy.
  - Direct visualization allows for excellent accuracy, making this the gold standard of diagnosis.
- 2D Echo:
  - Noninvasive, rapid, accurate
  - Higher sensitivity if no concurrent hemothorax
- Ultrasound as part of FAST
- Thoracoscopy/laparoscopy
- Suspicious clinical findings or mechanism in relatively stable patient

Management
- Prompt transport to ED is key.
- ABCs.
- If patient unstable or borderline but fails fluid resuscitation, pericardiocentesis or thoracotomy indicated.
- In stable patient, begin fluid resuscitation. Use Echo to determine need for OR pericardial window or thoracotomy.

Operative Keys
- Relieve tamponade.
- Aim for volume expansion.
- Correct acidosis.
- Maintain coronary perfusion.
- Avoid hypothermia.

Prognosis
- Of stable patients taken to OR, survival for stab wounds is 97%, for gunshot wounds 71%.
- Survival tends to be higher for single-chamber injuries, stab wounds, lack of significant intracardiac defect, hemodynamic stability on arrival.
- Unfavorable prognostic signs include presence of significant associated injuries, gunshot wound, coronary vessel lacerations, multichamber injuries, delayed diagnosis or treatment.

Complications (Occur in up to 50% of Patients)
- Intracardiac shunt
- Valvular lesion
- Ventricular aneurysm
- Retained foreign body
- Postpericardiotomy syndrome (Dressler's syndrome)

1. Pericardium should be opened anterior and parallel to phrenic nerve (longitudinally).
2. Lacerations are repaired with 3-0 nonabsorbable suture and pledgets.
3. A Foley catheter with inflated balloon may be used as a temporizing measure to gain control for large defects.

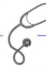

Postpericardiotomy syndrome is a self-limited syndrome of unknown etiology, presenting with fever, chest pain, pericardial effusion, rub, ECG abnormalities. Treatment is with acetylsalicylic acid (ASA) or indomethacin, and occasionally steroids.

Blunt Cardiac Trauma

Usually secondary to MVC, fall from heights, crush injury, blast injury, direct violent trauma.

Types
- Pericardial tears: Due to direct injury or increased intra-abdominal pressure
- Injury to valves, papillary muscles, chordae tendineae, septum
  - Especially likely if preexisting disease present
  - Aortic valve most frequently involved, followed by mitral valve
- Injury to coronary vessels
- Cardiac rupture
- Cardiac contusion
  - Occurs frequently but is rarely significant
  - ECG and enzyme abnormalities nonspecific and don't correlate with outcome

Pneumothorax

DEFINITION

Air in the pleural space.

SIGNS AND SYMPTOMS

- Chest pain
- Dyspnea
- Hyperresonance of affected side
- Decreased breath sounds of affected side

DIAGNOSIS

Upright chest x-ray is ~83% sensitive, demonstrates an absence of lung markings where the lung has collapsed (see Figure 6-13).

TREATMENT: TUBE THORACOSTOMY

Procedure
1. Elevate the head of the bed at least 30 degrees to reduce the chances of injury to abdominal organs.
2. Identify the fourth intercostal space in the midaxillary line.
3. Prep and sterilize the area.
4. Anesthetize the skin, muscle, periosteum, and parietal pleura through which the tube will pass by utilizing a local anesthetic such as lidocaine. If time permits to do intercostal blocks above and below, this provides better anesthesia.
5. Estimate the distance from incision to apex of the lung on the chest tube, ensuring that the distance is enough to allow the last drainage hole of the chest tube to fit inside the pleura. Place a clamp at this point of the chest tube.
6. Make a 2- to 4-cm skin incision over the rib below the one the tube will pass over. The incision should be big enough for the tube and one finger to fit through at the same time. Use blunt dissection to penetrate down to the fascia overlying the intercostal muscles.
7. Insert a closed heavy clamp over the rib and push through the muscles and parietal pleura. Spread the tips of the clamp to enlarge the opening.

Typical scenario: A 19-year-old male who was stabbed in the chest with a knife presents complaining of dyspnea. Breath sounds on the left are absent. *Think:* Pneumothorax.

The neurovascular bundle runs on the inferior margin of each rib.

When the clamp enters the pleura, a rush of air or fluid should be obtained.

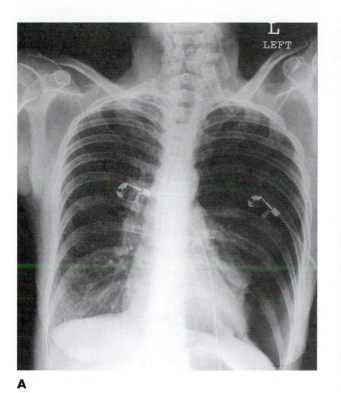
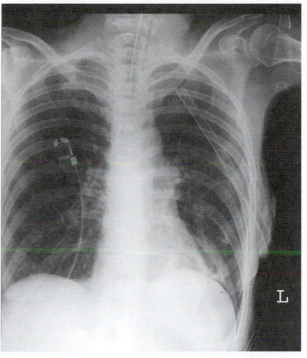

A   **B**

FIGURE 6-13. A. CXR demonstrating left-sided pneumothorax. Note lack of lung markings. **B.** Same patient, after tube thoracostomy and endotracheal intubation.

8. Close the clamps and insert one finger next to the clamp into the pleural space. Sweep the finger around to ensure that you are in the pleural space and there are no adhesions. While leaving your finger in, remove the clamp and insert the chest tube by clamping the tip with a curved clamp and following the path of your finger.
9. Remove the clamp and guide the chest tube in a superior and posterior direction.
10. Insert the tube until your previously placed marker clamp is against the skin.
11. Attach the tube to a water seal.
12. Secure the tube by using suture material to close the skin and then wrapping it around the chest tube tightly enough to prevent slipping (the two ends of the suture are wrapped in opposite directions; a purse-string stitch also works nicely).
13. Place an occlusive dressing over the area.
14. Chest tube placement should be confirmed by chest x-ray

Complications
- Subcutaneous (vs. intrathoracic) placement
- Bleeding from intercostal vessels
- Injury to intercostal nerves
- Infection
- Lung laceration
- Diaphragm injury
- Liver injury

Size of chest tube to use:
For adult large hemothorax: 36 to 40 French

For adult pneumothorax: 24 French or pigtail catheter

For children: Four times the size of appropriate endotracheal tube (ETT)

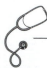

A diagnosis of tension pneumothorax via x-ray is a missed diagnosis. Do not delay treatment of a suspected tension pneumothorax in order to confirm your suspicion (i.e., tension pneumothorax is a clinical diagnosis).

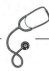

Remember to confirm appropriate chest tube placement with CXR.

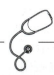

- One fourth of hemothorax cases have an associated pneumothorax.
- Three fourths of hemothorax cases are associated with extrathoracic injuries.

Bleeding usually stops spontaneously for low-velocity gunshot wounds and most stab wounds.

Tension Pneumothorax

- Life-threatening emergency caused by air entering the pleural space (most often via a hole in the lung tissue) but being unable to escape.
- Causes total ipsilateral lung collapse and mediastinal shift (away from injured lung), impairing venous return and thus decreased cardiac output, eventually resulting in shock.

SIGNS AND SYMPTOMS

Same as for pneumothorax, *plus* tracheal deviation *away* from affected side (in tension pneumothorax)

TREATMENT

- Requires immediate needle decompression followed by tube thoracostomy.
  - Needle decompression involves placing a needle or catheter over a needle into the second intercostal space, midclavicular line, over the rib on the side of the tension pneumothorax, followed by a tube thoracostomy (chest tube).
- Persistent air leak may indicate iatrogenic lung injury from chest tube placement—if unresolved, may require thoracoscopic repair.

Hemothorax

The presence of blood in the lungs.
- More than 200 cc of blood must be present before blunting of costophrenic angle will be seen on CXR.
- Treatment involves chest tube placement and drainage, and control of bleeding.

Indications for Thoracotomy
- 1,500 cc initial drainage from the chest tube
- 200 cc/hr for 4 hours continued drainage
- Patients who decompensate after initial stabilization

Thoracic Great Vessel Injury

- May affect aorta, brachiocephalic branches of aorta, pulmonary arteries and veins, superior vena cava (SVC), inferior vena cava (IVC), innominate vein, and azygos veins.
- More than 90% are caused by penetrating trauma.
- Vessels most susceptible to blunt trauma: Innominate artery, pulmonary veins, SVC, IVC, thoracic aorta.
  - Susceptibility increased by ligamentous attachments (pulmonary veins and venae cavae to atria, aorta with ligamentum arteriosum and diaphragm)
  - Mechanisms: Deceleration (shear force), compression between bones, intraluminal hypertension

ER Evaluation

History:
- Severity of deceleration
- Amount of energy transferred
- Patient position during event

Signs and Symptoms

- Hypotension
- Retrosternal chest pain
- Dyspnea
- New systolic murmur
- Unequal blood pressures or pulses in extremities
- External evidence of major chest trauma
- Palpable sternal or thoracic spine fractures
- Left flail chest

CXR Findings

- Widened mediastinum (see Figure 6-14)
- Tracheal or NG tube deviation to the right
- Depression of left mainstem bronchus
- Large hemothorax
- Indistinct aortic knob (most consistent finding)
- Indistinct space between pulmonary artery and aorta
- Presence of left apical cap
- Multiple rib fractures
- Foreign bodies:
  - Located near great vessels
- Out of focus compared to rest of film; may be intracardiac
- "Missing missile"; possible intra-arterial embolization

■ Initial Management

- IV access and fluid resuscitation as usual.
- ER thoracotomy is indicated in some patients (see section on ED thoracotomy)
- Chest tube may be placed when CXR reveals hemothorax.
  - Initial large volume of blood or ongoing hemorrhage may indicate great vessel injury and need for thoracotomy.
- May consider moderate permissive hypotension with limited fluids as temporizing measure prior to OR.

Diagnostic Modalities

- Angiography to localize injury and plan appropriate operation.
- CT for patients with normal initial CXR but suspicious mechanism and requiring CT for other reasons. If CT identifies injury, angiography still required for precise delineation of injury.
- TEE:
  - Fast, no contrast required, concurrent evaluation of cardiac function, versatile in terms of location
  - Contraindicated if potential airway problem or C-spine injury
  - Not as sensitive or specific as angiography or CT scan
  - User dependent

Potential causes of *iatrogenic* great vessel injury:
- CVP line or chest tube placement
- Intra-aortic balloon pump (IABP) placement
- Use of nonvascular clamp during ED thoracotomy
- Overinflation of Swan–Ganz balloon

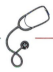

Traumatic aortic rupture is a high-mortality injury: Almost 90% die at the scene, and another 50% die within 24 hours.

- Pseudocoarctation syndrome: Increased BP in upper extremities with absent or decreased femoral pulses
- Injury to innominate or subclavian arteries will result in absent or decreased upper extremity pulses and BP with increased lower extremity BP.

Trauma

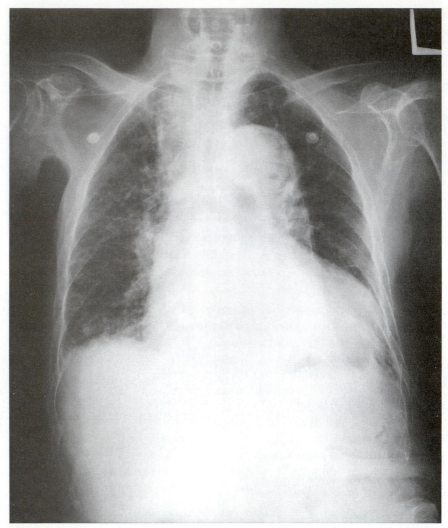

FIGURE 6-14. CXR illustrating wide mediastinum due to penetrating trauma of the ascending aorta.

- Patient should be prepped and draped from sternum to knees to allow alternate access from the groins in the event of an emergency.
- Traditional approach (i.e., left anterolateral sternotomy) is used for the unstable patient with an undiagnosed injury.
- Angiography in the stable patient may dictate an alternate operative approach based on the location of injury.

DEFINITIVE TREATMENT

- Surgical:
    - Clamp/control bleeding.
    - Reconstruction, with graft if needed.
    - Control proximal hypertension pharmacologically.
    - Cardiac bypass as needed.
- Nonoperative:
    - May be indicated in some cases
    - Close observation
    - Pharmacologic treatment
- Endovascular:
    - Stenting (still an investigative therapy)
- Postoperative management:
    - Continued hemodynamic monitoring
    - Pulmonary toilet

COMPLICATIONS

- Pulmonary: Atelectasis, acute respiratory distress syndrome (ARDS), pneumonia
- Infection
- Hemorrhage:
  - Secondary to technical mishap
  - Coagulopathy
- Paraplegia:
  - Associated with perioperative hypotension
  - Injury of intercostal arteries
  - Duration of clamp time

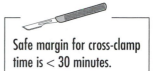

Safe margin for cross-clamp time is < 30 minutes.

HIGH-YIELD FACTS

Sucking Chest Wound

- Also known as a communicating pneumothorax.
- Caused by an open defect in the chest wall, often due to shotgun injuries.
- If the diameter of the defect is greater than two thirds the diameter of the trachea, air will preferentially enter through the defect.
- The affected lung will collapse on inspiration as air enters through the defect and expand slightly on expiration. This mechanism seriously impairs ventilation.
- Initial treatment involves covering wound with an occlusive dressing sealed on three sides. This will convert it to a closed pneumothorax while the unsealed side will allow air escape, preventing conversion into a tension pneumothorax.

Chest tube should **not** be placed through original wound.

Pulmonary Parenchymal Injuries

DEFINITIONS

- Laceration: Damage to the lung parenchyma
- Contusion: Direct injury without laceration leading to alveolar hemorrhage and edema
  - Penetrating trauma (stab wound, gunshot wound) manifests in minutes to hours.
  - Blunt trauma (deceleration) manifests in 48 to 72 hours.

MECHANISMS OF PHYSIOLOGIC DISRUPTION

- Pleural space problem interferes with lung function.
- Hemorrhage.
- Parenchymal injury impairs ventilation and oxygen exchange.

SIGNS AND SYMPTOMS

- Dyspnea
- Tachypnea
- Local ecchymosis

ARTERIAL BLOOD GAS (ABG) FINDINGS

- Hypoxemia
- Widened A-a gradient

Typical scenario: A 25-year-old female presents after a high-speed MVC with dyspnea and tachycardia. There is local bruising over right side of her chest. CXR shows a right upper lobe consolidation. *Think:* Pulmonary contusion.

Trauma

CXR Findings

- Local irregular patchy infiltrate corresponding to site of injury. This usually develops immediately, and always within 6 hours.
- Fluid density in lung field.

Treatment

Involves supplemental oxygen, pulmonary toilet, judicious fluid management, and aggressive pain control.
- Most frequent complication is pneumonia.
- Thoracic epidural is helpful for pain control.

ED Thoracotomy

Indications

- Salvageable patient with postinjury cardiac arrest
- Persistent severe hypotension secondary to tamponade, intrathoracic hemorrhage, or air embolism

Basics

- Left anterolateral incision: Fourth to fifth intercostal space
- Rib retractor
- Pericardiotomy:
  - Evacuation of blood and clots.
  - Control bleeding with digital pressure and/or partially occluding vascular clamp on atria or great vessels.
- In a nonbeating heart, may suture lacerations with 3-0 nonabsorbable suture.
- In a beating heart, delay repair of defects until initial resuscitation is completed and patient is in OR.

Outcome

- Overall survival for penetrating trauma— 20%
- Success rate for patients with signs of life—30–57%
- Success rate if no signs of life—13%
- Success rate for blunt injuries—1–2%

Thoracotomy

- Ten to 20% of all penetrating chest trauma ultimately requires thoracotomy.
- Decisions based on physical finding, imaging, and clinical course.

Acute Indications
- Tamponade
- Acute hemodynamic decompensation or in-hospital arrest
- Penetrating truncal trauma
- Thoracic outlet vascular injury
- Traumatic thoracotomy
- Massive air leak from chest tube
- Significant missile embolus to heart or pulmonary artery
- Endoscopic or radiographic evidence of tracheal, bronchial, or esophageal injury

Because of the low success rate for blunt injuries, ED thoracotomy is **not** indicated for blunt thoracic trauma.

- Great vessel injury
- Penetrating object that traverses mediastinum

Nonacute Indications
- Presence of clotted hemothorax
- Chronic traumatic diaphragmatic hernia
- Intracardiac injuries
- Traumatic pseudoaneurysms
- Nonclosing thoracic duct fistula
- Chronic post-traumatic empyema
- Infected intrapulmonary hematoma
- Missed tracheal or bronchial injury
- Tracheoesophageal fistula

Thoracoscopy

Use is increasing. Has been used successfully to:
- Remove clotted blood
- Evaluate diaphragm
- Look for hemopericardium
- Remove foreign body
- Control chest wall or internal mammary artery bleeding

> Trocar may be placed through chest tube site, with replacement of tube at conclusion of case.

Delayed Problems

- Clotted hemothorax: Leads to fibrosis, which will decrease functional lung capacity and serves as a nidus for infection.
  - Causes:
    - Failure to recognize hemothorax
    - Failure of proper chest tube placement
    - Failure of chest tube maintainence
    - Use of chest tube that is too small
  - Indications for intervention:
    - Volume loss > 25% on CXR
    - Secondary infection
  - Thoracoscopy may be used but becomes more difficult as time passes. After 1 week, thoracotomy more likely to be successful.
- Persistent air leak:
  - Failure of reexpansion
  - Main airway disruption
  - Lung laceration (may be stapled with mini-thoracotomy or thoracoscopy if persistent for > 7–10 days)
- Empyema:
  - Iatrogenic, primary, or secondary infection
  - More common with penetrating trauma
- Attempt chest tube or CT-guided drainage; thoracotomy if other methods fail

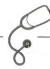

The most frequently injured solid organ associated with penetrating trauma is the **liver.**

The most frequently injured solid organ associated with blunt trauma is the **spleen** followed by the **liver.**

General

Penetrating abdominal injuries (PAIs) resulting from a gunshot wound create damage via three mechanisms:

1. Direct injury by the bullet itself
2. Injury from fragmentation of the bullet
3. Indirect injury from the resultant "shock wave"

PAIs resulting from a stabbing mechanism are limited to the direct damage of the object of impalement.

Blunt abdominal injuries (BAIs) also have three general mechanisms of injury:

1. Injury caused by the direct blow
2. Crush injury
3. Deceleration injury

Anatomy

- Anterior abdominal wall:
  - Bordered laterally by the midaxillary lines, superiorly by a horizontal line drawn through the nipples, and inferiorly by the symphysis pubis and inguinal ligaments.
  - The "thoracoabdominal region" is that region below the nipples and above the costal margins, and is the area within which the diaphragm travels. Penetrating injuries to this region are more likely to involve injury to the diaphragm.
- Flank: Area between the anterior and posterior axillary lines
- Back: Area posterior to the posterior axillary lines, bordered superiorly by a line drawn through the tips of the scapulae, and inferiorly by the iliac crests
- Diaphragm: Dome-shaped musculoaponeurotic division between thorax and abdomen
  - Three openings:
    - T8: IVC
    - T10: Esophagus, with vagus nerves
    - T12: Aorta (also thoracic duct, azygos vein)
  - Abundant blood supply: Pericardiophrenic, phrenic, and intercostal arteries
  - Innervated by phrenic nerves
- Peritoneal viscera: Liver, spleen, stomach, small bowel, sigmoid and transverse colon
- Retroperitoneal viscera: Majority of the duodenum (fourth part is intraperitoneal), pancreas, kidneys and ureters, ascending and descending colon, and major vessels such as the abdominal aorta, inferior vena cava, renal and splenic vessels
- Pelvic viscera: Bladder, urethra, ovaries and uterus in women, prostate in men, rectum, and iliac vessels

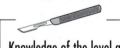

Knowledge of the level at which the aorta passes through the diaphragm helps to control bleeding in a trauma laparotomy by guiding digital compression or clamp placement.

Signs

- **Seat-belt sign**—ecchymotic area found in the distribution of the lower anterior abdominal wall and can be associated with perforation of the bladder or bowel as well as a lumbar distraction fracture (Chance fracture).
- **Cullen's sign** (periumbilical ecchymosis) is indicative of intraperitoneal hemorrhage.
- **Grey–Turner's sign** (flank ecchymoses) is indicative of retroperitoneal hemorrhage.
- **Kehr's sign**—left shoulder or neck pain secondary to splenic rupture. It increases when patient is in Trendelenburg position or with left upper quadrant (LUQ) palpation (caused by diaphragmatic irritation).

General

- Inspect the abdomen for evisceration, entry/exit wounds, impaled objects, and a gravid uterus.
- Check for tenderness, guarding, and rebound.

DIAGNOSIS

- Perforation: AXR and CXR to look for free air
- Diaphragmatic injury: CXR to look for blurring of the diaphragm, hemothorax, or bowel gas patterns above the diaphragm (at times with a gastric tube seen in the left chest).

Focused Abdominal Sonography for Trauma (FAST)

Positive if free fluid is demonstrated in the abdomen.

Advantages

- A rapid bedside screening study
- Noninvasive
- Not time consuming
- 80–95% sensitivity for intra-abdominal blood

Disadvantages

- Operator dependent
- Low specificity for individual organ injury

Four views are utilized to search for free intraperitoneal fluid (presumed to be blood in the trauma victim) that collects in dependent areas and appears as hypoechoic areas on ultrasound (see Figures 6-15 and 6-16):

- Morrison's pouch (RUQ): Free fluid can be visualized between the liver and kidney.
- Splenorenal recess (LUQ): Free fluid can be visualized between the spleen and kidney.
- Pouch of Douglas lies above the rectum (probe is placed in the suprapubic region).
- Subxiphoid and parasternal views to look for hemopericardium.

Peritonitus and guarding in a neurologically intact patient obviate the need for much diagnostic workup. Trauma laparotomy is indicated in this setting.

In a stable patient with neurologic dysfunction, whether from drugs, alcohol, head trauma, or baseline dementia, exam findings have a limited ability to direct care. These patients often require additional diagnostic tests.

Serial abdominal examinations can and should be performed.

HIGH-YIELD FACTS

Trauma

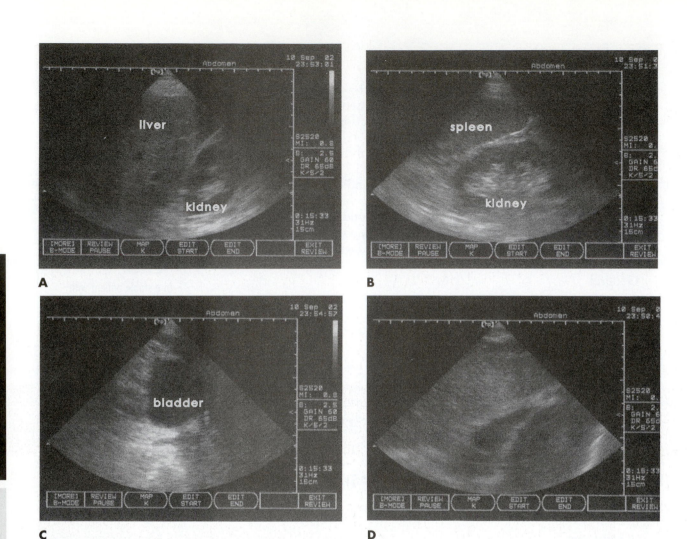

FIGURE 6-15. Normal focused sonography for trauma (FAST) views. **A.** Liver–kidney view. **B.** Spleen–kidney interface. **C.** Bladder view. **D.** Pericardial view.

DPL is especially useful in marginal or unstable patients with equivocal ultrasounds and for patients with hollow viscus injuries.

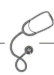

DPL should be undertaken only after gastric and urinary decompression.

Diagnostic Peritoneal Lavage (DPL)

Advantages
- Performed bedside
- Widely available
- Highly sensitive for hemoperitoneum
- Rapidly performed

Disadvantages
- Invasive
- Risk for iatrogenic injury (<1%)
- Low specificity (many false positives)
- Does not evaluate the retroperitoneum

OPEN DPL

Make vertical incision carefully from the skin to the fascia. Grasp the fascial edges with clamps, elevate, then incise through to the peritoneum. Insert the peritoneal catheter and advance toward the pelvis.

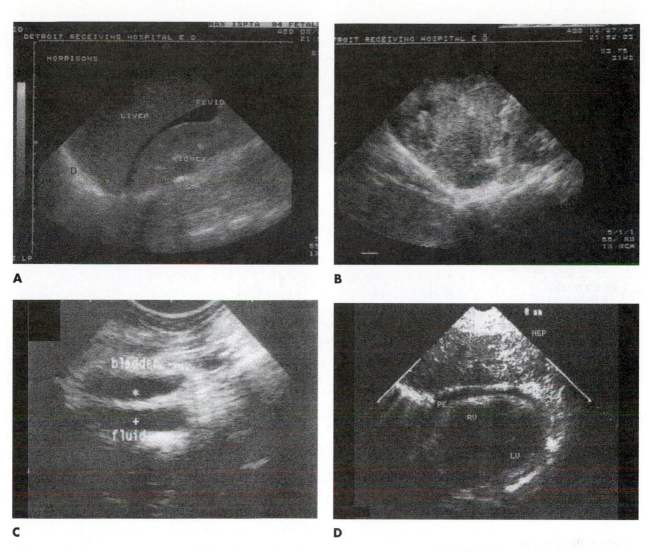

FIGURE 6-16. Abnormal FAST views. **A.** Liver–kidney view demonstrating presence of fluid (black stripe) in Morrison's pouch compared to Figure 6-15B. **B.** Fluid in splenoral recess. **C.** Free fluid in the pelvis. **D.** Pericardial effusion (denoted as PE). (A, B, and D reproduced, with permission, from Jones R, et al. *Trauma Ultrasonography.* [VC5]: Haines International, 1999. C reproduced, with permission, from Melanson SW, Heller M. *Emerg Med Clin N Amer* 16:1, 1998.)

CLOSED DPL

- Using skin clamps or an assistant's sterile gloved hands, elevate the skin on either side of the site of needle placement and make a "nick" with a #11 blade.
- Insert the needle (usually an 18-gauge needle comes with the kit) angled slightly toward the pelvis, through the skin and subcutaneous tissue and into the peritoneum. Most often three areas of resistance are met (felt as "pops") as the needle is passed through linea alba, transversalis fascia, and peritoneum.
- Using the Seldinger technique, a guidewire is placed through the needle and advanced into the peritoneum.
- The needle is removed, leaving the guidewire in place.
- The peritoneal catheter is then threaded over the wire, and the wire removed.
- Much faster and equally safe as open DPL.

If pelvic fracture is suspected, a supraumbilical approach should be used.

If the patient is pregnant, a suprafundal approach should be used.

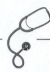

Criteria for a positive DPL:
- > 10 mL gross blood on initial aspiration
- > 100,000 red blood cells (RBCs)
- > 500 white blood cells (WBCs)
- Gram stain with bacteria or vegetable matter
- Amylase > 20 IU/L
- Presence of bile

Contraindications to DPL:
Absolute:
- Clear indication for laparotomy
Relative
- Coagulopathy
- Previous abdominal surgeries
- Morbid obesity
- Gravid uterus

CT is the most sensitive test for retroperitoneal injury.

- The peritoneal catheter is in a syringe and is connected to the catheter and aspiration is performed. If gross blood appears (> 5 to 10 cc) the patient should be taken to the OR for exploratory laparotomy.
- If the aspiration is negative, instill 15 cc/kg of warmed normal saline or lactated Ringer's solution into the peritoneum through IV tubing connected to the catheter.
- Let the solution stand for up to 10 minutes (if the patient is stable), then place the IV bag from which the solution came on the floor for drainage via gravity.
- A sample of the returned solution should be sent to the lab for stat analysis.

CT Scanning

- Useful for the hemodynamically stable patient.
- Has a greater specificity than DPL and ultrasound (US).
- Noninvasive
- Relatively time consuming when compared with DPL and US
- Diagnostic for specific organ injury; however, may miss diaphragmatic, colonic, and pancreatic injury

Angiography

- May be used to identify and embolize pelvic arterial bleeding secondary to pelvic fractures, or to assess blunt renal artery injuries diagnosed by CT scan.
- Otherwise limited use for abdominal trauma.

Serial Hematocrits

Serial hematocrits (every 4 to 6 hours) should be obtained during the observation period of the hemodynamically stable patient.

Laparoscopy

- Usage is increasing (mainly to identify peritoneal penetration from gun shot/knife wound), especially for the stable or marginally stable patient who would otherwise require a laparotomy
- Helpful for evaluation of diaphragm
- May help to decrease negative laparotomy rate
- However, may miss hollow organ injuries, and does not assess retroperitoneal injuries

Indications for Exploratory Laparotomy

- Abdominal trauma and hemodynamic instability
- Bleeding from stomach (not to be confused with nasopharyngeal bleeding)
- Evisceration
- Peritoneal irritation
- Suspected/known diaphragmatic injury

- Free intraperitoneal or retroperitoneal air
- Intraperitoneal bladder rupture (diagnosed by cystography)
- Positive DPL
- Surgically correctable injury diagnosed on CT scan
- Removal of impaled instrument
- Rectal perforation (diagnosed by sigmoidoscopy)
- Transabdominal missile (bullet) path (e.g., a gunshot wound to the buttock with the bullet being found in the abdomen or thorax)

Types of Injury: General Approach

DIAPHRAGMATIC INJURY

- May result from penetrating or blunt trauma.
- Left hemidiaphragm more frequently injured.
- History: Mechanism, severity of other injuries.

Signs and Symptoms
- Thoracic: Chest pain, dyspnea, worsening respiratory distress, decreased breath sounds, rib fractures, flail chest, hemo/pneumothorax
- Abdominal: Pain and tenderness

Diagnosis
- Noninvasive: CXR, upper GI series, barium enema, ultrasound, CT, magnetic resonance imaging (MRI)
- CXR findings (see Figure 6-17):
  - Initially normal in up to 50% of cases
  - Pneumo/hemothorax
  - Delayed films: Viscera in chest, obscured diaphragmatic shadow, elevated diaphragm, irregular diaphragmatic contour, pleural fluid
- Invasive: DPL, laparoscopy, thoracoscopy

Treatment
- OR: Achieve hemostasis, evaluate diaphragm, repair laceration with horizontal mattress sutures of 1-0 monofilament for small defects, or a running suture for larger defects.

Prognosis
- Mortality (~14%) usually due to other injuries.
- Morbidity is generally pulmonary (pneumonia, atelectasis) but may be secondary to technical mishap.

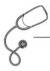

Contrast use:
- Noncontrast to look for intraparenchymal hematomas
- PO contrast to assess location and integrity of upper gastrointestinal (GI) tract
- IV contrast to look for organ or vascular injury

Trauma laparotomy:
- Midline incision.
- Pack all four quadrants with laparotomy pads.
- Evacuation of gross blood and clot.
- Control bleeding.
- Resuscitate as needed.
- Systematically remove pads and inspect for source(s) of injury.
- Definitive repair based on stability of patient and type of injury.

Any wound from the nipple line to the gluteal crease can cause peritoneal or retroperitoneal injury.

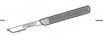

Maintain low threshold for conversion to laparotomy during laparoscopy.

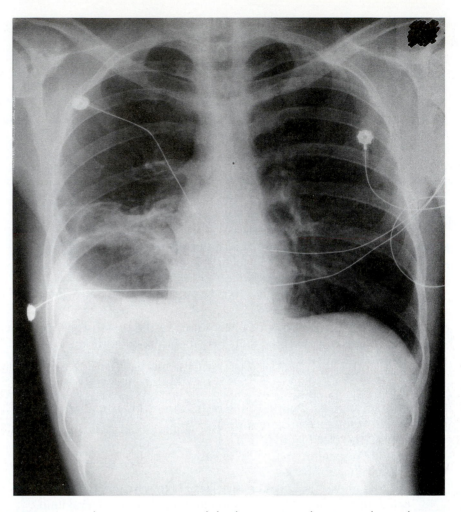

FIGURE 6-17. CXR demonstrating ruptured diaphragm. Note elevation and irregular contour of diaphragm, and viscera in chest.

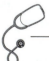

Diaphragmatic trauma is rarely an isolated injury. Look for it especially when the following injuries are present:
- Head trauma
- Fractures (pelvic, rib)
- Thoracic aorta
- Pneumo/hemothorax
- Intra-abdominal injury

- Do not force NGT; diaphragmatic hernia may result in kinking or unusual twisting of esophagus.
- Use caution in placing chest tubes if viscera are in the chest.

LIVER INJURY

See Table 6-2.

Anatomy
- Divided into eight segments (see Figure 6-18).
  - Right lobe: Posterolateral segments VI and VII, anteromedial segments V and VIII
  - Left lobe: Anterior segments III and IV, posterior segment II
  - Segment I
- Hepatic veins:
  - Middle hepatic vein joins left hepatic vein.
  - Right and left veins then drain into IVC.
- Portal vein (formed by superior mesenteric vein and splenic vein) accounts for 75% of hepatic blood flow.
- Liver has ligamentous attachments to the diaphragm.

Initial Treatment
- ABCs.
- Ascertain details about mechanism of injury.

TABLE 6-2. American Association for Surgery of Trauma (AAST) Liver Injury Scale (1994 revision).

Grade*	Type of Injury	Description of Injury
I	Hematoma	Subcapsular, < 10% surface area
	Laceration	Capsular tear, < 1 cm parenchymal depth
II	Hematoma	Subcapsular, 10–50% surface area; intraparenchymal < 10 cm in diameter
	Laceration	Capsular tear, 1–3 parenchymal depth, < 10 cm in length
III	Hematoma	Subcapsular, > 50% surface area of ruptured subcapsular or parenchymal hematoma; intraparenchymal hematoma > 10 cm or expanding 3-cm parenchymal depth
	Laceration	Parenchymal disruption involving 25–75% hepatic lobe or 1–3 Couinaud's segments
IV	Laceration	Parenchymal disruption involving > 75% of hepatic lobe or > 3 Couinaud's segments within a single lobe
V	Vascular	Juxtahepatic venous injuries (i.e., retrohepatic vena cava/central major hepatic veins)
	Vascular	Hepatic avulsion

*Advance one grade for bilateral injuries up to grade III.
Reproduced, with permission, from the American Association for Surgery of Trauma, *www.aast.org/injury/injury.html*.

- Further diagnostic strategies may be undertaken as previously discussed; specific concerns with liver injuries are as follows:
  - DPL: May be positive due to liver injury; however, not all liver injuries require an operation. Use caution (and additional modalities) in determining further course of action in this setting.

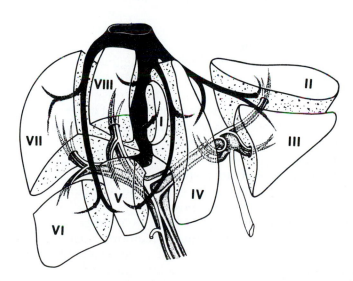

FIGURE 6-18. Liver segments. (From Schwartz.)

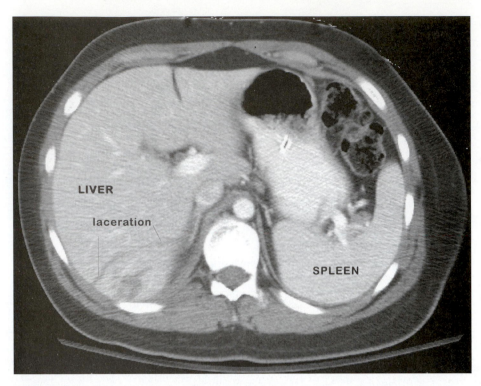

FIGURE 6-19. CT demonstrating liver laceration.

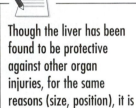

Though the liver has been found to be protective against other organ injuries, for the same reasons (size, position), it is very vulnerable to injury itself.

Use stability as the deciding factor in choosing operative or nonoperative management.

Imaging of the liver: If contrast pool or blush is noted on CT and patient remains stable, consider an **angiogram.**

- CT: Will detect blood and solid organ damage; is useful for grading injury. CT is *contraindicated* in the unstable or marginal patient (see Figure 6-19).
- Ultrasound, if accessible, should be performed initially as FAST, and may then be used for serial examinations following delineation of injury on CT.
- Diagnostic laparoscopy is still evolving in its use for liver injuries. Diagnosis and successful repair have been reported, but it has not become the standard of care as it remains difficult to correctly identify liver injuries.

Nonoperative Management
- Approximately one half of patients are eligible
- 96% success rate
- Penetrating trauma:
  - Operative management remains standard of care.
  - Select patients with stab wounds may warrant a trial of observation after CT and/or DPL.
- Blunt trauma:
  - May attempt trial of observation if:
    - Patient is stable or stabilizes after fluid resuscitation.
    - There are no peritoneal signs.
    - The injury can be precisely delineated and graded by CT scan.
    - There are no associated injuries requiring laparotomy.
    - There is no need for excessive hepatic-related blood transfusions.
- Complications: Hemorrhage (< 5%), biloma, abscess.
- Repeat CT scan in 2 to 3 days to look for expansion or resolution of injury.
- Patients may resume normal activities after 2 months.

Operative Management

- Generally needed for 20% of patients with grade III or higher injuries who present with hemodynamic instability due to hemorrhage.
- Laparotomy is undertaken through a long midline incision.
- The primary goal is the control of bleeding with direct pressure and packing.
- Patient should then be resuscitated as needed, with attention to temperature control, volume status, and acid–base balance.
- Once adequately resuscitated, the operation may proceed.
- Specifics of trauma liver surgery include:
  - Pringle maneuver.
  - Finger fracture of liver to expose damaged vessels and bile ducts.
  - Debridement of nonviable tissue.
  - Placement of an omental pedicle (with its blood supply) at the site.
  - Closed suction drainage.
  - Major hepatic resection is indicated when the parenchyma was totally destroyed by the trauma, the extent of injury is too great for packing, the injury itself caused a near-resection, or resection is the only way to control life-threatening hemorrhage.
  - Packing the perihepatic space with a planned reoperation in 24 to 36 hours is indicated when the patient is severely coagulopathic, there is bilobar bleeding that cannot be controlled, there is a large expanding hematoma, other methods to control bleeding have failed, or the patient requires transfer to a level I trauma center.
- Complications:
  - Hemorrhage (5%):
    - Due to inadequate OR hemostasis or coagulopathy.
    - If the patient remains hemodynamically stable, with corrected acidosis, hypothermia, and coagulopathy, consider angiogram for diagnosis and possible embolization.
    - If the patient is unstable, a return to the OR is indicated.
  - Hemobilia (1%):
    - Signs and symptoms: Upper GI bleed, RUQ pain, positive fecal occult blood, and jaundice.
    - Attempt angioembolization.
  - Hyperpyrexia:
    - Self-limited to 3 to 5 days
    - Etiology unknown
  - Abscess
  - Biliary fistula (7–10%):
    - Definition: > 50 mL/d drainage for > 14 days.
    - Will generally close spontaneously with adequate drainage.
- Prognosis: Overall, 10% mortality.
  - Of those requiring operation, 8–55% (This rate is thought to vary based on the experience of the surgeon.)

SPLEEN INJURY

See Figure 18-1 in spleen chapter for spleen and its relationships.

Anatomy

- Related to the diaphragm (superiorly and posterolaterally), to the stomach (medially and anterolaterally), to the left adrenal and kidney (posteromedially), to the chest wall (laterally), and to the phrenocolic ligament (inferiorly).
- Ligaments: Gastrosplenic and splenorenal (major); splenophrenic, presplenic fold, pancreaticosplenic, phrenicocolic, pancreaticocolic (minor).

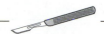

Pringle maneuver: Occlusion of the portal triad manually or with an atraumatic vascular clamp. Occlusion should not exceed 20 minutes if feasible.

If the Pringle maneuver fails to stop hemorrhage, consider an injury to the retrohepatic IVC.

Watch for increasing abdominal distention with decreasing hematocrit as potential indicators of postop bleeding.

The spleen is the most commonly injured organ in blunt abdominal trauma, and trauma is the most common reason for splenectomy.

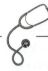

Transverse lacerations often stop bleeding spontaneously because they are parallel to blood vessels and not likely to disrupt them.

- Continues to increase in size until adolescence, after which it regresses up to 30%.
- The spleen receives 5% of cardiac output.
- See spleen chapter for details regarding function and physiology of the spleen.

Signs and Symptoms
- History: Check for preexisting diseases that cause splenomegaly (these patients are more vulnerable to splenic injury), details of injury mechanism.
- Exam: Look for peritoneal irritation, Kehr's sign, left-sided lower rib fractures, external signs of injury.

Initial Treatment
- ABCs.
- Patients who are stable or who stabilize with fluid resuscitation, may be considered for selective management.
- Further diagnostic tools:
  - CT scan: Able to define injury precisely. Figure 6-20 depicts a splenic hematoma.
  - Ultrasound: May be used for initial assessment to detect hemoperitoneum
  - DPL: Not specific for splenic injury; likely to get positive result for splenic injuries that do not require operation
  - Laparoscopy: Difficult to fully visualize and examine spleen; difficult to evacuate blood and clots
  - Angiogram: May be able to use therapeutically in the stable patient (embolization of CT-identified injury)

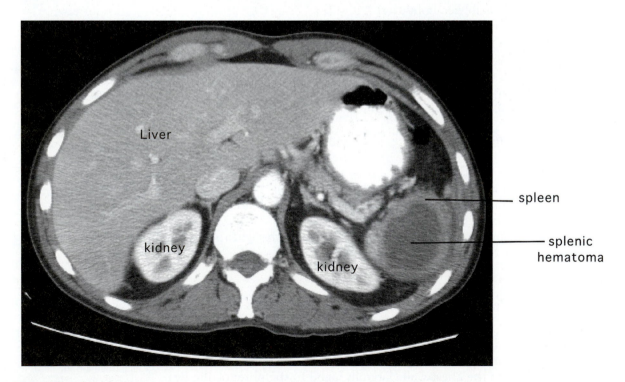

FIGURE 6-20. Splenic hematoma.

Definitive Treatment
- Nonoperative management:
  - Criteria:
    - Stable
    - No evidence of injury to other intra-abdominal organs
    - No coagulopathy
    - No impairment to physical exam (i.e., head injury)
    - Injury grade I or II (see Table 6-3)
  - Course:
    - Bed rest (2 to 3 days)
    - NGT decompression
    - Monitored setting
    - Serial exam
    - Serial hematocrit
    - Resume diet once potential for laparotomy decreased (when bed rest finished)
    - Follow-up CT at 3 to 5 days, or sooner if deterioration
    - Activity restrictions for 3 months
- Operative management:
  - Indications:
    - Signs and symptoms of ongoing hemorrhage
    - Failure of nonoperative management
    - Injury ≥ grade III
  - Preparation:
    - Have blood available.
    - Make sure the patient has multiple large-bore IVs. Consider a central line and arterial line.

Thirty percent of patients with splenic injury will present with hypotensive shock.

Radiographic signs of splenic injury:
- CT: Low-density mass or intrasplenic accumulation of contrast
- US: Perisplenic fluid, enlarged spleen, irregular borders, abnormal position, increase in size over time

TABLE 6-3. AAST Spleen Injury Scale (1994 revision).

Grade*	Injury Type	Description of Injury
I	Hematoma	Subcapsular, < 10% surface area
	Laceration	Capsular tear, < 1 cm parenchymal depth
II	Hematoma	Subcapsular, 10–50% surface area; intraparenchymal, < 5 cm in diameter
	Laceration	Capsular tear, 1–3 cm parenchymal depth that does not involve a trabecular vessel
III	Hematoma	Subcapsular, > 50% surface area or expanding; ruptured subcapsular or parenchymal hematoma ≥ 5 cm or expanding
	Laceration	> 3 cm parenchymal depth or involving trabecular vessels
IV	Laceration	Laceration involving segmental or hilar vessels producing major devascularization (> 25% of spleen)
	Laceration	Completely shattered spleen
V	Vascular	Hilar vascular injury with devascularized spleen

*Advance one grade for bilateral injuries up to grade III.
Reproduced, with permission, from the American Association for Surgery of Trauma, *www.aast.org/injury/injury.html.*

Patients with a vascular blush on CT scan are likely to fail nonoperative management.

Patients who fail nonoperative management usually do so within 48 to 72 hours.

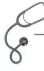

Indications for splenectomy:
- Source of exsanguination
- Pulverized organ
- Shock
- Associated life-threatening injuries
- Contraindications to prolonged surgery (severe coagulopathy, hypothermia)

Pneumococcal vaccine will be needed for patients undergoing splenectomy. It may be given on the day of hospital discharge.

Because of a common mechanism, Chance fractures and blunt small bowel injury are strongly associated. If one is present, you should look for the other.

- Laparotomy:
  - In situ inspection.
  - Palpation.
  - Perform splenectomy if the spleen is the primary source of exsanguinating hemorrhage.
  - If not, pack the area and search for other, more life-threatening injuries; address those first.
  - Subsequently, return to inspection of spleen. Mobilize fully unless the only injury is a minor nonbleeding one.
  - Minor nonbleeding injury: No intervention.
  - Capsular bleeding and most grade II injuries: Apply direct pressure ± topical hemostatic agent.
  - Persistently bleeding grade II or III injuries: Suture lacerations.
  - Multiple injuries: Consider mesh.
  - Complex fractures: Perform anatomic resection if possible, based on demarcation after segmental artery ligation.
  - Perform splenectomy (see indications).
- Complications:
  - Bleeding
  - Pulmonary complications (pneumonia, atelectasis)
  - Pancreatitis
  - Postsplenectomy thrombocytosis

BOWEL INJURY

Stomach, Jejunum, and Ileum
- Gastric perforation may be considered "clean-contaminated" rather than contaminated:
  - In a normal state, free of bacteria.
  - However, gastric juice can cause a chemical peritonitis.
- Small bowel is vulnerable to injury because it takes up a lot of space within the abdomen
- Isolated leaks from penetrating trauma lead to minimal contamination and patients usually do well if diagnosis is not delayed.
  - Increased concentration of organisms distally; terminal ileum injuries more closely resemble colonic injuries in terms of contamination.
- Blunt injuries are "blowouts" resulting frequently from lap belts, and occur near the ligament of Treitz and the ileocecal valve.
  - Mesentery can be significantly injured following blunt trauma.
- Diagnosis:
  - If the patient is awake and reliable, the exam is important to look for peritoneal irritation.
  - If the exam is not reliable, DPL or laparoscopy may be required.
  - CT scan has a high false-negative rate for small bowel injuries.
  - Look for free air on CXR.
- Laparotomy for gastric or small bowel injury.

OR Plan
- Obtain control of leak.
- Explore abdomen.
- Control bleeding.

- Gastric injury:
  - Mobilize stomach.
  - Pyloric injury—pyloroplasty.
  - Body injury—repair (if severe gastroesophageal junction injury, may need to anastomose and do a pyloroplasty).
  - Major injury—resection.
- Small bowel injury:
  - Expose injury site.
  - Bowel injury (small)—repair.
  - Short segment destroyed (with one or more injuries)—resection, primary anastomosis.
  - Severe associated injuries or unstable or coagulopathic—resect; plan for second look with delayed anastomosis.
  - Mesentery injured, without ischemia—repair.
  - Mesentery injured, with short segment of ischemia—resection, primary anastomosis.
  - Mesentery injured, with long segment ischemic—resect or close with plan for second look.
- Complications:
  - Leak
  - Fistula
  - Short gut syndrome (depends on amount of bowel resected)

Duodenum
- Mechanisms:
  - Three fourths of injuries result from penetrating trauma.
- Anatomy:
  - Duodenum begins at the L1 level.
  - Length: 25 to 30 cm to the ligament of Treitz.
  - Blood supply: Pancreaticoduodenal arteries, branches from the celiac axis and the superior mesenteric artery (SMA).
- Diagnosis:
  - Upper GI series with water-soluble contrast.
- CT will miss many injuries.
- DPL may miss isolated duodenal injuries; is better when there are associated injuries.
- Treatment:
  - Eighty percent of patients are able to undergo a primary repair.
  - Repair may be protected with an omental patch and/or gastric diversion.
- More complex operations:
  - Pyloric exclusion
  - Duodenoduodenostomy
  - Pancreaticoduodenectomy
- Prognosis:
  - Directly attributable mortality: 2–5%
  - Directly attributable morbidity: 10–20%
  - Complications: Dehiscence, sepsis, multiple organ failure, and duodenal-cutaneous fistula
  - Indications of late morbidity or mortality:
    - Presence of pancreatic injury
    - Blunt or missile mechanism
    - Size of defect > 75% of wall
    - First or second portions of duodenum
    - > 24-hour delay to treatment
    - Concurrent CBD injury

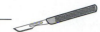

To determine viability of the bowel in the OR, inject fluorescein dye IV, and use a Wood's lamp to inspect the bowel. Nonviable bowel will have patchy or no fluorescence.

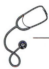

Duodenal hematoma may result from an MVC, but has been found to be associated with child abuse in the pediatric population. Patients present with signs and symptoms of small bowel obstruction, and require CT/upper GI series for diagnosis. Treatment is nonoperative and includes NGT decompression, total parental nutrition (TPN), reevaluation with upper GI series after about 1 week.

Large Bowel

- Injuries generally occur via a penetrating mechanism (75% gunshot wound, 25% stab wound). Blunt injuries are rare but result from MVCs. Iatrogenic transanal injuries may also occur.
- Signs and symptoms:
  - Abdominal distention, tenderness
  - Peritoneal irritation
  - Guaiac-positive stool
- Diagnosis:
  - In an awake and reliable patient, exam findings are of paramount importance in determining whether there has been a bowel injury (or, more relevantly, a need to go to the OR).
  - CXR may show free air.
  - CT may also show free air, but may miss the specific injury.
- In a patient with a flank injury but without clear peritoneal signs, consider a contrast enema.
- If in the OR for another reason, the smell or sight of feces is a good clue.
- Treatment:
  - Primary repair: For small or medium-sized perforations, repair the perforation or, if needed, resect the affected segment, close with primary anastomosis.
  - Anastomosis is contraindicated in the setting of massive hemorrhage.
- Prognosis:
  - Mortality is usually due to exsanguinations from associated injuries, or from sepsis or multiple organ failure.
- Complications: Abscess, suture line failure, fistula.

Rectum

- Two thirds extraperitoneal
- Mechanism:
  - 80% gunshot wound
  - 10% blunt
  - 6% transanal
  - 3% stab wound or impalement
- Diagnosis:
  - DRE/guaiac: Suspicion increased by blood in stool or palpation of defect or foreign body on exam.
  - Rigid proctoscopy: May be done in OR if needed; mandatory for patients with known trajectory of knife or gunshot wound across pelvis or transanal; if patient is unstable, may be delayed until after resuscitation.
  - X-ray to look for missiles or foreign bodies.
- Treatment:
  - Loop colostomy.
  - Loop colostomy with distal limb closure.
  - End colostomy/mucus fistula.
  - Extraperitoneal injuries must be diverted via colostomy but may not need to be repaired (if not too big and not easily accessible).
- Outcome:
  - Death secondary to sepsis, multisystem organ failure (MSOF): 0–5%
  - Complications: Abscess, fistula
  - Colostomy may be closed in 3 to 4 months

Thirty percent of patients with rectal injury will have an associated injury to the bladder.

Anus

- Mechanisms same as rectal injuries.
- Reconstruct sphincter as soon as patient is stabilized.
- Divert with sigmoid colostomy.

PANCREATIC INJURY

General

- Mechanism: Largely penetrating (gunshot wound >> stab wound).
- Seventy-five percent of patients with penetrating injury to the pancreas will have associated injuries to the aorta, portal vein, or IVC.

Anatomy

- Relationships (see Figure 17-1 in pancreas chapter):
  - Posterior: IVC, aorta, left kidney, renal vein, splenic vein, splenic artery, SMA, SMV
  - Lateral: Spleen
  - Medial: Duodenum
- Ducts:
  - Main (Wirsung): Traverses length of gland, slightly closer to superior edge than inferior edge; ends by joining CBD and emptying into duodenum.
  - Accessory (Santorini): A branch from the pancreatic duct in the neck of the pancreas; has its own entry into duodenum.

Diagnosis

- Inspect pancreas during laparotomies performed for other indications.
- Check amylase (may be elevated); consider CT, endoscopic retrograde cholangiopancreatography (ERCP).
- CT: Look for parenchymal fracture, intraparenchymal hematoma, lesser sac fluid, fluid between splenic vein and pancreatic body, retroperitoneal hematoma or fluid.
- ERCP: May be used in the stable patient if readily available or available intraoperatively; also may be used to evaluate missed injuries.

Treatment

- Nonoperative: May follow with serial labs and exam if patient can be reliably examined.
- Operative:
  - No ductal injury: Hemostasis and external drainage.
  - Distal transection, parenchymal injury with ductal injury: Distal pancreatectomy with duct ligation.
  - When duodenum or pancreatic head is devitalized, consider Whipple or total pancreatectomy.
  - Proximal transection/injury with probable ductal disruption:
    - If duct is spared, external drainage.
    - If duct is damaged, external drainage and pancreatic duct stenting may be considered.
    - There is no ideal operation for this type of injury.

Minimizing the time from injury to treatment is important in minimizing morbidity and mortality associated with pancreatic injury.

Eighty percent of pancreas can be resected without endocrine or exocrine dysfunction.

Outcome

- Average mortality 19%
  - Primary cause of death is exsanguination from commonly associated vascular injuries, or splenic and liver injuries. Pancreatitis is also common and sometimes severe.
  - Late deaths usually due to infection or multiple system organ failure.
- Average morbidity 30–40%; morbidity directly attributable to pancreatic injury 5%.

VASCULAR INJURY

- Retroperitoneum divided into four zones (see Figure 6-19)
- Zone I (middle): Aorta, celiac axis, proximal SMA, proximal renal artery, SMV, IVC
- Zone II (upper lateral): Renal artery and vein
- Zone III (pelvic): Iliac arteries and veins
- Zone IV (portal-retrohepatic): Portal vein, hepatic artery, IVC
- Incidence of major abdominal vessel injury in blunt trauma—5–10%
- Incidence of major abdominal vessel injury from penetrating trauma:
  - Stab wound—10%
  - Gunshot wound—25%
- Diagnosis: Shock, hemorrhage
  - Renal artery injury: Flank pain and hematuria.
  - Contained hematoma: Usually fluid responsive, distended abdomen, hypotensive, decreased pulses in LE, fluid on FAST, missiles on abdominal x-ray (AXR).
  - If stable, obtain CT scan and/or one-shot IVP.
- Treatment:
  - Basic resuscitation.
  - Prep patient from chin to thigh.
  - Keep patient warm.
  - Obtain control of bleeding.
    - If tamponaded, obtain proximal and distal control prior to opening hematoma.
    - Active hemorrhage: Use direct compression to obtain control based on specific injury, suture defect, resect and repair, or use graft.
- Outcome:
  - Survival: Suprarenal aorta—35%, infrarenal aorta—46%, portal vein—50%
    - Complication: Vasculoenteric fistula

GENITOURINARY (GU) TRAUMA

General

- Often overlooked in the initial evaluation of the multiply injured trauma victim.
- Diagnostic evaluation of the GU tract is performed in a "retrograde" fashion (i.e., work your way back from the urethra to the kidneys and renal vasculature).

Anatomy

The GU tract injury is divided into the upper (kidney and ureters) and lower tract (bladder, urethra, and genitalia) injury.

Suspect GU trauma with:
- Straddle injury
- Penetrating injury to lower abdomen
- Falls from height
- Hematuria noted on Foley insertion.

Signs and Symptoms

- Flank or groin pain
- Blood at the urethral meatus
- Ecchymoses on perineum and/or genitalia
- Evidence of pelvic fracture
- Rectal bleeding
- A "high-riding" or superiorly displaced prostate

Placement of Urethral Catheter

- A Foley or Coude catheter should be placed in any trauma patient with a significant mechanism of injury in the absence of any sign of urethral injury.
- Partial urethral tears warrant one careful attempt of a urinary catheter. If any resistance is met or a complete urethral tear is diagnosed, suprapubic catheter placement will be needed to establish urinary drainage.

Urinalysis

- The presence of gross hematuria indicates GU injury and often concomitant pelvic fracture.
- Urinalysis should be done to document presence or absence of microscopic hematuria.
- Microscopic hematuria is usually self-limited.

Retrograde Urethrogram

- Should be performed in any patient with suspected urethral disruption (before Foley placement).
- A preinjection KUB (kidneys, ureters, bladder) film should be taken.
- A 60-cc Toomey syringe (vs. a Luer-lock syringe) should be filled with the appropriate contrast solution and placed in the urethral meatus.
- With the patient in the supine position, inject 20 to 60 cc contrast over 30 to 60 seconds.
- A repeat KUB is taken during the last 10 cc of contrast injection.
- Retrograde flow of contrast from the meatus to the bladder without extravasation connotes urethral integrity and Foley may then be placed.
- May be performed in the OR in patients requiring emergency surgery for other injuries.

Bladder Rupture

Intraperitoneal
- Usually occurs secondary to blunt trauma to a full bladder.
- Treatment is surgical repair.

Extraperitoneal
- Usually occurs secondary to pelvic fracture.
- Treatment is nonsurgical management by Foley drainage.

Retrograde Cystogram

- Should be performed on patients with gross hematuria or a pelvic fracture.

Blood at the urethral meatus is virtually diagnostic for urethral injury and demands early retrograde urethrogram before Foley placement.

Do not probe perineal lacerations as they are often a sign of an underlying pelvic fracture and disruption of a hematoma may occur.

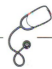

History of enlarged prostate, prostate cancer, urethral stricture, self-catheterization, or previous urologic surgery may make Foley placement difficult or can be confused with urethral disruption.

- Obtain preinjection KUB.
- Fill the bladder with 400 cc of the appropriate contrast material using gravity at a height of 2 ft.
- Obtain another KUB.
- Empty the bladder (unclamp the Foley), then irrigate with saline and take another KUB ("washout" film).
- Extravasation of contrast into the pouch of Douglas, paracolic gutters, and between loops of intestine is diagnostic for intraperitoneal rupture and requires operative repair of the bladder.
- Extravasation of contrast into the paravesicular tissue or behind the bladder as seen on the 'washout' film is indicative of extraperitoneal bladder rupture.

Ureteral Injury

- Least common GU injury
- Must be surgically repaired
- Diagnosed at the time of IVP or CT scan during the search for renal injury

Renal Contusion

- Most common renal injury.
- Renal capsule remains intact.
- IVP is usually normal, and CT scan may show evidence of edema or micro-extravasation of contrast into the renal parenchyma.
- Often associated with a subcapsular hematoma.
- Management is conservative and requires admission to the hospital.
- Recovery is usually complete unless there is underlying renal pathology.

Renal Laceration

- Classified as either minor (involving only the renal cortex) or major (extending into the renal medulla and/or collecting system).
- Diagnosed by CT scan or IVP.
- Minor renal lacerations are managed expectantly.
- Management of major renal lacerations are varied and depend on the surgeon, hemodynamic stability of the patient, and the extent of injury and its coincident complications (ongoing bleeding and urinary extravasation).

Renal Fracture ("Shattered Kidney")

- Involves complete separation of the renal parenchyma from the collecting system.
- Usually leads to uncontrolled hemorrhage and requires surgical intervention.

EXTREMITY TRAUMA

SIGNS AND SYMPTOMS

- Tenderness to palpation

- Decreased range of motion
- Deformity or shortening of extremity
- Swelling
- Crepitus
- Laceration or open wound over extremity (open fracture)
- Temperature or pulse difference in one extremity compared to the other
- Loss of sensation in extremity
- Abnormal capillary refill

TREATMENT

- Reduction of fracture or dislocation under sedation.
- Splint extremity.
- Irrigation, antibiotics, and tetanus prophylaxis for open fractures.

COMPLICATIONS

- Compartment syndrome
- Neurovascular compromise
- Fat embolism
- Osteomyelitis
- Rhabdomyolysis (with prolonged crush injuries)
- Avascular necrosis
- Malunion
- Nonunion

PEDIATRIC TRAUMA

Airway

- Smaller airway
- Relatively large tongue
- Anterior larynx
- Narrowest portion is below the vocal cord at the level of cricoid

$$\text{ET tube size} = \frac{\text{age} + 16}{4}$$

$$\text{Depth} = \frac{\text{age (years)}}{2} + 12$$

$$\text{Depth} = \text{Internal diameter} \times 3$$

Breathing

Infants: 40 breaths/min
Children: 20 breaths/min
Tidal volume: 7 to 10 mL/kg

Circulation

Child blood volume 80 mL/kg:
- One fourth of blood volume must be lost before hypotension occurs.

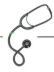

Signs of compartment syndrome: The 6 Ps
Pain
Pallor
Paresthesias
Pulse deficit
Poikilothermia
Paralysis

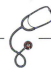

Rhabdomyolysis causes myoglobin release, which can cause renal failure. Maintaining a high urine output together with alkalinization of the urine can help prevent the renal failure by reducing precipitation of myoglobin in the kidney.

Endotracheal (ET) tube size based on size of cricoid ring rather than glottic opening because narrowest part of the child's airway is beyond the glottic opening.

Systolic BP = 80 mm Hg + 2 (age in years)

	INFANT	CHILD	
Eye opening	Spontaneously	Spontaneously	4
	To speech	To speech	3
	To pain	To pain	2
	No response	No response	1
Best motor response	Spontaneous	Obeys command	6
	Withdraws from touch	Localizes pain	5
	Withdraws from pain	Same	4
	Decorticate	Same	3
	Decerebrate	Same	2
	No response	Same	1
Best verbal response	Coos, babbles, smiles	Oriented	5
	Crying, irritable	Confused	4
	Cries, screams to pain	Inappropriate words	3
	Moans, grunts	Incomprehensible	2
	No response	No response	1
TOTAL			15

FIGURE 6-21. Pediatric Glasgow Coma Scale.

- Hypovolemia causes tachycardia long before it causes hypotension.
- Intraosseous cannulation < 6 years
- Adequate urine output must be maintained:
  - Infant—2 mL/kg/hr
  - Child—1.5 mL/kg/hr
  - Adolescent—1 mL/kg/hr

Neurologic

- Separate Glasgow Coma Scale for infants and children (see Figure 6-21).
- CT head without contrast for any child with decreased level of consciousness or suspected loss of consciousness.
- Increased intracranial pressures may be masked in infants because cranium can expand via open fontanelles.

Thermal Injury

BURN INJURY BASICS

Incidence

- U.S. incidence: 1.5 to 2 million burn injuries per year
- Highest-risk populations: Infants and children, elderly, low socioeconomic status

Causes

- Most common: **Scald** (of which 80% may be treated as outpatient)
- Most common cause requiring admission to burn center: **Flame,** due to house fire or clothing ignition

American Burn Association Criteria for Admission to a Burn Center

- Second- or third-degree burns of > 10% body surface area (BSA) in patients under 10 or over 50 years old
- Second- or third-degree burns of > 20% BSA in patients of other ages
- Significant burns to face, hands, feet, genitalia, perineum, or skin over major joints
- Full-thickness burns of > 5% BSA at any age
- Significant electrical injury (including lightning)
- Significant chemical injury
- Lesser burn injury in conjunction with inhalational injury, trauma, or preexisting medical conditions
- Burns in patients requiring special social, emotional, or rehabilitation assistance (i.e., child or elder abuse)

ASSESSMENT

At the Scene

1. Remove patient from source of heat, electric current, or chemical substance (without contacting current or chemical).
2. Extinguish burning clothing/remove clothing.

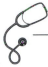

Incidence of burns is higher during winter months.

Seventy-five percent of burn-related deaths can be attributed to **house fires.**

Typical scenario: A 4-year-old child is brought to your emergency department (ED) with a 14% total body surface area (TBSA) burn, including both second and third degree. It looks as if he had been seated in scalding water. Where should this child be cared for? *Think:* This patient is under 10 years old, with > 10% TBSA burned, including the perineum and genitalia, and may require special social assistance (due to likelihood of child abuse). He should be transferred to a burn center.

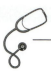

Typical scenario: An adult male is brought to the ED with second-degree burns of his chest and abdominal wall, anterior right leg, and perineum. What percentage TBSA does he have? *Think:* Rule of Nines says 18% for anterior torso, 9% for anterior leg, and 1% for perineum = 28%.

3. ABCs; intubate patient if indicated.
   - If carbon monoxide inhalation is suspected, administer 100% oxygen by nonrebreather mask (accelerates dissociation).
4. Lavage when appropriate to dilute chemical agents.

ER

1. Follow through with above if not completed at scene.
2. Apply cold saline soaks for analgesia if burns are < 25% BSA (watch for hypothermia).
3. Cover burns with clean sheet and then warm blanket.
4. Elevate burned areas when possible to minimize edema.
5. Basic laboratories: Arterial blood gas (ABG), complete blood count (CBC), electrolytes, carboxyhemoglobin.
6. Weigh patient.
7. Begin fluid resuscitation.
8. Insert Foley catheter in patients requiring fluid resuscitation or with significant perineal burns.
9. Electrocardiogram (ECG).
10. Continue to monitor vital signs. (Patients with high-voltage electrical injury require cardiac monitor, as do any intubated or otherwise unstable patients.)

Assessment of Extent and Severity of Burns

- Consider only second- and third-degree burns when stating %BSA burned.
- The Rule of Nines may be used to estimate the area burned (see Figure 7-1).
- The palm of the patient's hand is roughly equivalent to 1% BSA.
- Percent BSA burned (see Table 7-1) is used to determine need for fluid resuscitation (see below).

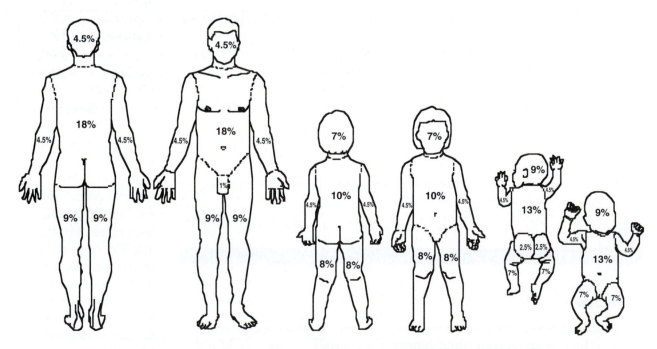

FIGURE 7-1. Rule of Nines for estimating body surface area burned in adults, children, and infants. (Reproduced, with permission, from Stead LG, *BRS Emergency Medicine.* Philadelphia: Lippincott Williams and Wilkins, 2000: 558.)

- Patients not requiring admission to any hospital should receive appropriate management and follow-up, including cleansing of burned areas; debridement of loose, nonviable skin; application of topical antimicrobial/nonadherent dressing or of biologic dressing (described below).
- Assess need for escharotomy or fasciotomy (see below).

Deciding Who May Be Treated as Outpatient

- Most first-degree burns
- Superficial and intermediate second-degree burns of < 10% BSA (excluding most burns of face, eyes, hands, perineum)
- Patients with acceptable social situations amenable to providing a safe and helpful environment at home

Basics

- More than maintenance for all patients with > 15% BSA burn (oral resuscitation should be avoided in these patients because of likely ileus).
- Note that the following fluid requirements will be further increased in patients with fever or requiring intubation (increased insensible loss).

Parkland Formula

For first 24 hours:
- Lactated Ringer's (LR) at rate of 4 mL/kg/%BSA burn.
- Give half of 24-hour requirement in first 8 hours from the time of burn, and the remainder over the next 16 hours.
- In second 24-hour period, change fluid to $D_5 1/2NS$, and give albumin if albumin is < 1.5 or < 3.0 and patient is also hypotensive.

Choosing Fluid Type

- Colloid vs. crystalloid:
  - Use crystalloid as described above unless fluid requirement based on urine output is > 2 times estimated in first 12 hours; then use colloid.

Typical scenario: How much fluid should a 60-kg female with a 25% TBSA burn receive during the first 24 hours? *Think:* Parkland formula. At 4 mL/kg/%, 4 × 60 × 25 = 6,000 mL required over the next 24 hours, at a rate of 375 mL/hr for the first 8 hours, and 188 mL/hr for the next 16 hours.

	INFANTS/CHILDREN				ADULTS
	BIRTH	**1 Year**	**5 Years**	**10 Years**	**15 Years+**
Head/Neck	19%	17%	13%	11%	9%
Arm (each)	9%	9%	9%	9%	9%
Trunk (anterior)	18%	18%	18%	18%	18%
Trunk (posterior)	18%	18%	18%	18%	18%
Leg (each)	12%	15%	17%	17%	18%
Perineum	1%	1%	1%	1%	1%

TABLE 7-1. BSA.

- By 48 hours, both are equally effective at restoring intravascular volume and cardiac output, but colloid is associated with more late pulmonary complications and higher mortality.
  - *Sugar or no sugar:*
    - Endocrine response to burn is hyperglycemia, so euglycemic patients do not need sugar initially.

Pediatric Patients

- First 24 hours:
  - Under 15 years old, estimate need as LR at 3 mL/kg/%BSA, and give as in adults, first half over 8 hours and second half over next 16 hours.
  - Additional need should be given as electrolyte-free water.
- Second 24 hours:
  - Use colloids as in adults, except for small children in whom $D_5 1/4NS$ may be more appropriate.
- Additional needs met with D_5W

Monitoring Fluid Status

- Resuscitation is adequate when urine output is 30 to 50 cc/hr in adults and 1 cc/kg/hr in children < 30 kg.
  - Adjust fluids when urine output is more than 33% different (in either direction) from recommended over 2 to 3 hours.
- Swan–Ganz catheter may be required to assess cardiac function in sicker patients.
- Use inotropes as needed to maintain blood pressure (BP).
- Monitor daily weights.
- Oliguria: Usually secondary to insufficient fluid resuscitation:
  - Consider diuretics when concerned about **myoglobinuria:** Seen with high-voltage injury, associated soft-tissue mechanical injury, deep burns involving muscle, extensive burns with excess fluid and still oliguric.
  - If mannitol (an osmotic diuretic) is used, the patient will require a central venous pressure (CVP) line because urine output ceases to be an adequate assessment of fluid status.

Variations in Fluid Requirements

Increased
- High-voltage electrical injury
- Inhalational injury
- Delayed resuscitation
- Intoxicated at time of injury

Decreased
- Patients > 50 years old
- Patients < 2 years old
- Patients with cardiac or pulmonary disease

Daily

- ABCs (airway, breathing, circulation), physiologic resuscitation.
- Cleanse wounds, trim nonviable skin.
- Daily burn care in shower or tank if possible; otherwise at bedside.

Definitive Therapy

- For definitive nonexcisional therapy, continue daily cleansing and debridement until granulation tissue is present with minimal or no necrotic debris, at which time a biologic dressing is applied.
- For operative therapy, see Operations section.

The risk of infection of burned tissue is increased because the wound is protein rich and moist, and is thus a good culture medium. The neoeschar and lack of vascularity limit antibiotic delivery.

PHYSIOLOGIC EFFECT ON BODY SYSTEMS

Cardiovascular

Pre-resuscitation

- **Increased microvascular permeability** secondary to release of vasoactive materials (via arachidonic acid pathway, substance P, interleukin-1 (IL-1), IL-6, IL-8, histamine)
- **Decreased cardiac output** but overall hyperdynamic state with **increased ejection fraction**
- **Increased hematocrit** due to decreased blood volume, increased blood viscosity
- **Increased peripheral vascular resistance**
- **Oliguria** because decreased blood volume and cardiac output (CO) lead to decreased renal blood flow and decreased glomerular filtration rate (GFR)

After Resuscitation

- Persistent hyperdynamic state:
  - CO increases, leading to increased renal blood flow and increased GFR.
  - Elevated metabolic requirements.
  - Elevated catecholamines and glucagon.
  - Decreased levels of insulin and thyroxin.
  - Result in catabolic state.
- **Edema** (peaks at 8 to 12 hours) as fluid is lost from intravascular compartment.

Hypovolemia and hemoconcentration can lead to an elevated hematocrit and decreased left ventricular end diastolic volume that result in decreased CO and low-flow state.

Pulmonary

- In the absence of thoracic burns or inhalation injury, hypovolemia may result in rapid but **shallow respirations.**
- After resuscitation, **hyperventilation** occurs with or without modest parenchymal dysfunction, leading to a mild respiratory alkalosis.

HIGH-YIELD FACTS

Thermal Injury

- **Increased pulmonary vascular resistance,** but no change in pulmonary capillary permeability.
- With circumferential thoracic burns, the constricting eschar and edema cause a **restrictive defect** and may necessitate escharotomy.

Hematologic

- **Plasma loss**
- **Red blood cell (RBC) destruction** in proportion to extent of burn:
  - Cell lysis secondary to heat
  - Microvascular thrombosis in areas with tissue damage
- Early:
  - Decrease in platelets
  - Decrease in fibrinogen
  - Increase in fibrin degradation products
- Later, levels return to normal and then become elevated, though **antithrombin III (ATIII)** and **protein C** are decreased.

Gastrointestinal (GI)

Burn patients are susceptible to Curling's ulcer, which is due to lack of the normal mucosal barrier.

- Most patients with > 25% TBSA will have an **ileus** that typically resolves between day 3 and 5.
- GI permeability is increased, with **increased bacterial translocation.**
- Patients generally require an NG tube and GI prophylaxis with an H_2 blocker.

Endocrine

- Increased glucagon, cortisol, catecholamines
- Decreased insulin, triiodothyronine (T_3)

Immunologic

- Loss of skin barrier function
- > 20% BSA, cell-mediated immunity decreases in proportion to burn size
- Early decrease in white blood count (WBC) (especially lymphocytes), then granulocytosis and B-lymphocytosis, with T-cell activation
- Decreased IL-2, immunoglobulin G (IgG), natural killer (NK) cells
- Increased IL-6, tumor necrosis factor-alpha (TNF-α)
- Polymorphonuclear neutrophil (PMN) dysfunction: Immunosuppression, increased susceptibility to infection, decreased chemotaxis, dysfunction related to size of burn

Metabolism and Nutrition

- Hypermetabolism: Increased oxygen consumption, increased CO, increased minute ventilation volume, increased temperature, increased urinary nitrogen
- Greatly increased blood flow to wound
- Catecholamine release, especially norepinephrine

- Increased UUN [VC1] secondary to breakdown of muscle protein to glucose because of greatly increased need for glucose
- Increased protein and calorie needs
- Start PO supplementation by nasogastric tube (NGT) day 3 or 4 if no oral intake, but ileus resolved
- Total parenteral nutrition (TPN) if needed

Escharotomy

- Areas of concern: Circumferential burns of extremities (including penis) or thorax.
- Indications:
    - Impairment or failure of peripheral circulation or ventilatory exchange, manifested by cyanosis
    - Impaired capillary refill
    - Paresthesias
    - Pain
    - Elevated compartment pressure > 30 mm Hg
- No anesthesia is needed.
- Technique:
    - Make an incision through the eschar and the superficial fascia so that the edges of the eschar separate.
- The incision should be in the mid-lateral or mid-medial area from the proximal to distal margin of burn, and across any involved joints.
- The opposite side may also need to be incised.

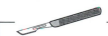

Need for escharotomy may be decreased by maintaining limb elevation and by enforcing active motion at least 5 minutes per hour.

Fasciotomy

- Escharotomy may fail, especially when the burn is from high-voltage electrical injury or is associated with soft tissue, bone, or vascular injury.
- If compartment syndrome persists after escharotomy, incision of the fascia is also required.
- General anesthesia is required.

The most common compartment requiring fasciotomy is the anterior tibial compartment.

Debridement and Skin Grafting

- Excisional treatment is indicated for most deep second- and third-degree burns once the patient is stabilized.
- Advantages: Decreased length of stay, earlier return to work, decreased incidence of infection, decreased complications, improved survival.
- Technique:
    - Full-thickness burns require debridement to the investing fascial layer using the scalpel and bovie.
    - Tangential excision may be used for deep partial burns of < 20% BSA and for staged excision of more extensive partial- and full-thickness burns.
- A Goulian knife, which takes off sequential thin layers, can be used for partial- and some full-thickness excisions; requires debridement until uniform capillary bleeding.

Limit burn excision operations to excision of < 20% BSA at one trip to the OR or to a set time limit of 2 hours.

Burn debridement with the Goulian knife is frequently accompanied by a significant amount of blood loss, which can be minimized by using topical thrombin spray and infiltration with epinephrine or vasopressin.

- Once debridement is complete, the wound is covered with split-thickness skin graft (STSG), full-thickness graft, or biologic dressing.
- Wound closure.
- STSG may be applied when the burn is excised or there is no residual nonviable tissue, no pooled secretions, and surface bacterial count is < 10^5/cm^2
- Autograft should be 0.010 to 0.015 inches thick:
  - Donor sites may be reharvested (after 2 to 3 weeks when reepithelialization is complete), but the quality decreases each time as dermis is thinner.
  - Grafts may be meshed at a ratio of 1.5:1 to increase coverage, unless burns are on face or joints.
- If the risk of mortality is anticipated to be < 50%, first graft hands, feet, face, and joints.
- If > 50%, graft flat surfaces first to decrease uncovered surface area.
- Biologic dressings: Bilaminate; outer layer with pores to permit water vapor but not liquid or bacterial passage, and inner layer that permits ingrowth of fibrovascular tissue from wound surface.

Options for Biologic Dressings

- Allograft:
  - Cadaveric
  - Prevents wound desiccation
  - Promotes maturation of granulation tissue
  - Limits bacterial proliferation
  - Prevents exudative loss of protein and RBC
  - Decreases wound pain
  - Increases movement
  - Decreases evaporation
  - Decreases heat loss
- Xenograft:
  - Porcine
  - Less effective
  - More subgraft bacteria
- Biobrane:
  - Synthetic collagen dermal analog, with silastic epidermal analog
  - Partial-thickness burns
- Pain is reduced
- Comes off on its own when reepithelialization occurs

INFECTION

Signs

- Degeneration of second degree to full thickness
- Focal color change to dark brown and black
- Degeneration of wound with neoeschar formation
- Rapid eschar separation
- Hemorrhagic discoloration of subeschar fat

- Erythematous or violaceous edematous wound margin
- Crusted margin
- Metastatic septic lesions in unburned tissue

Biopsy Reveals

- Microorganisms in unburned tissue
- Hemorrhage in unburned tissue
- Heightened inflammatory reaction in adjacent viable tissue
- Small-vessel thrombosis or ischemic necrosis or unburned tissue
- Perineural and lymphatic migration of organisms
- Vasculitis with perivascular cuffing
- Intracellular viral inclusion

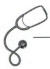

Infection is more likely in patients with > 30% BSA burn without complete excision or grafting. Apparently infected wounds need to be examined daily and biopsied, including eschar and underlying unburned tissue.

Stages of Infection

1. Colonization: Superficial, penetrating, proliferating
2. Invasion: Microinvasion, deep invasion, microvascular invasion

Treatment

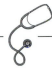

Mafenide acetate (Sulfamylon) penetrates eschar well and should therefore be used when infection is present.

1. For invasive infection, change to Sulfamylon and start systemic antibiotics.
2. For pseudomonal or pediatric infections, infuse subeschar piperacillin, and plan for emergent operative debridement within 12 hours.
3. For candidal infections, start antifungal creams; if that treatment fails, start systemic therapy with amphotericin B.
4. *Aspergillus* may infect subcutaneous tissues late in the course, and if it crosses the fascia, amputation of the extremity is required.
5. Viral infections with herpes simplex virus, type 1 (HSV-1), though uncommon, may occur, and require 7 days of acyclovir 5% ointment.

Other Infections in the Burned Patient

PNEUMONIA

- Cause of death in over half of fatal burns.
- Agent is usually *Staphylococcus aureus* or gram negatives such as *Escherichia coli* and *Enterococcus*.
- Average time frame: Onset after day 10.
- Hematogenous pneumonia may occur later, around the 17th day, from a remote septic focus; appears as a round infiltrate on chest x-ray (CXR). Treatment is to remove source and treat with antibiotics. This type is more often fatal than bronchopneumonia.

SUPPURATIVE THROMBOPHLEBITIS

- Prevent by changing peripheral IVs every 3 days.
- Usual signs may not exist because of burned skin or immunosuppression.
- For an occluded peripheral vein, explore and surgically remove involved vein, and start antibiotics.

ACUTE ENDOCARDITIS

- Likelihood increased because of long-term need for IV.
- Culprit typically *S. aureus*
- Systemic antibiotic therapy

SUPPURATIVE SINUSITIS

- Due to nasal intubation or long-term NGT
- Confirm with computed tomography (CT)
- Treat with antibiotics
- Drain if treatment fails

BACTEREMIA AND SEPSIS

- Decreased incidence with use of perioperative antibiotics.
- Use antibiotics only when there is documented infection.

BURN SCAR CANCER

Characteristics

- Rare
- Called Marjolin's ulcer
- Usually squamous cell carcinoma, which metastasizes via lymph nodes
- Diagnosis made by biopsy
- Treatment: Wide excision of all involved tissue

INHALATIONAL INJURY

DESCRIPTION

- Consists of a chemical tracheobronchitis and acute pneumonitis.
- Inhalation of smoke and products of incomplete combustion.
- Suspect inhalational injury in patients burned in closed spaces or who have impaired mentation.
- Extent of injury is determined by composition of inhaled gases, size of particles, duration of toxic exposure, and quantity of fluid administration.

SIGNS AND SYMPTOMS

Patients may have hoarse voice, cough, wheeze, bronchorrhea, hypoxemia, carbonaceous sputum, head and neck burns, singed nose hairs.

DIAGNOSIS

- Often delayed but is made with the use of CXR, bronchoscopy, and ventilation–perfusion (V/Q) scan.
- Bronchoscopy reveals edema and ulceration.
- V/Q scanning will demonstrate carbon particle deposition on endobronchial mucosa.

TREATMENT

- Mild injury: Use warm humidified oxygen and an incentive spirometer.
- Half-life of carbon monoxide decreased from 4 hours on room air to 60 minutes with 100% oxygen.
- Moderate: Repeated bronchoscopy when there is continued mucosal sloughing and the patient is unable to clear it.
- Severe, with progressive hypoxemia: Intubation

COMPLICATIONS

Most commonly, pneumonia

Carbon Monoxide (CO) Poisoning

- In closed space burns.
- Impairs tissue oxygenation by decreasing oxygen-carrying capacity of blood, shifting oxygen–hemoglobin dissociation curve to the left, binding myoglobin and terminal cytochrome oxidase.
- Symptoms do not correlate well with carboxyhemoglobin levels.
- Measure carboxyhemoglobin with ABG.
- Treatment is hyperbaric oxygen.
  - Decreases half-life to 30 minutes (2 atm).

ELECTRICAL INJURY

DEFINITION

- Extent of injury depends on voltage of current:
  - Up to 1,000 volts—increased resistance limits further passage of current and heating of tissue.
  - > 1,000 volts—passage of current is not limited and tissue injury can continue.
- Deeper tissue may be more severely injured because it cools more slowly.

MECHANISM

- Tissue damaged via conversion to thermal energy.
- Damage occurs in skin and underlying tissues along the course of current.
- Skin at the point of contact is often severely charred.

SIGNS AND SYMPTOMS

- Charring at point of contact.
- Myoglobinuria (with muscle damage).
- Hyperkalemia (due to tissue necrosis).
- High-voltage or lightning injury may cause cardiac arrest.
- Neuropathy (immediately following injury, likely to resolve over time).
- Compartment syndrome: Swelling of injured extremity with pain, paresthesia, pallor, pulselessness, poikilothermia.

Mortality of burns with inhalational injury is increased compared to burns without inhalational injury.

Carbon monoxide has an affinity for hemoglobin 200 times that of oxygen.

Normal carboxyhemoglobin:
3–5% nonsmokers
7–10% smokers

Extent of damage from electrical injury depends on both current density and tissue conduction. The surface wound usually underestimates the extent of damage to deeper tissues.

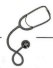

5 Ps of compartment
syndrome:
- **Pain**
- **Paresthesia**
- **Pallor**
- **Pulselessness**
- **Poikilothermia**

TREATMENT

- Patients with loss of consciousness or abnormal ECG require cardiac monitoring for 48 hours even if there are no further arrhythmias or ECG changes.
- Electrical injury is more likely than other types of burn injury to necessitate fasciotomy because deep tissue edema may be extensive, causing compartment syndrome.

LATE COMPLICATIONS

- Delayed hemorrhage because of inadequate wound exploration, debridement, or exposure of vessel
- Cataracts

LIGHTNING INJURY

- Fatal in one third of victims
- Likely to cause cardiopulmonary arrest
- Can cause transient coma or other neurologic deficits
- Can cause rupture of tympanic membrane
- Can cause myoglobinuria

CHEMICAL INJURY

Strong acid burns may
leave a deceptively healthy
appearance of tan smooth
skin.

MECHANISM

- General: Protein denaturation and precipitation, with release of thermal energy
- Liquefaction necrosis (alkali)
- Delipidation (petroleum products)
- Vesicle formation (vesicant gas)

SEVERITY

Determined by:
- Concentration
- Amount of agent in contact
- Duration of contact (Tissue injury continues to occur as long as the agent remains in contact with the skin.)

Chemical wound irrigation
should be with *water* only.
Attempts to neutralize the
agent may cause further
release of thermic injury,
thereby causing further
damage.

PRIORITIES IN TREATMENT

- Remove all clothing to prevent further contact.
- Copious water lavage: Irrigation should continue for at least 30 minutes for acid burns, and longer for alkali burns (because they penetrate deeper into the tissue).
- Check pulmonary status (for edema, mucosal desquamation, bronchospasm).

Sunburn

- Characteristics:
  - Pain and erythema reach peak within 10 to 24 hours, and resolve in 3 to 4 days.
  - Watch for postural hypotension with severe sunburns.
- Treatment:
  - Cool showers
  - Topical analgesics
  - Antihistamines
  - Ensure adequate hydration (usually PO fluids are sufficient)
- Severe sunburns should be treated as partial-thickness burns.

Heat Shock

DEFINITION

- Loss of thermoregulation that occurs when demands for maintenance of blood pressure are greater than demands for maintaining temperature.

SIGNS AND SYMPTOMS

- Temperature > 105°F or 40.6°C
- Hypotension
- Hypovolemia
- Acid–base disturbance
- Anhidrosis
- CNS dysfunction
- Disorientation
- Bizarre behavior

TREATMENT

- Cool the patient.
- Cardiac monitoring.
- Correct acid–base disturbance.
- Ensure adequate hydration.

PROGNOSIS

Mortality is 18%.

People at Risk

- Military personnel
- Winter sport athletes
- Elderly
- Homeless
- People with impaired mental status or consciousness

Risk of cold injury is further increased with wet clothes, air movement, and peripheral vascular disease.

HIGH-YIELD FACTS

Thermal Injury

Ambient tissue temperature must be at least −2°C for freezing to occur.

Frostbite sequelae to watch for in your patients: Hyperhidrosis, paresthesia, cool extremities, cold sensitivity, edema.

Vascular system damage in frostbite occurs during thawing. Platelet aggregates form, occluding the microvasculature, and decreasing flow to the frozen extremity.

Frostbite

- Affects exposed parts first.
- Rare, but worse, is contact with liquid petroleum or metal at subfreezing temperatures, which causes rapid and extensive tissue freezing.
- Physiology of tissue necrosis:
  - Freezing disrupts cellular architecture, leading to cell death via intracellular ice crystallization, cellular dehydration, and microvascular thrombosis.
- Thawing causes extracellular loss of high-protein fluid, vasospasm at a narrow border of frozen tissue with surrounding vasodilatation.

CHARACTERISTICS

See Table 7-2.

- Sensation is lost at tissue temperatures ≤ 10°C.
- *Hunting reaction:* Alternating vasoconstriction and vasodilation of the cutaneous microvasculature that helps protect extremities while sacrificing core temperature. This mechanism fails once hypothermia is systemic.
- Nerves and blood vessels are more sensitive than skin.
- Vascular changes become evident upon thawing.

APPEARANCE

- Mild frostbite: Bright red, warm, painful, with paresthesia, rapid edema, large vesicles, late superficial eschar (resolves in 1 to 2 weeks)
- Deep frostbite: Deep purple, cool, minimally painful, small hemorrhagic vesicles, slow edema, mummification of deep structures

TREATMENT

1. Remove wet and restrictive clothing.
2. **Wrap in warm blankets and give warm fluid.**

TABLE 7-2. Severity of frostbite injury.	
First Degree	■ Hyperemia ■ Edema ■ Superficial epidermal freezing ■ Minimal necrosis ■ No vesicles
Second Degree	■ Hyperemia ■ Edema ■ Vesicles ■ Sensation intact
Third Degree	■ Full-thickness necrosis ■ Variable depth of subcutaneous involvement ■ Small vesicles
Fourth Degree	■ Full-thickness necrosis of skin into muscle and bone ■ Gangrene ■ Usually requires amputation

3. ***Immediate* rewarming of frozen parts: Place in circulating water at 40°C until pink and perfused.**
   - Should not take longer than 20 to 30 minutes.
   - Patient will not be able to judge temperature of water so it must be kept steady.
   - Do not thaw until you are certain that no further freezing will occur.
4. Bed rest.
5. Use a bed cradle to keep wounds exposed to air and vesicles intact.
6. Daily wound care with gentle whirlpool cleansing.
7. No debridement until demarcation has occurred (which may take several weeks or even months).
   - Mummified tissue over a frostbitten area provides protection for the damaged tissue and should not be debrided early.
8. Antibiotics only for infection.

Nonfreezing Cold Injury

- More common than frostbite.
- Physiologic damage: Microvascular injury, endothelial damage, capillary stasis, vascular occlusion.
- Varieties:
  - Trench foot.
  - Immersion foot.
  - Chillblain (pernio): Due to prolonged exposure to dry cold above freezing temperatures; affects women and mountain climbers; appears as small superficial ulcers, hemorrhagic bullae, localized cyanosis.
- Treatment: Same as for frostbite, but use soft dressings.
- Long-term sequelae: Same as for frostbite.

REWARMING FOR SYSTEMIC HYPOTHERMIA

Passive
- For temperatures 32 to 35°C: Remove clothes, warm blankets, allow to shower.
- For temperatures 28 to 32°C: Warm shower and then give intravenous fluids via fluid warmer.

Active
For temperatures < 28°C: Circulating water bath at 40°C.

The extent of frostbite injury can be determined only after demarcation and sloughing of gangrenous tissues.

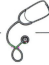

Rewarming at temperatures > 40°C can cause further tissue damage, particularly because the patient will not be likely to sense "burning."

Patients who are hypothermic cannot be pronounced dead. They must first be rewarmed. Remember, "You are dead only if you are warm and dead."

HIGH-YIELD FACTS

Thermal Injury

The Breast

SURGICALLY RELEVANT ANATOMY

Basic Structure

- Composed of glandular, fibrous, and adipose tissue.
- Lies within layers of superficial pectoral fascia.
- Each mammary gland consists of approximately 15 to 20 lobules, each of which has a lactiferous duct that opens on the areola.
- Has ligaments that extend from the deep pectoral fascia to the superficial dermal fascia that provide structural support referred to as *Cooper's ligaments*.
- Frequently extends into axilla as the *axillary tail of Spence*.
- Is partitioned into 4 quadrants by vertical and horizontal lines across the nipple: Upper inner quadrant (UIQ), lower inner quadrant (LIQ), upper outer quadrant (UOQ), and lower outer quadrant (LOQ).

BOUNDARIES FOR AXILLARY DISSECTION

See Figure 8-1.
- *Superior:* Axillary vein
- *Posterior:* Long thoracic nerve
- *Medial:* Either lateral to, underneath, or medial to the medial border of the pectoralis minor muscle, depending on the level of nodes taken
- *Lateral:* Latissimus dorsi muscle

Blood Supply

- Arterial: Axillary artery via the lateral thoracic and thoracoacromial branches, internal mammary artery via its perforating branches, and adjacent intercostal arteries.
- Venous: Follows arterial supply; axillary, internal mammary, and intercostal veins; axillary vein responsible for majority of venous drainage.

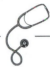

Skin dimpling in breast cancer is due to traction on Cooper's ligaments.

Typical scenario: A female with one or more risk factors for breast cancer presents with a mass in the upper outer quadrant of the breast. *Think:* She's at risk for cancer, and 50% of breast cancers occur in the upper outer quadrant. Therefore, the mass is likely to be malignant.

Venous drainage is largely responsible for metastases to the spine through **Batson's plexus.**

Lymph node involvement by tumor tends to progress from level I to III. The higher the level, the worse the prognosis.

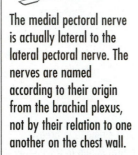

The medial pectoral nerve is actually lateral to the lateral pectoral nerve. The nerves are named according to their origin from the brachial plexus, not by their relation to one another on the chest wall.

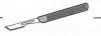

The anesthesiologist should not paralyze the patient at surgery because the major nerves (long thoracic and thoracodorsal) are identified by observing muscle contraction when stimulating them with a forcep.

Perform breast self-examination at same time each month (one week after menstrual period is ideal).

The smallest mass palpable on physical exam is 1 cm.

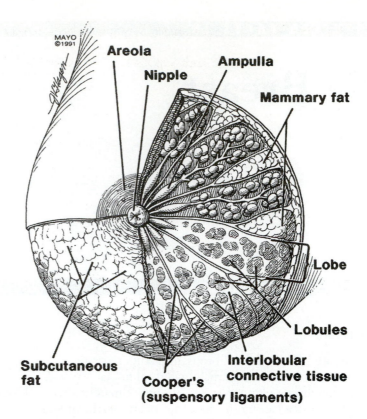

MAYO ©1991

FIGURE 8-1. Normal breast anatomy.

Lymphatic Drainage

- Level I: Lateral to lateral border of pectoralis minor.
- Level II: Deep to pectoralis minor.
- Level III: Medial to medial border of pectoralis minor.
- *Rotter's* nodes lie between the pectoralis major and pectoralis minor muscles.
- The axillary and internal mammary lymph nodes drain the lateral and medial aspects of the breast, respectively.

Nerves

See Table 8-1.

INITIAL EVALUATION OF PATIENTS WITH POSSIBLE BREAST DISEASE

- Complete medical history, including risk factors for breast cancer (see below). Be sure to inquire about any history of nipple discharge or any changes in the size, shape, symmetry, or contour of the breasts.
- Physical examination:
  - Inspection: Note color, symmetry, size, shape, and contour, and check for dimpling, erythema, edema, or thickening of skin with a porous appearance **(peau d'orange).**
  - Palpation: Palpate all four quadrants, the axillary lymph nodes, and the nipple–areolar complex for any discharge.

TABLE 8-1. Neural structures encountered during major breast surgery.

Nerves	Muscle(s)/Area Supplied	Functional Deficit if Injured
Long thoracic nerve (of Bell)	Serratus anterior	Winging of scapula
Thoracodorsal nerve	Latissimus dorsi	Cannot push oneself up from a sitting position
Medial and lateral pectoral nerves	Pectoralis major and minor	Weakness of pectoralis muscles
Intercostobrachial nerve	Crosses axilla transversely to supply inner aspect of arm	Area of anesthesia on inner aspect of arm

EVALUATION OF A PALPABLE BREAST MASS

Approach

- See Figure 8-2.
- If age < 30, serial physical examination with observation for 2 to 4 weeks or until next menstrual period is an option.

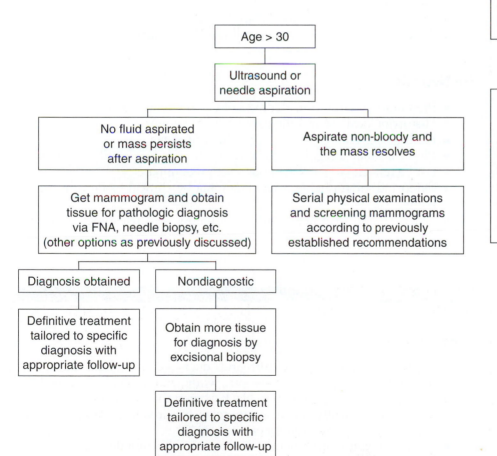

FIGURE 8-2. Evaluation of palpable breast mass.

Fine-needle aspiration (FNA) is not sensitive enough to rule out malignancy (10% false-negative rate).

All persistent breast masses require evaluation.

Typical scenario: A 42-year-old woman presents with an undiagnosed breast mass. *Think:* Evaluate without delay. Observation is not an option if age > 30.

Differential Diagnosis

- Infectious/inflammatory: Mastitis, fat necrosis, Mondor's disease
- Benign lesions: Fibroadenoma, fibrocystic changes, mammary duct ectasia, cystosarcoma phyllodes (occasionally malignant), intraductal papilloma, gynecomastia
- Premalignant disease: Ductal carcinoma in situ (DCIS), lobular carcinoma in situ (LCIS)
- Malignant tumors: Infiltrating ductal, infiltrating lobular, and inflammatory carcinoma; Paget's disease; and other less common histologic types of breast cancer

---

INFECTIOUS/INFLAMMATORY

Mastitis

- Usual etiologic agent: *Staphylococcus aureus* or *Streptococcus* spp.
- Most commonly occurs during early weeks of breast-feeding.
- Physical exam: Focal tenderness with erythema and warmth of overlying skin, fluctuant mass occasionally palpable.
- Diagnosis: Ultrasound can be used to localize an abscess; if abscess present, aspirate fluid for Gram stain and culture.
- Treatment: Continue breast-feeding and recommend use of breast pump as an alternative.
- Cellulitis: Wound care and IV antibiotics.
- Abscess: Incision and drainage followed by IV antibiotics.

Fat Necrosis

- Presentation: Firm, irregular mass of varying tenderness
- History of local trauma elicited in 50% of patients
- Predisposing factors: Chest wall or breast trauma
- Physical exam: Irregular mass without discrete borders that may or may not be tender; later, collagenous scars predominate
- Often indistinguishable from carcinoma by clinical exam or mammography
- Diagnosis and treatment: Excisional biopsy with pathologic evaluation for carcinoma

---

BENIGN DISEASE

Fibroadenoma

- Definition: Fibrous stroma surrounds duct-like epithelium and forms a benign tumor that is grossly smooth, white, and well circumscribed.
- Risk factors: More common in black women than in white women.
- Incidence: Typically occurs in late teens to early 30s; estrogen-sensitive (increased tenderness during pregnancy).
- Signs and symptoms: Smooth, discrete, circular, mobile mass.
- Diagnosis: FNA.

Typical scenario: A female presents complaining of nipple pain during breast-feeding with focal erythema and warmth of breast on physical exam. *Think:* Mastitis ± breast abscess. Incise and drain if fluctuance (abscess) present.

Typical scenario: A 25-year-old female presents with a painful breast mass several weeks after sustaining breast trauma by a seat belt in a car accident. *Think:* The most common cause of a persistent breast mass after trauma is fat necrosis.

Typical scenario: A 20-year-old female presents with a well-circumscribed mass in her left breast. It is mobile, nontender, and has defined borders on physical exam. *Think:* Fibroadenoma until proven otherwise.

- Treatment:
  - If FNA is diagnostic for fibroadenoma and patient is under 30, may observe depending on severity of symptoms and size (< 3 cm).
  - If FNA is nondiagnostic, patient is over 30, or is symptomatic, must excise mass. The mass is well encapsulated and can be shelled out easily at surgery.

Mondor's Disease

- Definition: Superficial thrombophlebitis of lateral thoracic or thoracoepigastric vein.
- Predisposing factors: Local trauma, surgery, infection, repetitive movements of upper extremity.
- Presentation: Acute pain in axilla or superior aspect of lateral breast.
- Physical exam: Tender cord palpated.
- Diagnosis: Confirm with ultrasound.
- Treatment:
  - Clear diagnosis by ultrasound: Salicylates, warm compresses, limit motion of affected upper extremity. Usually resolves within 2 to 6 weeks.
  - If persistent, surgery to divide the vein above and below the site of thrombosis or resect the affected segment.
  - Ultrasound nondiagnostic or an associated mass present: Excisional biopsy.

Fibrocystic Changes

- Usually diagnosed in 20s to 40s.
- Presentation: Breast swelling (often bilateral), tenderness, and/or pain.
- Physical exam: Discrete areas of nodularity within fibrous breast tissue.
- Evaluation: Serial physical examination with documentation of the fluctuating nature of the symptoms is usually sufficient unless a persistent discrete mass is identified; definitive diagnosis requires aspiration or biopsy with pathologic evaluation.
- Symptoms thought to be of hormonal etiology and tend to fluctuate with the menstrual cycle.
- Associated with a group of characteristic histologic findings, each of which has a variable relative risk for the development of cancer.
- Not associated with an increased risk for breast cancer unless biopsy reveals lobular or ductal hyperplasia with atypia.
- Treatment:
  - For cases with a classic history or absence of a persistent mass: Conservative management; options include nonsteroidal anti-inflammatory drugs (NSAIDs), oral contraceptive pills (OCPs), danazol, or tamoxifen; advise patient to avoid products that contain xanthine (e.g, caffeine, tobacco, cola drinks).
  - If single dominant cyst, aspirate fluid; may discard if green or cloudy but must send to cytology and excise cyst if bloody.

Mammary Duct Ectasia (Plasma Cell Mastitis)

- Definition: Inflammation and dilation of mammary ducts
- Most commonly occurs in the perimenopausal years
- Presentation: Noncyclical breast pain with lumps under nipple/areola with or without a nipple discharge

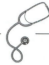

Mondor's disease most commonly develops along the course of a single vein.

Typical scenario: A female presents complaining of acute pain in her axilla and lateral chest wall, and a tender cord is identified on physical exam. *Think:* Mondor's disease vs. chest wall infection. Confirm with ultrasound.

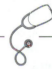

Ten percent of all women develop clinically apparent fibrocystic changes.

Typical scenario: A 35-year-old female presents with a straw-colored nipple discharge and bilateral breast tenderness that fluctuates with her menstrual cycle. *Think:* Fibrocystic changes. Consider a trial of OCPs or NSAIDs.

Typical scenario: A 45-year-old female presents with breast pain that does not vary with her menstrual cycle with lumps in her nipple—areolar complex and a history of a nonbloody nipple discharge. *Think:* Mammary duct ectasia.

There is no need for axillary node dissection in cystosarcoma phyllodes, as lymph node metastases rarely occur.

Typical scenario: A 35-year-old female presents with a 1-month history of a spontaneous unilateral bloody nipple discharge. Radial compression of the involved breast results in expression of blood at the 12 o'clock position. *Think:* Intraductal papilloma.

Causes of gynecomastia:
- Increased estrogen (tumors, endocrine disorders, liver failure, nutritional imbalances)
- Decreased testosterone (aging, testicular failure primary or secondary, renal failure)
- Drugs (e.g., spironolactone)

- Exam: Palpable lumps under areola, possible nipple discharge
- Diagnosis: Based on exam; excisional biopsy required to rule out cancer
- Treatment: Excision of affected ducts

Cystosarcoma Phyllodes

- A variant of fibroadenoma.
- Majority are benign.
- Patients tend to present later than those with fibroadenoma (> 30 years).
- Characteristics: Indistinguishable from fibroadenoma by ultrasound or mammogram. The distinction between the two entities can be made on the basis of their histologic features (phylloides tumors have more mitotic activity). Most are benign and have a good prognosis.
- Exam: Large, freely movable mass with overlying skin changes.
- Diagnosis: Definitive diagnosis requires biopsy with pathologic evaluation.
- Treatment:
  - Smaller tumors: Wide local excision with at least a 1-cm margin
  - Larger tumors: Simple mastectomy

Intraductal Papilloma

- Definition: A benign local proliferation of ductal epithelial cells.
- Characteristics: Unilateral serosanguineous or bloody nipple discharge.
- Presentation: Subareolar mass and/or spontaneous nipple discharge.
- Evaluation: Radially compress breast to determine which lactiferous duct expresses fluid; mammography.
- Diagnosis: Definitive diagnosis by pathologic evaluation of resected specimen.
- Treatment: Excise affected duct.

Gynecomastia

- Definition: Development of female-like breast tissue in males.
- May be physiologic or pathologic.
- At least 2 cm of excess subareolar breast tissue is required to make the diagnosis.
- Treatment: Treat underlying cause if specific cause identified; if normal physiology is responsible, only surgical excision (subareolar mastectomy) may be effective.

PREMALIGNANT DISEASE

See Table 8-2.

TABLE 8-2. Premalignant disease.

Disease	DCIS	LCIS
Cell of origin	Inner layer of epithelial cells in major ducts	Cells of terminal duct–lobular unit
Definition	Proliferation of ductal cells that spread through the ductal system but lack the ability to invade the basement membrane	A *multifocal* proliferation of acinar and terminal ductal cells
Age	> ½ of cases occur after menopause	Vast majority of cases occur prior to menopause
Palpable mass	Sometimes	*Never*
Diagnosis	Clustered microcalcifications on mammogram, malignant epithelial cells in breast duct on biopsy	Typically a clinically occult lesion; undetectable by mammogram and **incidental on biopsy**
Lymphatic invasion	< 1%	Rare
Risk of invasive cancer	Increased risk in ipsilateral breast, usually same quadrant; infiltrating ductal carcinoma most common histologic type; comedo type has the worst prognosis	Equally increased risk in either breast, *infiltrating ductal carcinoma* also most common histologic type (counterintuitive); associated with simultaneous LCIS in the contralateral breast in over ½ of cases
Treatment	■ If small (< 2 cm): Lumpectomy with either close follow-up or radiation ■ If large (> 2 cm): Lumpectomy with 1-cm margins and radiation ■ If breast diffusely involved: Simple mastectomy	■ None; bilateral mastectomy an option if patient is high risk

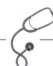

Tumors Running and Leaping Promptly to Bone
- **Thyroid**
- **Renal**
- **Lung**
- **Prostate**
- **Breast**

MALIGNANT TUMORS

Infiltrating Ductal Carcinoma

- Most common invasive breast cancer (80% of cases).
- Most common in perimenopausal and postmenopausal women.
- Ductal cells invade stroma in various histologic forms described as scirrhous, medullary, comedo, colloid, papillary, or tubular.
- Metastatic to axilla, bones, lungs, liver, brain.

Infiltrating Lobular Carcinoma

- Second most common type of invasive breast cancer (10% of cases)

Twenty percent of infiltrating lobular breast carcinoma have simultaneous contralateral breast cancer.

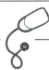

Greater than 75% of patients have axillary metastases at time of diagnosis of inflammatory breast carcinoma, and distant metastases are common.

Typical scenario: A 45-year-old female presents with enlargement of her left breast with nipple retraction, erythema, warmth, and induration. *Think:* Inflammatory breast carcinoma.

Fibrocystic changes of the breast alone is not a risk factor for breast cancer.

Despite all known risk factors, most women with breast cancer (75%) present without any identifiable risk factors.

- Originates from terminal duct cells and, like LCIS, has a high likelihood of being bilateral
- Presents as an ill-defined thickening of the breast
- Like LCIS, lacks microcalcifications and is often multicentric
- Tends to metastasize to the axilla, meninges, and serosal surfaces

Paget's Disease (of the Nipple)

- 2% of all invasive breast cancers
- Usually associated with underlying LCIS or ductal carcinoma extending within the epithelium of main excretory ducts to skin of nipple and areola
- Presentation: Tender, itchy nipple with or without a bloody discharge with or without a subareolar palpable mass
- Treatment: Usually requires a modified radical mastectomy

Inflammatory Carcinoma

- Two to 3% of all invasive breast cancers.
- Most lethal breast cancer.
- Vascular and lymphatic invasion commonly seen at pathologic evaluation.
- Frequently presents as erythema, "peau d'orange," and nipple retraction.
- Treatment: Consists of **chemotherapy** followed by surgery and/or radiation, depending on response to chemotherapy.

BREAST CANCER

Epidemiology

- One in eight women will develop breast cancer in their lifetime.
- Second most common cause of cancer death among women overall (lung cancer number 1).
- Incidence increases with increasing age.
- One percent of breast cancers occur in men.

Risk Factors

- Early menarche (< 12)
- Late menopause (> 55)
- Nulliparity or first pregnancy > 30 years
- White race
- Old age
- History of breast cancer in mother or sister (especially if bilateral or premenopausal)
- Genetic predisposition (BRCA1 or BRCA2 positive, Li–Fraumeni syndrome)
- Prior personal history of breast cancer
- Previous breast biopsy
- DCIS or LCIS
- Atypical ductal or lobular hyperplasia

- Postmenopausal estrogen replacement (unopposed by progesterone)
- Radiation exposure

Breast Cancer in Pregnant and Lactating Women

- Three breast cancers are diagnosed per 10,000 pregnancies.
- A FNA should be performed. If it identifies a solid mass, then it should be followed by biopsy.
- Mammography is possible as long as proper shielding is used.
- Radiation is not advisable for the pregnant woman. Thus, for stage I or II cancer, a modified radical mastectomy should be done rather than a lumpectomy with axillary node dissection and postoperative radiation.
- If lymph nodes are positive, delay chemotherapy until the second trimester.
- Suppress lactation after delivery.

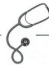

Breast Cancer in Males

- Predisposing factors: Klinefelter's syndrome, estrogen therapy, elevated endogenous estrogen, previous irradiation, and trauma.
- Infiltrating ductal carcinoma most common histologic type (men lack breast lobules).
- Diagnosis tends to be late, when the patient presents with a mass, nipple retraction, and skin changes.
- Stage by stage, survival is the same as it is in women. However, more men are diagnosed at a later stage.
- Treatment for early-stage cancer involves a modified radical mastectomy and postoperative radiation.

Males with breast cancer often have direct extension to the chest wall at diagnosis.

Genetic Predisposition

- Five to 10% of breast cancers are associated with an inherited mutation.
- p53: A tumor suppressor gene; Li–Fraumeni syndrome results from a p53 mutation.
- BRCA1: On 17q21, also associated with ovarian cancer.
- BRCA2: On chromosome 13; not associated with ovarian cancer.
- Somatic mutation of p53 in 50% and of Rb in 20% of breast cancers.

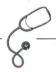

Genetic syndromes associated with breast cancer:
Autosomal dominant:
- Li–Fraumeni
- Muir–Torre
- BRCA1 and BRCA2 Cowden's syndrome
- Peutz–Jeghers syndrome
Autosomal recessive:
- Ataxia–telangiectasia

Screening Recommendations (from the American Cancer Society)

- Screening reduces mortality by 30–40%.
- Begin monthly breast self-examinations at age 20.
- First screening mammogram at age 35.
- Consult MD for individualized recommendations regarding mammograms between ages 40 and 50.
- Annual mammograms after age 50.

Start yearly mammograms 10 years before the age at which first-degree relative was diagnosed with breast cancer.

Diagnostic Options

Mammography
See below.

Ultrasound
(++) No ionizing radiation
(+) Good for identifying cystic disease and can also assist in therapeutic aspiration
(+) Results easily reproducible
(−) Resolution inferior to mammogram
(−) Will not identify lesions < 1 cm

FNA (Aspiration of Tumor Cells with Small-Gauge Needle)
(+) Low morbidity
(+) Cheap
(+) Only 1–2% false-positive rate
(−) False-negative rate up to 10%
(−) Requires a skilled pathologist
(−) May miss deep masses

Needle Localization Biopsy
(+) Locates occult cancer in > 90%

Core Biopsy
(−) Chance of sampling error

Stereotactic Core Biopsy
(+) Fewer complications compared to needle localization biopsy
(+) Less chance of sampling error than core biopsy alone
(+) No breast deformity

Mammography

See Figures 8-3 and 8-4.

- Identifies 5 cancers/1,000 women.
- Sensitivity 85–90%.
- False positive 10%, false negative 6–8%.
- If cancer is first detected by mammogram, 80% have negative lymph nodes (vs. 45% when detected clinically).

Suspicious Findings
- Stellate, speculated mass with associated microcalcifications

Reporting Mammogram Results
I: No abnormality
II: Benign abnormality
III: Probably benign finding
IV: Suspicious for cancer
V: Highly suspicious for cancer

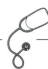

Benign cysts should not be bloody. A bloody aspirate usually indicates malignancy.

Five to 10% of palpable masses have a negative mammogram.

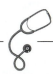

Mammography is more useful if age > 30 because the large proportion of fibrous tissue in younger women's breasts make mammograms more difficult to interpret.

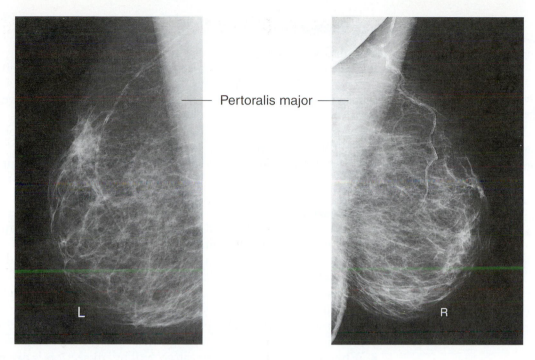

Pertoralis major

FIGURE 8-3. Normal mammogram.

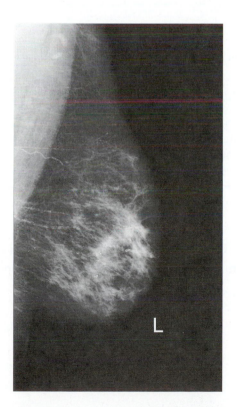

FIGURE 8-4. Abnormal mammogram. Note paranchymal assymmetric denstiy in subareolar area. Suspicious for malignancy.

Recommended chemotherapy for breast cancer is CAF (cyclophosphamide, adriamycin, 5-FU) or CMF (methotrexate instead of adriamycin).

Prognosis depends more on stage than on histologic type of breast cancer.

Lumpectomy with postoperative radiation is a viable treatment option only in stages I and II.

Treatment Decisions

Types of Operations

- *Radical mastectomy:* Resection of all breast tissue, axillary nodes, and pectoralis major and minor muscles (rarely preferred)
- *Modified radical mastectomy:* Same as radical mastectomy except pectoralis muscles left intact
- *Simple mastectomy:* Same as radical mastectomy except pectoralis muscles left intact and no axillary node dissection
- *Lumpectomy and axillary node dissection:* Resection of mass with rim of normal tissue and axillary node dissection—good cosmetic result
- *Sentinel node biopsy:* Recently developed alternative to complete axillary node dissection:
  - Based on the principle that metastatic tumor cells migrate in an orderly fashion to first draining lymph node(s).
  - Lymph nodes are identified on preoperative scintigraphy and blue dye is injected in the periareolar area.
  - Axilla is opened and inspected for blue and/or "hot" nodes identified by a gamma probe.
  - When sentinel node(s) is positive, an axillary dissection is completed.
  - When sentinel node(s) is negative, axillary dissection is not performed unless axillary lymphadenopathy identified.

TNM System for Breast Cancer

Tx: Cannot assess primary tumor
T0: No evidence of primary tumor
T1: ≤ 2 cm
T2: ≤ 5 cm
T3: > 5 cm
T4: Any size, with direct extension to chest wall or with skin edema or ulceration
Nx: Cannot assess lymph nodes
N0: No nodal mets
N1: Movable ipsilateral axillary nodes
N2: Fixed ipsilateral axillary nodes
N3: Ipsilateral internal mammary nodes
Mx: Cannot assess mets
M0: No mets
M1: Distant mets or supraclavicular nodes

Staging System for Breast Cancer and 5-Year Survival Rates (from the American Joint Committee on Cancer Staging)

- See Table 8-3.
- 5-year survival rates by stage:

Stage	5-Year Survival Rate
I	92%
II	87%
III	75%
IV	13%

TABLE 8-3. Staging system for breast cancer.	
Stage 0	DCIS or LCIS
Stage I	Invasive carcinoma ≤ 2 cm in size (including carcinoma in situ with microinvasion) without nodal involvement and no distant metastases.
Stage II	Invasive carcinoma ≤ 5 cm in size with involved but movable axillary nodes and no distant metastases, or a tumor > 5 cm without nodal involvement or distant metastases
Stage III	Breast cancers > 5 cm in size with nodal involvement; or any breast cancer with fixed axillary nodes; or any breast cancer with involvement of the ipsilateral internal mammary lymph nodes; or any breast cancer with skin involvement, pectoral and chest wall fixation, edema, or clinical inflammatory carcinoma, if distant metastases are absent
Stage IV	Any form of breast cancer with distant metastases (including ipsilateral supraclavicular lymph nodes)

Hormone Receptor Status and Response to Therapy

Hormone Receptor Status	Response to Therapy
ER+/PR+	80%
ER−/PR+	45%
ER+/PR−	35%
ER/PR−	10%

Hormonal Therapy: Tamoxifen

- Selective estrogen receptor modulator that blocks the uptake of estrogen by target tissues
- Side effects: Hot flashes, irregular menses, thromboembolism, increased risk for endometrial cancer
- Survival benefit for pre- and postmenopausal women, but benefit greater for ER+ patients
- May get additional benefit by combining tamoxifen with chemotherapy

Recurrence

- 5–10% local recurrence at 10 years
- Metastases in < 10% of cases
- Local chest wall recurrence most common within 2 to 3 years, if at all

Metastasis

- Median survival 2 years.
- Palliative therapy indicated.
- Doxorubicin in this setting has a response rate of 50% with a 1-year survival of 60%.

Endocrine System

HORMONES

DEFINITION

A chemical substance secreted by cells in one part of the body that acts on distant organs or tissues.

CLASSES

- Steroid:
    - Adrenal cortical: Cortisol, aldosterone
    - Ovarian, testicular, and placental hormones (not discussed here)
- Tyrosine-derived:
    - Thyroid: triiodothyronine (T_3), thyroxine (T_4)
    - Adrenal medulla: Epinephrine, norepinephrine
- Protein/peptide:
    - Pituitary:
        - Anterior: Growth hormone (GH), adrenocorticotropic hormone (ACTH), thyroxine-stimulating hormone (TSH), follicle-stimulating hormone (FSH), luteinizing hormone (LH), prolactin (PRL)
        - Posterior: Antidiuretic hormone (ADH), oxytocin
    - Parathyroid: Parathyroid hormone
    - Pancreas: Insulin, glucagon, somatostatin

All **protein** hormones are produced in locations starting with **p**:
Pituitary
Parathyroid
Pancreas

MECHANISMS OF ACTION

See Table 9-1.

TABLE 9-1. Summary of endocrine hormones and their functions.

Endocrine Organ	Hormone	Functions	Stimulated By	Inhibited By
Anterior pituitary	Growth hormone (GH)	■ Opposes insulin ■ Stimulates amino acid uptake ■ Stimulates release of fatty acid from storage sites ■ Mediates immunoglobulin F (IGF) synthesis ■ Stimulates growth of nearly all tissues	■ Growth hormone–releasing hormone (GHRH) ■ Hypoglycemia ■ Arginine ■ Exercise ■ L-dopa ■ Clonidine ■ Propranolol	Somatostatin
	Adrenocorticotropic hormone (ACTH)	■ Stimulates secretion of adrenocortical hormones	■ Corticotropin-releasing hormone (CRH) ■ Stress	Cortisol (negative feedback)
	Thyroid-stimulating hormone (TSH)	■ Regulates secretion of triiodothyronine (T_3) and thyronine (T_4)	■ Thyrotropin-releasing hormone (TRH)	Negative feedback
	Follicle-stimulating hormone (FSH)	■ Stimulates ovarian follicular growth (female) ■ Stimulates spermatogenesis and testicular growth (male)	■ Gonadotropin-releasing hormone (GnRH)	Negative feedback
	Luteinizing hormone (LH)	■ Ovulation (female) ■ Luteinization of follicle (female) ■ Stimulates production of estrogen and progesterone (female) ■ Promotes production of testosterone (male)	■ GnRH	Negative feedback
	Prolactin (PRL)	■ Facilitates breast development in preparation for milk production	■ TRH ■ Estrogen ■ Stress ■ Exercise	Bromocriptine
Posterior pituitary	Antidiuretic hormone (ADH, vasopressin)	■ Promotes water absorption in collecting ducts of kidney ■ Vasoconstriction of peripheral arterioles, increasing blood pressure	■ Increased plasma osmolality ■ Decreased plasma volume	
	Oxytocin	■ Increases frequency and strength of uterine contractions ■ Stimulates breast milk ejection	■ Suckling ■ Vaginal stimulation	
Thyroid	T_3, T_4	■ Increase basal metabolic rate (BMR), oxygen consumption	■ TSH	Negative feedback

TABLE 9-1. Summary of endocrine hormones and their functions. (continued)

Thyroid (continued)		<ul><li>Increase protein synthesis, lipolysis, glycogenolysis, gluconeogenesis</li><li>Increase heart rate and contractility</li><li>Increase catecholamine sensitivity</li><li>Stimulate release of steroid hormones</li><li>Stimulate erythropoiesis and 2,3-diphosphoglycerate (DPG) production</li><li>Increase bone turnover</li></ul>		
	Calcitonin	<ul><li>Increases serum calcium (by inhibiting osteoclasts)</li><li>Increases phosphate excretion</li></ul>	<ul><li>High serum calcium</li></ul>	<ul><li>Low serum calcium</li></ul>
Parathyroid	Parathyroid hormone (PTH)	<ul><li>Kidney: Increases calcium resorption in proximal convoluted tubule</li><li>Rapid</li><li>Also increased excretion of sodium, potassium, phosphate, and bicarbonate</li><li>Bone: Increases calcium mobilization</li><li>Rapid phase: Equilibration with extracellular fluid (ECF)</li><li>Slow phase: Enzyme activation (promoting bone resorption)</li><li>GI tract (indirect): Increases absorption via vitamin D</li></ul>	<ul><li>Low serum calcium</li></ul>	<ul><li>High serum calcium</li></ul>
Pancreas	Insulin (B-cell)	Effects on liver:<ul><li>Glycogenesis, glycolysis, synthesis of protein, triglycerides, cholesterol, very low-density lipoprotein (VLDL)</li><li>Inhibits glycogenolysis, ketogenesis, gluconeogenesis</li></ul>Effects on muscle:<ul><li>Protein synthesis, glycogen synthesis</li></ul>Effects on fat:<ul><li>Promotes triglyceride storage</li></ul>	Hyperglycemia	Hypoglycemia
	Glucagon (A-cell)	Metabolic effects:<ul><li>Glycogenolysis, gluconeogenesis, ketogenesis (liver); lipolysis (adipose tissue); insulin secretion</li></ul>	Hypoglycemia	Hyperglycemia

(continues)

151

		Effects on gastrointestinal (GI) secretion: ■ Inhibition of gastric acid and pancreatic exocrine secretion Effects on GI motility: ■ Inhibition of peristalsis Cardiovascular effects: ■ Increase in HR and force of contraction		
	Somatostatin (D-cell)	■ Inhibition of gastric acid, pepsin, pancreatic exocrine secretion ■ Inhibition of ion secretion ■ Inhibition of motility ■ Reduction of splanchnic blood flow ■ Inhibition of insulin, glucagons, pancreatic polypeptide secretion		
	Pancreatic polypeptide (F-cell)	■ Function not known, but level rises after a meal (possible inhibition of pancreatic exocrine secretion)		
Adrenal cortex	Cortisol (zona fasciculate and reticularis)	■ Stimulation of hepatic gluconeogenesis, inhibition of protein synthesis, increased protein catabolism, lipolysis, inhibition of peripheral glucose uptake ■ Inhibition of fibroblast activity, inhibition of bone formation, reduction of GI calcium absorption ■ Inhibition of leukocytes, decreased migration of inflammatory cells to site of injury, decreased production of mediators of inflammation	■ ACTH circadian rhythm ■ Stress	■ Negative feedback
	Androgens (zona fasciculate and reticularis)	■ Dehydroepiandrosterone (DHEA), DHEA sulfate are converted to testosterone and dihydrotestosterone in the periphery ■ Adrenal androgens make up < 5% of total testosterone production in the normal male		

	Aldosterone (zona glomerulosa)	<ul><li>Stimulates renal tubular sodium absorption in exchange for potassium and hydrogen</li><li>Net effect: Fluid reabsorption and intravascular volume expansion</li></ul>	
Adrenal medulla	Epinephrine and norepinephrine	<ul><li>Increased oxygen consumption</li><li>Increased heat production</li><li>Stimulation of glycogenolysis, lipolysis, inhibition of insulin secretion</li></ul>	Stress Receptors α: Vasoconstriction β_1: Cardiac inotropic and chronotropic stimulation β_2: Noncardiac smooth muscle relaxation (vessels, uterus, bronchi)

MULTIPLE ENDOCRINE NEOPLASIA (MEN)

General

Autosomal dominant disorders resulting in multiple (metachronous or synchronous) tumors in different endocrine organs.

MEN I

- Chromosomal defect: 11q12–13 (deletion)
- Pituitary adenomas
- Parathyroid hyperplasia
- Pancreatic islet cell tumors
- Involvement:
  - Two glands: 50%
  - Three glands: 20%
- Age at presentation:
  - Without known affected family members: 20s to 30s
  - With known affected members: Prior to age 20 (through screening)

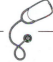

All tumors associated with MEN I occur in endocrine glands that start with P:
Pituitary
Parathyroid
Pancreas

MEN IIA

- RET oncogene mutation on chromosome 10q11.2; missense mutations on chromosome 1
- Parathyroid hyperplasia
- Medullary thyroid carcinoma
- Pheochromocytoma

MEN IIB

- RET oncogene mutation on chromosome 10q11.2
- Medullary thyroid carcinoma
- Pheochromocytoma
- Mucosal neuroma
- Marfanoid habitus

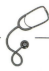

MEN IIA and IIB comprise the medullary thyroid carcinoma/pheochromocytoma syndrome. The additional components differ: Another **p** in MEN IIA (parathyroid), and **m** in MEN IIB (mucosal neuromas and Marfanoid habitus).

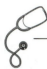

Persistence of the thyroid–pharynx connection may occur via a sinus or cyst, called a thyroglossal duct cyst. Thyroglossal duct cysts present as midline neck masses in children or adolescents, and should be excised because of the risk of infection.

THYROID

Development

- Third week of gestation: Thyroid forms at the base of the tongue between the first pair of pharyngeal pouches, in an area called the foramen cecum.
- It then descends to its usual location where it develops into the bilobed organ with an isthmus. It remains connected to the floor of the pharynx through the second month, via the thyroglossal duct, which subsequently obliterates.
- As it descends, the thyroid acquires the parafollicular cells (calcitonin secretion) from the ultimobranchial bodies.
- Iodine trapping and T_4 synthesis begin by the third or fourth month of gestation.

Anatomy

See Figure 9-1.

Gross Anatomy
- Two lobes, isthmus, pyramidal lobe (pyramidal lobe is present in 80%)
- Suspended from larynx, attached to trachea (cricoid cartilage and tracheal rings)
- Weighs 20 to 25 g in adults
- Relationships:
  - Anterior: Sternohyoid, sternothyroid, thyrohyoid, omohyoid muscles
  - Posterior: Trachea
  - Posterolateral: Common carotid arteries, internal jugular veins, vagus nerves
  - Parathyroid glands on posterior surface of thyroid, and may be within capsule

Histology
- Follicles with a cuboidal epithelium and central colloid (secreted by epithelium) are surrounded by fibrovascular stroma.
  - Follicles store thyroglobulin.
- Within stroma are C-cells (secrete calcitonin).

Vasculature

See Figure 9-2.

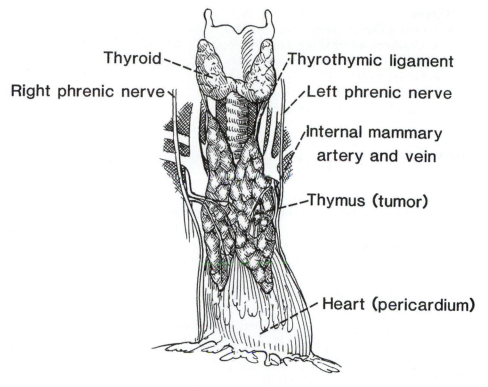

FIGURE 9-1. Thyroid anatomy. (Copyright 2003, Mayo Foundation.)

Arterial

- Superior thyroid arteries (on each side)
  - First branch of external carotid artery at the level of the carotid bifurcation
- Inferior thyroid artery (on each side)
  - From thyrocervical trunk of subclavian artery
- Ima (sometimes present)
  - From aortic arch or innominate artery

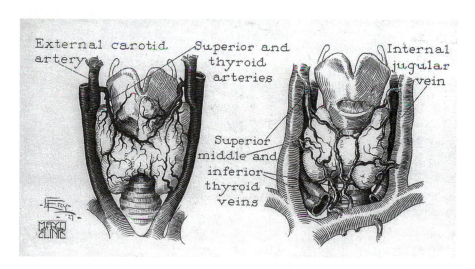

FIGURE 9-2. Thyroid blood supply. (Copyright 2003, Mayo Foundation.)

Lymphatics drain ultimately to internal jugular nodes. Intraglandular lymphatics connect both lobes, explaining the relatively high frequency of multifocal tumors in the thyroid.

The recurrent laryngeal nerve innervates all the intrinsic muscles of the larynx, except the cricothyroid, and provides sensory innervation to the mucous membranes below the vocal cord. It can be damaged during a thyroid operation, so the surgeon must know its course well. Damage produces ipsilateral vocal cord paralysis, and results in hoarseness or sometimes shortness of breath due to the narrowed airway.

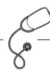

Thyroid follicles store enough hormone to last 2 to 3 months. Thus, there is no need to worry about your postop hypothyroid patients who are NPO for several days. They can resume taking their levothyroxine when they begin a PO diet.

Venous
- Superior thyroid vein (on each side)
  - Drains to internal jugular (IJ)
- Middle thyroid vein (on each side)
  - Drains to IJ
- Inferior thyroid vein (on each side)
  - Drains to brachiocephalic vein

Innervation

- The right recurrent laryngeal nerve (RLN) branches from the vagus nerve, loops under the right subclavian artery, and ascends to the larynx (posterior to the thyroid) between the trachea and esophagus. It may be anterior or posterior to the inferior thyroid artery. The left RLN branches from the vagus lateral to the ligamentum arteriosum, runs under the aortic arch, and then ascends along the tracheoesophageal groove to the larynx.
- Sympathetic: Superior and middle cervical sympathetic ganglia (vasomotor)
- Parasympathetic: From vagus nerves, via branches of laryngeal nerves

Hormones

FORMATION OF THYROID HORMONE

- Iodide in the extracellular fluid is actively transported into the epithelial cells of the thyroid follicles, where it is concentrated to 30 times its serum concentration.
- Iodide is oxidized to iodine and combined with tyrosine within the thyroglobulin molecule, resulting in mono- and di-iodinated tyrosines.
- These tyrosines couple to make thyroxine.
- Thyroglobulin is synthesized and secreted from the endoplasmic reticulum and Golgi complex.
- Each thyroglobulin contains 1 to 3 thyroxines.

HORMONE REGULATION

- TSH causes:
  - Thyroglobulin proteolysis, releasing hormone into circulation within 30 minutes
  - Iodide trapping
  - Increased iodination and coupling, forming more thyroid hormones
  - Increased size of and secretion from thyroid cells
  - A change in epithelium from cuboidal to columnar, with increased number of cells
- Increased thyroid hormone in blood causes **decreased TSH secretion** from pituitary, by an incompletely understood mechanism.

EFFECTS OF THYROID HORMONE

- Cardiovascular system: *Increased* heart rate (HR), cardiac output (CO), blood flow, blood volume, pulse pressure (no change in mean arterial pressure [MAP])
- Respiratory system: *Increased RR, depth of respiration*
- Gastrointestinal (GI) system: *Increased* motility

- Central nervous system (CNS): Nervousness, anxiety
- Musculoskeletal system: *Increased* reactivity up to a point, then response is weakened; fine motor tremor
- Sleep: Constant fatigue but decreased ability to sleep
- Nutrition: Increased basal metabolic rate (BMR), need for vitamins, metabolism of CHO, lipid, and protein; decreased weight

Examination of the Thyroid

1. Observe the anterior neck for masses or enlargement.
2. Because the thyroid is suspended from the larynx, it rises with swallowing. Have the patient swallow during your exam.
3. In addition, palpate for cervical lymph nodes.

Assessment of Function

- If T_4 production is increased, both tT_4 and fT_4 increase.
- If production decreases, both tT_4 and fT_4 decrease.
- If amount of thyroid-binding globulin (TBG) changes, only tT_4 changes, not fT_4.

Congenital Anomalies

- Complete failure to develop
- Incomplete descent: Lingual or subhyoid position (if gland enlarges, patient will have earlier respiratory symptoms)
- Excessive descent: Substernal thyroid
- Malformation of branchial pouch
- Persistent sinus tract remnant of developing gland: **Thyroglossal duct cyst**—may occur anywhere along course as a midline structure with thyroid epithelium, usually between the isthmus and the hyoid bone:
    - Most common congenital anomaly
    - Few symptoms but may become infected
    - Easier to see when tongue is sticking out
    - Surgical treatment: Excision of duct remnant and central portion of hyoid bone
- 1% contain calcium
- Lateral aberrant thyroid: Usually well-differentiated papillary cancer metastatic to cervical lymph nodes

Hyperthyroidism

CAUSES

- Graves' disease
- Toxic nodular goiter
- Toxic thyroid adenoma
- Subacute thyroiditis
- Functional metastatic thyroid cancer
- Struma ovarii

Palpation of the thyroid is easiest if you stand behind the patient and reach your arms around to the front of the neck. Expect the isthmus to be about one fingerbreadth below the cricoid cartilage.

In 70% of cases of lingual thyroid, it is the patient's only functioning thyroid tissue. The implication is that you must look for other functioning thyroid tissue prior to removing a lingual thyroid.

Ten percent of patients will have atrial fibrillation that may be refractory to medical treatment until hyperthyroidism is controlled.

Graves' Disease

- Affects nearly 2% of American women
- 6 times more common in women
- Onset age 20 to 40
- Signs and symptoms:
  - Present in > 90%: Nervousness, increased sweating, tachycardia, goiter, pretibial myxedema, tremor
  - Present in 50–90%: Heat intolerance, palpitations, fatigue, weight loss, dyspnea, weakness, increased appetite, eye complaints, thyroid bruit
  - Other: Amenorrhea, decreased libido and fertility
- Diagnosis:
  - Labs: Decreased TSH, increased T_3 and/or T_4, increased thyroid receptor antibodies (TrAb).
  - Histology: Hyperplastic columnar epithelium with less colloid than normal and more mitoses.
  - Thyroid scan shows diffusely increased uptake.
- Treatment:
  - Antithyroid drugs
  - Ablation with ^{131}I
  - Subtotal or total thyroidectomy
- Choosing a treatment:
  - Consider: Age, severity, size of gland, comorbidity
  - Radioablation is the most common choice in the United States:
    - Indicated for small or medium-sized goiters, if medical therapy has failed, or if other options are contraindicated.
    - Most patients become euthyroid in 2 months.
    - Most ultimately require thyroid hormone replacement.
    - Complications include exacerbation of thyroid storm initially.
    - Clearly contraindicated in pregnant patients.
  - Surgical treatment:
    - Indicated when radioablation is contraindicated—young or pregnant patients, for example.
    - Patients should be euthyroid first.
    - Advantage is immediate cure.
  - Medical therapy with β-blockers for symptom relief or antithyroid drugs (propylthiouracil [PTU], methimazole) that inhibit binding of I and coupling.
    - May cause side effects such as rash, fever, or peripheral neuritis.
    - Patients will relapse if meds are discontinued.

Toxic Nodular Goiter

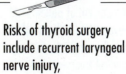

- Also called Plummer's disease.
- Also causes hyperthyroidism, but without the extrathyroidal symptoms.
- Treatment is **surgical,** as medical therapy may alleviate symptoms but is less effective than in Graves' disease, and ablation has a high failure rate.
  - Solitary nodule: Nodulectomy or lobectomy
  - Multinodular goiter: Lobectomy and contralateral subtotal lobectomy

Thyroid Storm

- Life-threatening extreme hyperthyroid state precipitated by infection, labor, surgery, iodide administration, or recent radioablation.

- Patient presents disoriented, febrile, and tachycardic, often reporting vomiting and diarrhea.
- Best way to treat this is to avoid it. Prophylaxis includes achieving euthyroid state preop.
- Treatment: Fluids, antithyroid medication, β-blockers, NaI or Lugol's solution, hydrocortisone, and a cooling blanket.

Hypothyroidism

CAUSES

- Autoimmune thyroiditis
- Iatrogenic: s/p thyroidectomy, s/p radioablation, secondary to antithyroid medications
- Iodine deficiency
- Dyshormonogenesis
- Signs and symptoms (differ, depending on age of diagnosis):
- Infants/peds: Characteristic Down's-like facies, failure to thrive, mental retardation
- Adolescents/adults (particularly when due to autoimmune thyroiditis):
  - 80% female
  - Complain of fatigue, weight gain, cold intolerance, constipation, menorrhagia, decreased libido and fertility
  - Less common complaints: Yellow-tinged skin, hair loss, tongue enlargement
  - Physiologic effects: Bradycardia, decreased cardiac output, hypotension, shortness of breath secondary to effusions

Immediate treatment (of infants) with thyroid hormone will help minimize the neurologic and intellectual deficits.

DIAGNOSIS

- History and physical exam findings
- Labs:
  - T_4, T_3: Decreased
- TSH:
  - Increased in primary hypothyroidism.
  - Decreased in secondary hypothyroidism.
  - Confirm with TRH challenge: TSH will not respond in secondary hypothyroidism.
  - Thyroid autoantibodies present in autoimmune thyroiditis
  - Low hematocrit (Hct)
- Electrocardiogram (ECG): Decreased voltage and flat or inverted T waves.

TREATMENT

Thyroxine PO, or IV emergently if patient presents in myxedema coma.

Thyroiditis

ACUTE

- Infectious etiology: *Streptococcus pyogenes*, *Staphylococcus aureus*, *Pneumococcus pneumoniae*
- Risk factors: Female sex, goiter, thyroglossal duct
- Signs and symptoms: Unilateral neck pain and fever, euthyroid state, dysphagia
- Treatment: IV antibiotics and surgical drainage

The bacteria that cause acute suppurative thyroiditis usually spread through lymphatics from a nearby locus of infection.

Ten percent of patients with subacute thyroiditis become permanently hypothyroid.

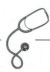

Twenty percent of patients with Hashimoto's thyroiditis will be hypothyroid at diagnosis. A euthyroid state is more common.

Typical scenario: A 35-year-old female who emigrated from Russia in 1990 is referred to you for a solitary right thyroid mass. On exam, you find a solitary mass, 2 × 1 cm, that is firm and fixed. There are no palpable lymph nodes. What is a likely diagnosis? *Think:* Papillary thyroid cancer, which is the most common variety. Eighty-five to 90% of patients report FNA that shows cuboidal cells with abundant cytoplasm, and psammoma bodies. Computed tomography (CT) shows no other foci of disease. What's your next step? *Think:* Near-total thyroidectomy.

SUBACUTE (DE QUERVAIN)

- Etiology: Post-viral upper respiratory infection (URI)
- Risk factors: Female sex
- Signs and symptoms: Fatigue, depression, neck pain, fever, unilateral swelling of thyroid with overlying erythema, firm and tender thyroid, transient hyperthyroidism usually preceding hypothyroid phase
- Diagnosis: Made by history and exam
- Treatment:
  - Usually self-limited disease (within 6 weeks).
  - Manage pain with nonsteroidal anti-inflammatory drugs (NSAIDs)

CHRONIC (HASHIMOTO'S THYROIDITIS)

- Etiology: Autoimmune
- Risk factors: Down's, Turner syndrome, familial Alzheimer's disease, history of radiation therapy as child
- Signs and symptoms: Painless enlargement of thyroid, neck tightness, presence of other autoimmune diseases
- Diagnosis: Made by history and physical, and labs
  - Labs: Circulating antibodies against microsomal thyroid cell, thyroid hormone, T_3, T_4, or TSH receptor
  - Pathology: Firm, symmetrical, enlargement; follicular and Hürthle cell hyperplasia; lymphocytic and plasma cell infiltrates
- Treatment:
  - Thyroid hormone (usually results in regression of goiter).
  - With failure of medical therapy, partial thyroidectomy is indicated.

RIEDEL'S FIBROSING THYROIDITIS

- Rare.
- Fibrosis replaces both lobes and isthmus.
- Risk factors: Associated with other fibrosing conditions, like retroperitoneal fibrosis, sclerosing cholangitis.
- Signs and symptoms: Usually remain euthyroid; neck pain, possible airway compromise; firm, nontender, enlarged thyroid.
- Diagnosis: Open biopsy required to rule out carcinoma or lymphoma.
  - Pathology: Dense, invasive fibrosis of both lobes and isthmus. May also involve adjacent structures.
- Treatment:
  - With airway compromise, isthmectomy
  - Without airway compromise, medical treatment with steroids

Workup of a Mass

GENERAL INFORMATION

- Fifteen percent of solitary thyroid nodules are malignant.
- 40 malignant tumors/1 million people/year.
- < 1% of all malignancies in the United States.
- Ninety to 95% present as well-differentiated cancer.

SIGNS AND SYMPTOMS

- History of previous head or neck irradiation, family history, age, gender, sudden enlargement of nodule, compressive complaints.

- Exam: Note size, mobility, quality, adherence of mass, and presence of lymphadenopathy. Concerning findings include hard, fixed gland, palpable cervical lymph node.

- DIAGNOSIS: FINE-NEEDLE ASPIRATION (FNA)

  - *Benign* (65%):
    - Ultrasound (US) for sizing.
    - Initial thyroglobulin level; follow over time.
  - *Suspicious* (15%): Usually follicular or Hürthle cell (20% will be malignant).
    - Obtain ^{123}I scan:
      - 85% cold nodule, with 10–25% chance malignancy
      - 5% hot nodule with 1% chance malignancy
    - Surgery is indicated if serial T_4 levels do not regress and biopsy is worrisome
  - *Malignant* (5%): Surgery.
  - *Nondiagnostic* (15%).
  - Cyst: Drain completely (curative in 75% of cases). If larger than 4 cm or complex, or if it recurs after three attempts at drainage, then evaluate for OR.

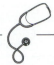

FNA of thyroid nodule has 1% false-positive rate and 5% false-negative rate.

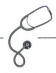

FNA is less reliable if patient has history of irradiation, and initial OR biopsy may be appropriate.

Thyroid Cancer

See Table 9-2.

TABLE 9-2. Thyroid cancer.

	Papillary	Follicular	Medullary	Anaplastic
Percent	80–85 75% of pediatric thyroid cancer	5–10	5–10	1
Risk factors	Radiation	Dyshormonogenesis	Associated with multiple endocrine neoplasia (MEN) in 30–40%	■ Prior diagnosis of well-differentiated thyroid cancer ■ Iodine deficiency
Age group	30–40	50s	50–60	60–70
Sex (F/M)	2/1	3/1	1.5/1	1.5/1
Signs and symptoms	■ Painless mass ■ Dysphagia ■ Dyspnea ■ Hoarseness ■ Euthyroid	■ Painless mass ■ Rarely hyperfunctional	■ Painful mass ■ Palpable lymph node (LN) (15–20%) ■ Dysphagia ■ Dyspnea ■ Hoarseness	■ Rapidly enlarging neck mass ■ Neck pain ■ Dysphonia ■ Dysphagia ■ Hard, fixed LN

(continues)

TABLE 9-2. Thyroid cancer. *(continued)*

	Papillary	Follicular	Medullary	Anaplastic
Diagnosis	■ Fine-needle aspiration (FNA) ■ Computed tomography (CT) or magnetic resonance imaging (MRI) (to assess local invasion)	■ FNA ■ CT or MRI (to assess local invasion)	■ FNA ■ Presence of amyloid is diagnostic ■ Check immunohisto-chemistry for calcitonin	■ FNA
Gross characteristics	■ Intrathyroidal ■ Partially encapsulated ■ Likely to be multifocal ■ Hard ■ White ■ Areas of necrosis ■ Cystic changes	■ Encapsulated tumor ■ Solitary	■ Unilateral ■ Mid–upper lobes ■ Familial tumors more likely multicentric and bilateral	■ Macroinvasion ■ Clinically + LN
Histologic characteristics	■ Papillary projections ■ Pale, abundant cytoplasm ■ Psammoma bodies ■ Orphan Annie eyes	■ Solitary ■ Encapsulated (90%)	■ Cell of origin: C cells ■ Sheets of cells ■ Amyloid ■ Collagen	■ Sheets of heterogeneous cells
Metastases	Lymphatic	Hematogenous	■ Lymphatic (local neck and mediastinal nodes) ■ Local (into trachea and esophagus)	■ Aggressive local disease ■ 50% have synchronous pulmonary mets at diagnosis
Treatment	■ Minimal ca: Lobectomy and isthmectomy ■ Other: Total or near-total thyroidectomy	■ Minimal ca: Lobectomy and isthmectomy ■ Other: Total or near-total thyroidectomy	■ Sporadic MTC Total thyroidectomy and central neck node dissection (modified radical neck dissection for + LN)	■ Debulking resection of thyroid and invaded structures ■ External radiation therapy (XRT)

TABLE 9-2. Thyroid cancer. *(continued)*

	Papillary	Follicular	Medullary	Anaplastic
Treatment (continued)	▪ For + LN, modified radical neck dissection ▪ ^{131}I ablation for patients with residual thyroid tissue or LN mets!	▪ For + LN, modified radical neck dissection ▪ ^{131}I ablation for patients with residual thyroid tissue or LN mets	▪ Familial MTC: Total thyroidectomy and central neck node dissection	▪ Doxorubicin-based chemotherapy
Prognosis	▪ Worse prognosis for older age patients and those with distant mets ▪ Presence of + LN not strongly correlated with overall survival	▪ Worse prognosis for older patients, those with distant mets, tumor size > 4 cm, high tumor grade ▪ Presence of + LN not strongly correlated with overall survival		Poor prognosis
Variants	**Sclerosis variant:** 100% incidence of LN metastases at diagnosis	**Hürthle cell tumors:** Bilateral, multifocal, spread to regional LN. Treatment: Ipsilateral lobectomy, isthmectomy, and central neck dissection. If pathology is carcinoma, total completion thyroidectomy indicated.		
Survival	10-year survival: 74–93%	10-year survival: 70%	10-year survival: 70–80%	Median survival: 4–5 months

PARATHYROID

Development

- Superior glands develop from fourth pharyngeal pouch.
  - Adult position fairly constant with respect to the superior lobes of thyroid.
- Inferior glands develop from third pharyngeal pouch, in conjunction with thymus.
  - Inferior glands have more variable position (intrathymic or even superior to superior glands).

Anatomy

- Weight < 50 mg/gland.
- 3 × 3 × 3 mm.
- Yellow-brown tissue similar to surrounding fatty tissue.
- Histology: Normal gland contains mainly chief cells, with occasional oxyphils.
- Vasculature: Inferior thyroid arteries; superior, middle, and inferior thyroid veins.

Of the half of serum calcium in an ionized, active form, 80% is bound to albumin, and 20% is found in a citrate complex.

Hypercalcemic crisis (calcium > 13 mg/dL and symptomatic): Treat with saline, diuretics, and if needed, antiarrhythmic agents.

Physiology/Calcium Homeostasis

Primary function: Endocrine regulation of calcium and phosphate metabolism.

- Regulators of calcium and phosphate metabolism: Parathyroid hormone (PTH), vitamin D, calcitonin
- Organ systems involved: Gastrointestinal (GI) tract, bone, kidney

PTH

- Synthesized in precursor form by the parathyroids (see Figure 9-3).
- Calcium levels regulate secretion of cleaved PTH (with negative feedback mechanism).
- Bone:
  - Stimulates osteoclasts
  - Inhibits osteoblasts
  - Stimulates bone resorption, releasing calcium and phosphate
- Kidney:
  - Increases reabsorption of calcium
  - Increases phosphate excretion
- GI tract:
  - Stimulates hydroxylation of 25-OH D

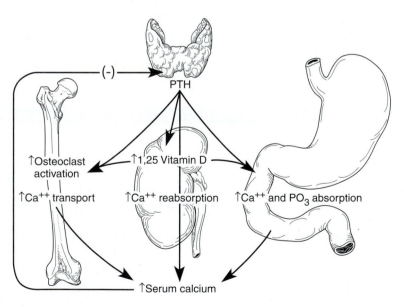

FIGURE 9-3. Actions of parathyroid hormone.

- 1,25 OH D, then increases absorption of calcium and phosphate
  - Promotes mineralization
  - Enhances PTH's effect on bone

Calcitonin
- Secreted by thyroid C-cells
- Inhibits bone resorption
- Increases urinary excretion of calcium and phosphate

Hyperparathyroidism

PRIMARY

Due to overproduction of PTH, causing increased absorption of calcium from intestines, increased vitamin D_3 production, and decreased renal calcium excretion, thereby raising the serum level.
- Incidence: 1/800 in the United States
- Signs and symptoms:
  - "Stones": Kidney stones
  - "Bones": Bone pain, pathologic fractures
  - "Groans": Nausea, vomiting, constipation, pancreatitis, peptic ulcer disease
  - "Moans": Lethargy, confusion, depression, paranoia
- Etiology:
  - Solitary adenoma 85–90%
  - Four-gland hyperplasia 10%
  - Cancer < 1%
- Preop localization: US, FNA of suspicious US findings, Sestamibi scan
- Diagnosis: Elevation of plasma PTH, with inappropriately high serum calcium
- Treatment:
  - Solitary adenoma: Solitary parathyroidectomy
  - Multiple gland hyperplasia: Remove three glands, or all four with reimplantation of one gland in forearm.
- Outcome:
  - First operation has 98% success rate.
- Reoperation has 90% success rate if remaining gland is localized preop.

SECONDARY

Due to chronic renal failure or intestinal malabsorption that causes hypocalcemia with appropriate increase in PTH.
- Signs and symptoms:
  - Bone pain from renal osteodystrophy and pruritus.
  - Patients are often asymptomatic.
- Diagnosis: Made by labs in asymptomatic patient
- Treatment:
  - Nonsurgical: In renal failure patients, restrict phosphorus intake, treat with phosphorus-binding agents and calcium/vitamin D supplementation. Adjust dialysate to maximize calcium and minimize aluminum.
  - Surgical: Indicated for intractable bone pain or pruritus, or pathologic fractures, with failure of medical therapy.
    - 3½-gland parathyroidectomy

Hyperparathyroidism. *Think:* Stones, bones, groans, and moans.

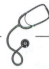

Not all patients with hypercalcemia have hyperparathyroidism. Hypercalcemia of malignancy (due to tumor-secreted PTH-related protein) must be ruled out. Malignancies commonly implicated include lung, breast, prostate, head, and neck.

Patients with familial hyperparathyroidism (i.e., MEN) have a high recurrence rate; total parathyroidectomy with forearm reimplantation is indicated to facilitate potential reoperation. Patients with sporadic four-gland hyperplasia may undergo total parathyroidectomy with reimplantation or three-gland excision.

TERTIARY

Due to autonomously functioning parathyroid glands, resistant to negative feedback, for example, persistent hypercalcemia following renal transplantation.

- Usually a short-lived phenomenon.
- If persistent, surgery is indicated (3½-gland parathyroidectomy).

Hypoparathyroidism

- Uncommon.
- Etiology:
  - Surgically-induced: Usually following total thyroidectomy; usually transient and treated if symptoms develop
  - Congenital absence of all four glands
  - DiGeorge syndrome: Absence of parathyroids and thymic agenesis
  - Functional: Chronic hypomagnesemia
- Signs and symptoms:
  - Numbness and tingling of circumoral area, fingers, toes
- Anxiety, confusion
- May progress to tetany, hyperventilation, seizures, heart block
- Treatment: Supplementation with calcium and vitamin D.
- Pseudohypoparathyroidism: Familial target tissue resistance to PTH. Patients remain hypocalcemic and hyperphosphatemic despite bone resorption from elevated PTH. Treatment consists of calcium and vitamin D supplementation.

Parathyroid Cancer

- Signs and symptoms:
  - Forty to 50% present with firm, fixed mass.
  - Extremely high calcium, PTH, and alkaline phosphatase.
  - Also associated bone disease, renal insufficiency, and renal stones.
- Pathology:
  - Pale, white, adherent mass, with a thick fibrous capsule and septa
  - Enlarged hyperchromatic nuclei and varied nuclear size
- Treatment: En bloc surgical resection of mass and surrounding structures, ipsilateral thyroid lobectomy, regional lymph nodes.
- Postop external radiation therapy (XRT) and chemotherapy are not usually beneficial.
- Five-year survival: 70%.

ADRENAL GLAND

Anatomy

- Retroperitoneal bilateral organs, anterior and medial to superior pole of kidneys
- At T11
- Size: 3 to 6 g each, 5 × 2.5 cm (normal, nonpregnant adult)
- Vasculature: Branches of aorta, inferior phrenic, and renal arteries; venous drainage to central vein to inferior vena cava (IVC) (right), or to left renal vein (left)

> **Typical scenario:** A patient complains of tingling around her lips on postoperative day 1 s/p total thyroidectomy. *Think:* Hypoparathyroidism causing hypocalcemia. Supplement calcium and vitamin D. Continue to follow calcium levels.

> Hypocalcemia:
> *Chvostek:* Contraction of facial muscles when tapping on facial nerve
> *Trousseau:* Development of carpal spasm by occluding blood flow to forearm

- Histology:
  - Cortex:
    - Glomerulosa: 15%; aldosterone synthesis
    - Fasciculata: 75%; cells in linear configuration perpendicular to gland surface; steroids and cortisol synthesis
    - Reticularis: 10%; cholesterol storage; cortisol, androgen, and estrogen secretion
  - Medulla: Polyhedral cells in cords

Physiology

See section on endocrine organs and Figure 9-4.

Hyperplasia

- Zona reticularis widens, with an increased number of cells that hyperfunction.
- Weight: 6 to 12 g.
- If ectopic production of ACTH, pathology is similar, but weight is 12 to 30 g.

Adenoma

- Consists of cortical cells, causes hypercortisolism and hyperaldosteronism, but rarely androgen-related symptoms
- Not > 5 cm, weight < 100 g
- Homogeneous cell population, tumor necrosis, low mitotic activity

Adrenal Cortical Carcinoma

DEFINITION

Very rare adrenal tumor.

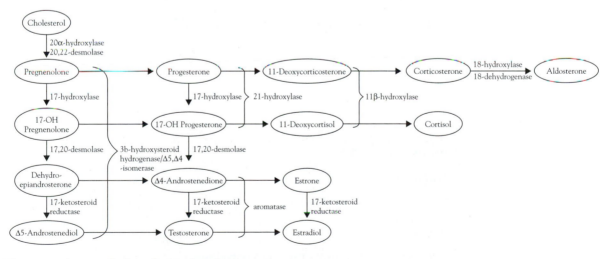

FIGURE 9-4. Pathways of adrenal steroid synthesis.

EPIDEMIOLOGY

- Affects women more than men, peak < 5 years old or 30 to 40 years old.

SIGNS AND SYMPTOMS

- Vague abdominal complaints (due to enlarging retroperitoneal mass)
- Symptoms related to overproduction of a steroid hormone (most tumors are functional)

PATHOLOGY

- > 6 cm, weight 100 to 5,000 g
- Necrotic and hemorrhagic tumor
- Hard to distinguish malignant tumor unless positive lymph nodes or distant metastases
- If vascular invasion has occurred, will see desmoplasia and mitoses
- Large hyperchromatic nuclei with enlarged nucleoli

DIAGNOSIS

- 24-hour urine collection for cortisol, aldosterone, catecholamines, metanephrine, vanillylmandelic acid, 17-OH corticosteroids, 17-ketosteroids
- CT (lesions > 7 mm) or magnetic resonance imaging (MRI) (especially for assessing IVC invasion)
- Chest x-ray (CXR) to rule out pulmonary metastases

TREATMENT

- Radical en bloc resection.
- If cannot completely resect, debulk to reduce amount of cortisol-secreting tissue.
- Bone metastases should be palliated with XRT.
- No role for chemotherapy.
- Monitor steroid hormone levels postop.
- Recurrence also warrants resection.
  - Recurrence: Lungs, lymph nodes, liver, peritoneum, bone

PROGNOSIS

- Seventy percent present in stage III or IV.
- Five-year survival 40% for complete resection.
- If local invasion, median survival is 2.3 years.
- Tumors with high mitotic activity, high DNA ploidy, or excessive production of androgens or 11-deoxysteroids are more likely to recur or metastasize.

Cushing Syndrome

DEFINITION

Excessive cortisol production.

CAUSES

- Iatrogenic administration of corticosteroids
- Pituitary tumor that secretes ACTH

> Fifty percent of adrenal cortical carcinomas secrete cortisol, resulting in Cushing's syndrome.

- Adrenal tumor that secretes cortisol
- Ectopic ACTH secretion by tumor elsewhere

SIGNS AND SYMPTOMS

Appearance
- Weight gain
- Truncal obesity
- Extremity wasting
- Buffalo hump
- Moon facies
- Striae
- Hirsutism

Physiologic
- Mild glucose intolerance
- Amenorrhea
- Decreased libido
- Depression
- Impaired memory
- Muscle weakness

DIAGNOSIS

See Table 9-3.
- Confirm presence of hypercortisolism:
  - Low-dose dexamethasone test
  - 24-hour urinary cortisol
- Determine whether pituitary-dependent or independent:
  - High-dose dexamethasone test
- CT (adrenals):
  - Can distinguish cortical hyperplasia from tumor with sensitivity > 95%, but lacks specificity
- MRI (sella).
- Petrosal sinus sampling.
- Adrenal source: Tumor or hyperplasia seen on CT or MRI, low plasma ACTH, no suppression with high-dose dexamethasone suppression test.
- Ectopic ACTH production: CT shows bilateral adrenal hyperplasia, increased plasma ACTH, no suppression, negative petrosal sinus sampling.
- Pituitary tumor: CT shows bilateral adrenal hyperplasia, mild elevation ACTH, + suppression, + petrosal sinus sampling

TREATMENT

- Cushing disease: Transsphenoidal resection of pituitary adenoma.
- Adrenal adenoma: Laparoscopic adrenalectomy.
- Adrenal carcinoma: Open adrenalectomy.
- Ectopic ACTH: Resection of primary lesion.
- Unresectable lesions and recurrence should be debulked for palliation.
- Medical treatment to suppress cortisol production: Metyrapone, aminoglutethimide, mitotane.

Typical scenario: A young male presents with weight gain, especially in the trunk; loss of muscle mass; and a buffalo hump. He has recently been noted to be mildly glucose intolerant. His past medical history is significant for severe asthma, for which he is chronically on steroids. **Think:** Cushing's syndrome secondary to exogenous administration of steroids.

Most common cause of ectopic ACTH production is small cell lung cancer.

Low-dose dexamethasone suppression test: Single dose of steroid at 11 P.M., followed by measurement of serum and urinary cortisol levels at 8 A.M. Normal: < 5 μg/dL (because evening dose suppresses further release) Abnormal: > 5 μg/dL High-dose dexamethasone (8 mg) distinguishes pituitary cause (suppression) from adrenal or ectopic cause (no suppression).

TABLE 9-3. Assays in the workup of Cushing syndrome.

Test	Result	Interpretation
24-hour urinary free cortisol *or* single dose dexamethasone suppression test	Normal	Hypercortisolism can be ruled out: ■ Low-dose dexamethasone (2 mg) normally decreases urinary 17-ketosteroids. Lack of suppression confirms hypercortisolism ■ High-dose dexamethasone (8 mg) decreases urinary cortisol to < 50% if pituitary-dependent Cushing syndrome, but does not decrease it at all if cause is primary adrenal or ectopic adrenocorticotropic hormone (ACTH) production
Plasma ACTH	Very high	Ectopic ACTH production
	Intermediate value	Pituitary tumor
	Low or undetectable	Adrenal source: Either adenoma, hyperplasia, or very rarely, cancer
Urinary 17-ketosteroids	< 10 mg/day	Adenoma
	> 60 mg/day	Cancer
	In between	Likely hyperplasia
Metyrapone test	Increased ACTH	Pituitary cause
Petrosal sinus sampling	Sinus/plasma ACTH ratio > 3 after corticotropin-releasing hormone (CRH) administration	Identifies Cushing's disease with 100% sensitivity

Addison's Disease

DEFINITION

Adrenal insufficiency:
- Primary: Due to destruction of adrenal cortex with sparing of medulla
- Secondary: Failure due to hypothalamic or pituitary abnormalities

ETIOLOGY

Primary
- Autoimmune adrenalitis
- Tuberculosis (TB)
- Fungal infection
- Acquired immune deficiency syndrome (AIDS)
- Metastatic cancer
- Familial glucocorticoid deficiency

Most common cause of secondary adrenal insufficiency is iatrogenic due to long-term glucocorticoid therapy.

- Post-adrenalectomy
- Bilateral adrenal hemorrhage

Secondary
- Craniopharyngioma
- Pituitary surgery or irradiation
- Empty sella syndrome
- Exogenous steroids

SIGNS AND SYMPTOMS

- Nausea
- Vomiting
- Weight loss
- Weakness
- Fatigue
- Lethargy
- Hyperpigmentation

DIAGNOSIS

- Hyponatremia, hyperkalemia.
- ACTH stimulation test: Give ACTH and measure cortisol level after 30 minutes. If adrenal failure is present, there will be no increase in cortisol.
- Baseline ACTH level is elevated in patients with primary failure.

TREATMENT

- Glucocorticoid therapy for primary and secondary causes
- Additional mineralocorticoid therapy for primary cause
- Addisonian crisis: Volume and glucocorticoids IV

Conn's Syndrome

DEFINITION

- Hyperaldosteronism
  - Primary
  - Secondary

ETIOLOGY

Primary (Due to Excessive Aldosterone Secretion)
- Aldosterone-secreting tumor
- Idiopathic adrenocortical hyperplasia

Secondary (Due to Elevated Renin)
- Renal artery stenosis
- Cirrhosis
- Congestive heart failure (CHF)
- Normal pregnancy

SIGNS AND SYMPTOMS

- Muscle weakness and cramping
- Polyuria
- Polydipsia

The sudden cessation of long-term glucocorticoid therapy can precipitate adrenal insufficiency because it suppresses the intrinsic control by the hypothalamus and pituitary. Six months may be required for the intrinsic controls to function properly.

Typical scenario: A patient with known Addison's disease presents with acute upper abdominal pain, with peritoneal signs, and confusion. *Think:* Addisonian crisis.

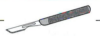

Patients with Addison's disease or who have been taking exogenous steroids for 6 months or longer are likely to require stress-dose steroids perioperatively. The timing and dose may vary depending on the planned procedure and baseline doses of the patient.

Renin is produced in the juxtaglomerular (JG) cells of the kidney. Angiotensinogen is synthesized in the liver and converted to angiotensin I in the kidney. Angiotensin I is converted to angiotensin II in the lung.

In working up a patient for suspected Conn's disease, make sure you don't have a patient with uncontrolled hypertension on potassium-wasting diuretics.

- Hypertension
- Hypokalemia

DIAGNOSIS

Primary
- Diastolic hypertension without edema
- Low renin
- Elevated aldosterone
- Hypokalemia, elevated urinary potassium (off antihypertensive medications)
- Plasma aldosterone
- Post-captopril plasma aldosterone:
  - Normally results in decreased aldosterone
  - Diagnostic of hyperaldosteronism if ratio > 50
- Imaging:
  - CT picks up tumors > 1 cm. If there is an aldosteronoma, opposite adrenal appears atrophied.
  - Iodocholesterol scan: Picks up 90% of aldosteronomas and shows how functional they are. Hyperplasia will present as bilateral hyperfunction vs. unilateral (for tumor).
  - If all imaging is nondiagnostic, then sample adrenal vein for aldosterone and cortisol pre- and post-ACTH.
    - Unilateral elevation of aldosterone or aldosterone/cortisol ratio indicates aldosterone-secreting adenoma.
    - Bilateral elevation of aldosterone is consistent with hyperplasia.

TREATMENT

Primary
- Hyperplasia: Medical treatment with spironolactone, nifedipine, amiloride and/or other antihypertensive
- Adenoma: Laparoscopic adrenalectomy
- Outcome:
  - Most patients become normotensive and normokalemic with treatment.
  - Twenty to 30% have recurrent hypertension (HTN) in 2 to 3 years, but for unknown reason.

Secondary
- Treat underlying cause.

Hypoaldosteronism

DEFINITION

Decreased aldosterone without a change in cortisol production.

ETIOLOGY

- Congenital error of aldosterone synthesis
- Failure of zona glomerulosa (autoimmune)
- s/p adrenalectomy
- Drug inhibition

SIGNS AND SYMPTOMS

- Postural hypotension
- Persistent severe hyperkalemia
- Muscle weakness
- Arrhythmia

TREATMENT

- Mineralocorticoid therapy

Congenital Adrenal Hyperplasia

DEFINITION

Inherited disease caused most commonly by a deficiency of 21 hydroxylase (autosomal recessive inheritance) in cortisol synthesis

PATHOPHYSIOLOGY

- Results in compensatory adrenal enlargement under influence of ACTH.
- Intermediate steroid metabolites accumulate and go into the androgen pathway instead.

SIGNS AND SYMPTOMS

- Ambiguous external genitalia (prenatal)
- Virilization (postnatal)
- Children: Increased rate of growth, premature development of secondary sex characteristics

DIAGNOSIS

- Twenty-four-hour urinary 17-ketosteroids, 17-hydroxysteroids, urinary free cortisol, serum testosterone or estrogen.
- CT is indicated to rule out adrenal neoplasm.

TREATMENT

- Glucocorticoid replacement
- Surgical reconstruction of ambiguous genitalia (clitoroplasty, vaginoplasty)

Incidentaloma

DEFINITION

Asymptomatic adrenal mass found on 0.6% abdominal/pelvic CTs done for other reasons, most of which end up to be benign, nonfunctioning adenomas (if < 5 cm)

DIAGNOSIS

- History and physical
- Check 24-hour urinary free cortisol, VMA, metanephrine, and urinary catecholamine.

Typical scenario: A 50-year-old male has an abdominal CT scan. Appendicitis is confirmed, and the patient undergoes a successful appendectomy and uneventful recovery. The CT scan also revealed a 2-cm adrenal mass. What's your next step? *Think:* Test for functionality. If the mass is functional, it should be resected regardless of its small size.

TREATMENT

- If > 5 cm or functional, surgical resection.
- If < 5 cm or nonfunctional, follow up in 6 months, and operate if there are any changes.
- Operation for adenoma is laparoscopic adrenalectomy.
- If cancer, check extent of disease; do en bloc resection.

MEDULLARY TUMORS

Neuroblastoma

DEFINITION

- Neural crest tumor occurring primarily in children (small round blue cell tumor)
- Fourth most common pediatric malignancy
- Can occur anywhere along sympathetic chain—40% in adrenal, 25% in paraspinal ganglia, 15% in thorax, 5% in pelvis
- May spontaneously differentiate and regress
- Aggressive tumor that commonly presents with distant metastases, in 50% of infants and two thirds of older children (to lymph node, bone, liver, subcutaneous tissue)

ASSOCIATED DISEASES

- Neurofibromatosis
- Beckwith–Wiedemann syndrome
- Trisomy 18

SIGNS AND SYMPTOMS

- Abdominal or flank mass
- Subcutaneous blue nodules (blueberry muffin sign)

DIAGNOSIS

- Imaging: CT for staging
- Urinary tumor markers: Elevated 24-hour homovanillylmandelic acid, VMA

TREATMENT

- Localized disease (stages I and II): Surgical resection.
- Lymph node mets warrant XRT.
- Chemotherapy for all except those with disease confined to primary location.

PROGNOSIS

- Mortality lower when diagnosed within first year of life
- Five-year survival 90% for disease confined to primary site; 20–40% for disseminated disease

Most common extra-adrenal location is organ of Zuckerkandl (to left of aortic bifurcation at IMA).

Pheochromocytoma

DEFINITION

Chromaffin cell tumor that can arise anywhere along the sympathetic chain, most common location is adrenal gland.

ASSOCIATED DISEASES

- MEN IIA and IIB
- Von Hippel–Lindau disease
- Neurofibromatosis

SIGNS AND SYMPTOMS

- HTN: May be sustained elevation, normal with paroxysmal hypertension, or sustained hypertension with acute elevations
- Anxiety, palpitations, pallor, diaphoresis

DIAGNOSIS

- 24-hour urinary: Catecholamines, VMA, metanephrine
- Clonidine test: Will suppress plasma catecholamine concentrations in normal patients but not in patients with pheochromocytoma
- CT or MRI, or nuclear scan

TREATMENT

- Preop alpha-adrenergic blockade, plus beta blockers for persistent tachycardia.
- Arterial blood pressure monitoring is essential because extreme changes in blood pressure may occur with manipulation.
- Laparoscopic approach has been used by some for small intra-adrenal tumors.
- Open operation uses a transabdominal approach to allow for exploration of entire abdomen. Adrenalectomy of involved gland is indicated.
- If malignant:
  - Resect recurrences and metastases when they occur.
  - Treat with catecholamine blockade.
  - Use XRT for bony mets.
  - Chemotherapy has a 60% response rate.

PROGNOSIS

- For malignant tumors: 5-year survival 36–60%

Pituitary

ANATOMY

See Figure 9-5.
- Ectodermal origin
- Relations:
  - Within sella turcica (floor of sella is roof of sphenoid sinus)
  - Surrounded by dura
  - Optic chiasm superior and anterior to pituitary stalk
  - Lateral cavernous sinuses
  - Superior: Diaphragma sella (meningeal tissue)

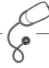

Pheochromocytoma:
- If extra-adrenal, then more likely malignant
- If bilateral, more likely familial

10% rule for pheochromocytoma:
10% malignant
10% familial
10% extra-adrenal
10% bilateral

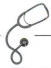

Alpha blockade must precede beta blockade in patients with pheochromocytoma. Beta blockers have negative inotropic and chronotropic effects and cause unopposed vasoconstriction, which may precipitate malignant hypertension and cardiac failure when given first.

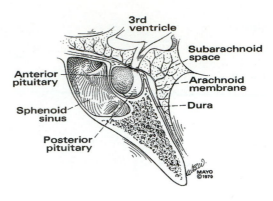

FIGURE 9-5. Pituitary anatomy. (Reproduced, with permission, from the Mayo Foundation. © 1979.)

- Size: $12 \times 9 \times 6$ mm, 500 to 600 mg
- Parts:
  - Adenohypophysis (embryologically from Rathke's pouch): Anterior lobe
  - Neurohypophysis (from neural primordial): Posterior lobe
    - Blood supply:
    - Anterior lobe lacks a direct supply. Portal channels from the hypothalamus and posterior pituitary supply it.
    - Posterior pituitary is supplied by middle and inferior hypophyseal arteries, branches of the ICA.
- Drains via cavernous sinuses to petrosal sinuses to jugular veins.
- For hormone actions, see section on endocrine organs.

Macroadenomas compress the pituitary stalk, preventing dopamine from traveling from hypothalamus to posterior pituitary gland where it normally inhibits prolactin production. Thus, compression results in hyperprolactinemia.

Adenoma

- Benign tumors arising from anterior lobe.
- Divided into two types based on size:
  - Macroadenoma: > 1 cm diameter
  - Microadenoma: < 1 cm diameter

SIGNS AND SYMPTOMS

- Macroadenomas: Visual loss (bilateral hemianopsia), hypopituitarism, headache, hyperprolactinemia due to compression of surrounding structures
- Microadenomas: Signs and symptoms depend on type of hormone overproduced.
  - Prolactinoma (most common): Secondary amenorrhea, galactorrhea
  - Growth hormone–producing tumor: Gigantism or acromegaly depending on age of patient; also, coarse facial features, thick finger and heel pads, cardiomegaly, hepatomegaly, enlarged mandible, increased teeth spaces, neuropathy, arthropathy, osteoporosis, HTN, diabetes mellitus (DM), goiter
  - ACTH: See adrenal section
  - Multihormonal

DIAGNOSIS

Imaging and clinical presentation.

- Preoperative: Complete endocrine assessment; electrolytes to look for borderline diabetes insipidus
- Surgery:
    - Transsphenoidal approach: Results in improved function of remaining pituitary gland
    - Transcranial approach: When transsphenoidal not possible due to location of carotid arteries, extra-sella tumor
- Perioperative glucocorticoids, serial visual field assessment, repeat endocrine assessment
- Postop XRT: For large lesions
- Primary radiation therapy: Consider when surgery contraindicated for other reasons in nonfunctioning tumor as primary therapy may worsen preexisting hypopituitarism
- Medical treatment:
    - For prolactinomas: Bromocriptine
    - For GH-secreting adenomas: Somatostatin, which decreases tumor size in 20–50%, normalizes GH in 50%, and normalizes IGF-1 in 40–80%

COMPLICATIONS

- Death due to direct hypothalamic injury (< 1%)
- Delayed mortality: Cerebrospinal fluid (CSF) leak, vascular injury
- Morbidity: Diabetes insipidus (2–17%), cerebrovascular accident (CVA), meningitis

Sheehan Syndrome

- Postpartum infarction and necrosis of pituitary leading to hormonal failure
- Etiology: Pituitary ischemia due to hemorrhage, hypovolemic shock, pituitary portal venous thrombosis

SIGNS AND SYMPTOMS

- Failure of lactation
- Amenorrhea
- Progressive decreased adrenal function and thyroid function

POSTERIOR PITUITARY DISORDERS

Syndrome of Inappropriate Antidiuretic Hormone (SIADH)

- Occurs in 15% of hospital patients.
- Impaired water secretion.
- Hypersecretion of ADH results in increased urinary sodium with elevation of urine osmolality.
- Causes: CNS injury, cancer, trauma, drugs

Diabetes Insipidus

- Decreased ADH secretion
- Impaired water conservation; large volumes of urine, leads to increased plasma osmolality and thirst
- One third idiopathic; two thirds due to tumor or trauma

Acute Abdomen

Definition

Abdominal pain accompanied by one or more peritoneal signs: Rigidity, tenderness (with or without rebound), involuntary guarding. May or may not be accompanied by hypotension and tachycardia, leading to imminent shock.

Risk Factors

The very young and the elderly are at increased risk for ruptured viscus, particularly appendicitis.

SIGNS AND SYMPTOMS

Precipitating or palliative factors may include:
- Change in position
- Association with food (better, worse)
- Pain that wakes one from sleep (significant)
- Association with vomiting

Quality of Pain
- Visceral pain is deep, dull, and poorly localized.
- Somatic pain is constant, sharp, and localized.

Radiation
- Biliary tract pain may radiate to the epigastrium, right shoulder, or right scapula (latter two due to right hemidiaphragmatic irritation).
- Splenic rupture and left lower lobe (LLL) pneumonia may radiate to left shoulder.
- Small bowel pain may radiate to the epigastrium and periumbilical area.
- Large bowel pain may radiate to suprapubic area
- Kidney pain may radiate to flank, groin, and genitalia.
- Pancreas pain may radiate to upper back, epigastrium, and left shoulder.

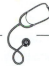

Assessment of pain should include PQRST:
Precipitating or palliative factors
Quality of pain: Stabbing, shooting, boring, dull
Radiation
Severity
Timing

Kehr's sign is pain referred to the left shoulder due to irritation of the left hemidiaphragm. Often seen with splenic rupture.

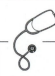

Hallmark of pain in mesenteric ischemia is pain out of proportion to physical findings.

Free air under the diaphragm on CXR or AXR is highly suggestive of a ruptured viscus.

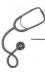

Most common cause by far (90%) of free air under diaphragm is perforated peptic ulcer. Other causes include hollow viscus injury secondary to trauma, aortic dissection, mesenteric ischemia (usually under left hemidiaphragm), and large bowel perforation.

Severity of Pain

May be assessed by several methods including:

- Verbal scale from 1 to 10
- Visual analog scale
- Pictoral scale (e.g., Wong–Baker faces)

Timing

- Does it come and go (colic) or is it constant?
- Colicky pain is associated with:
  - Biliary colic
  - Nephrolithiasis (renal colic)
  - Bowel obstruction
  - Mesenteric ischemia

PHYSICAL EXAM

Things to look for:

- Vital signs—explain any abnormalities
- General—appearance, attitude
- Chest—auscultation
- Abdomen:
  - Inspection: Distention, swelling, erythema
  - Percussion: Tympany, dullness, tenderness
  - Palpation: Muscle rigidity, tenderness, rebound pain, hyperesthesia
- Pelvis—bimanual exam, adnexal masses, cervical tenderness
- Rectal—tenderness, mass, blood

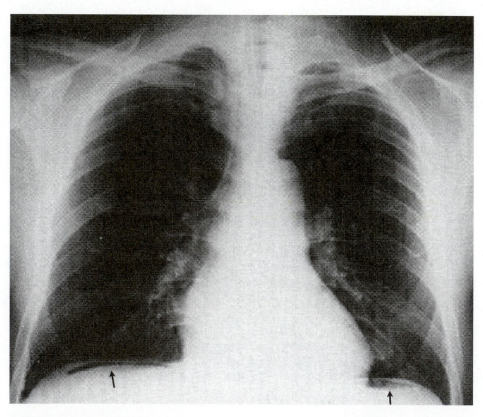

FIGURE 10-1. Upright CXR demonstrating free air under both hemidiaphragms (arrows). (Reproduced, with permission, from Billittier et al. *Emerg Med Clin of N Amer* 14:(4); November 1996, p. 795.)

DIAGNOSIS

Initial laboratory evaluation should include:

- CBC
- Electrolytes
- Amylase
- LFTs for right upper quadrant (RUQ) pain
- β-hCG (human chorionic gonadotropin) for all women of childbearing age
- Chest x-ray (CXR) and abdominal x-ray (AXR) to look for free air (can detect as little as 1 to 2 mL, easier to see under right hemidiaphragm. Presence of stomach bubble obscures it on the left). (See Figure 10-1.)
- Abdominal computed tomography (CT) is being used more often these days because often the cause of acute abdominal pain is difficult to decipher even with physical exam and labs. (See Figure 10-2.)

MANAGEMENT

- Early diagnosis improves outcome.
- Key is deciding whether surgical intervention is needed.

SURGICAL CAUSES OF ABDOMINAL PAIN

Right Upper Quadrant (RUQ)

Perforated duodenal ulcer
Cholecystitis
Hepatic abscess
Retrocecal appendicitis
Appendicitis in a pregnant woman

Right Lower Quadrant (RLQ)

Appendicitis
Cecal diverticulitis
Meckel's diverticulitis

Left Lower Quadrant (LLQ)

Sigmoid diverticulitis
Volvulus

Left Upper Quadrant (LUQ)

Splenic rupture
Splenic abscess

Diffuse

Bowel obstruction
Leaking aneurysm
Mesenteric ischemia

Contrast for abdominal CT:
For the most optimal imaging, both oral and IV contrast is used. In some cases (such as intractable vomiting or allergy to IV contrast) this is not possible. Noncontrast CT although suboptimal for most cases (except nephrolithiasis) still provides lots of information.

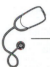

Serial abdominal exams and observation may be necessary in cases in which the etiology of abdominal pain is initially unclear.

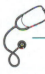

Pain of perforated ulcer is severe and of **sudden onset.**
Murphy's sign is seen in cholecystitis

Appendicitis is still the most common surgical emergency in the pregnant woman.

Periumbilical

Early appendicitis
Referred pain from small bowel

The pain of appendicitis localizes to **McBurney's point.**
Physical exam signs in appendicitis: Rovsing's, obturator, psoas (see chapter on the appendix)

Suprapubic

Ectopic pregnancy
Ovarian torsion
Tubo-ovarian abscess
Psoas abscess
Incarcerated groin hernia

NONSURGICAL CAUSES OF ABDOMINAL PAIN

RUQ

Right lower lobe (RLL) pneumonia
Biliary colic
Cholangitis
Hepatitis
Fitz-Hugh–Curtis syndrome

Patients with splenic rupture will have an elevated white count in the setting of trauma.

Midepigastric

Peptic ulcer disease (nonperforated)
Myocardial infarction
Esophagitis
Pulmonary embolism
Pancreatitis
Herpes zoster
Rectus sheath hematoma

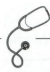

Patients with bowel obstruction will initially be able to take in fluids by mouth, and vomit a short time afterward.

RLQ or LLQ

Ureteral calculi
Regional enteritis
Inflammatory bowel disease
Pelvic inflammatory disease (PID)
Endometriosis
Prostatitis
Mittelschmerz
Urinary tract infection (UTI)
Ruptured ovarian cyst

AAA: Pulsatile mass on physical exam

LUQ

LLL pneumonia
Gastritis
Splenomegaly
Splenic infarct

Abscesses present with elevated white count and fever.

Diffuse

Abdominal wall hematoma
Black widow spider envenomation
Lead poisoning
Addisonian crisis
Sickle cell crisis
Diabetic ketoacidosis
Diabetic gastropathy
Opiate withdrawal
Hemorrhagic dengue fever
Nerve root compression

ABDOMINAL PAIN IN THE ELDERLY

Elderly patients who present with abdominal pain must be treated with particular caution. Common problems include:

- Difficulty communicating
- Comorbid disease
- Inability to tolerate intravascular volume loss
- Unusual presentation of common disease
- May not mount a white blood cell count or a fever
- Complaint often incommensurate with severity of disease

Note: Up to 2% of elderly patients with an MI will present with abdominal pain.

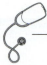

Fitz-Hugh–Curtis syndrome is perihepatitis associated with chlamydial infection of cervix.

Myocardial infarction (MI): Do an electrocardiogram (ECG) on all patients presenting with midepigastric pain.

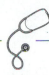

Pain of pancreatitis described as boring, radiating straight to the back

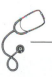

In elderly patients with abdominal pain, always consider vascular causes, including:
Abdominal aortic aneurysm (AAA)
Mesenteric ischemia (MI)

Most common cause of abdominal pain in the elderly is cholecystitis.

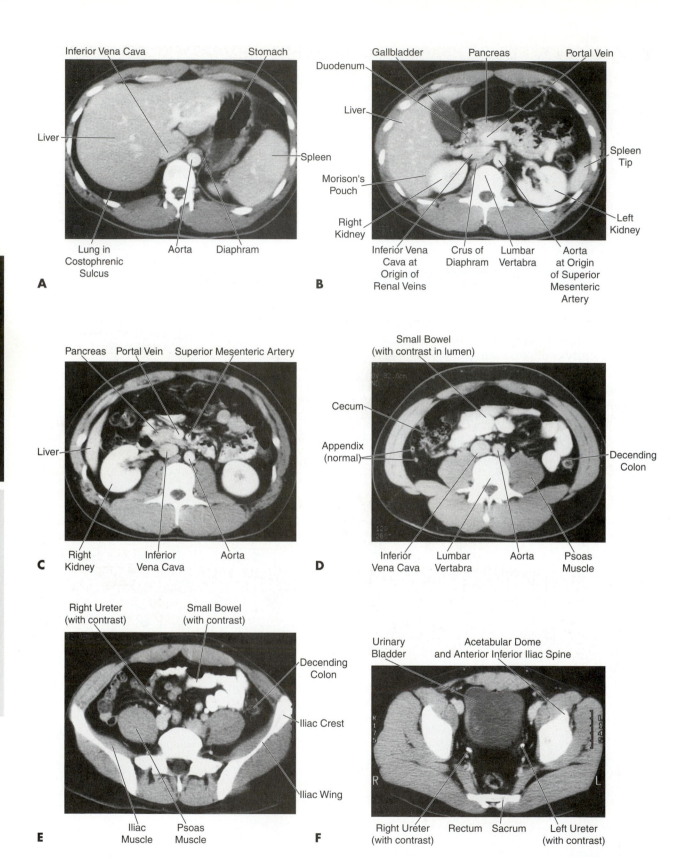

FIGURE 10-2. Abdominal CT anatomy. Normal abdominopelvic CT scan of a 26-year-old man. Both oral and intravenous contrast was administered. **A.** Liver (right and left lobes), stomach, and spleen. **B.** Liver, gallbladder, kidneys, and pancreas. **C.** Kidneys, pancreas, and intestines. **D.** Small bowel, cecum, ascending colon, and normal appendix. **E.** Intestines and ureters at level of iliac wings. **F.** Bladder, distal ureters, and rectum at the level of the acetabular domes. (Reproduced, with permission, from Schwartz DT, Reisdorff EJ, eds. *Emergency Radiology.* New York: McGraw-Hill, 2000: 519.)

The Esophagus

ANATOMY

- The esophagus is a muscular tube that begins at the pharynx, travels through the thorax in the posterior mediastinum, and empties into the cardia of the stomach.
- Superior third: Striated muscle only.
- Middle third: Both striated and smooth muscle.
- Inferior third: Smooth muscle only.
- Two sphincters are present which function as control points:
  - Upper esophageal sphincter (UES) prevents the passage of excess air into the stomach during breathing.
  - Lower esophageal sphincter (LES) prevents the reflux of gastric contents.

Recall the vertebral levels at which the following traverse the diaphragm:
T8 = inferior vena cava (IVC)
T10 = esophagus
T12 = aorta

The LES is not a true anatomical sphincter; however, it functions as one.

DYSPHAGIA

DEFINITIONS

- Dysphagia: Difficulty swallowing, occurs when there is obstruction to the passage of food from the mouth to the stomach.
- Odynophagia: Pain on swallowing. May or may not accompany dysphagia.

TYPES

- Mechanical: Patient typically reports difficulty swallowing solids more than liquids.
- Neuromuscular: Patient typically reports difficulty swallowing both solids *and* liquids.

CAUSES

Mechanical
- Foreign body
- Inflammation (infectious esophagitis, caustic exposure)
- Strictures (inflammatory, post-irradiation)
- Neoplasms

- Extrinsic compression (aortic aneurysm, retropharyngeal abscess, thyromegaly, etc.)

Neuromuscular
- Tongue paralysis
- Lesions of cranial nerves IX and/or X
- Disorders of the neuromuscular junction (NMJ) (e.g., myasthenia gravis)
- Primary disorders of muscle (e.g., polymyositis, dermatomyositis)
- Disorder of esophageal smooth muscle (scleroderma, achalasia, diffuse esohageal spasm)

Achalasia: *Gr.* Failure to relax

Classic triad of achalasia: Dysphagia, regurgitation, and weight loss

Gastroesophageal reflux produces a sour taste due to the presence of hydrochloride while achalasia does not.

Barium swallow:
- Bird's beak or steeple sign: Achalasia
- Corkscrew-shaped: Diffuse esophageal spasm

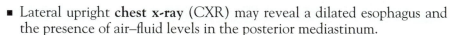

ACHALASIA

DEFINITION

Achalasia is the result of a primary or secondary derangement of the myenteric plexus, the network of neurons involved in the coordination of gastrointestinal (GI) motility. The resulting dysphagia is due to three mechanisms:

1. Nonperistaltic contrations
2. Incomplete relaxation of the LES after swallowing
3. Increased resting tone of the LES

SIGNS AND SYMPTOMS

- Dysphagia for both solids and liquids
- Regurgitation of food
- Severe halitosis (due to the decomposition of stagnant food within the esophagus

DIAGNOSIS

- Lateral upright **chest x-ray** (CXR) may reveal a dilated esophagus and the presence of air–fluid levels in the posterior mediastinum.
- **Barium swallow** will reveal the characteristic distal bird's beak sign due to the collection of contrast material in the proximal dilated segment and the passage of a small amount of contrast through the narrowed LES.
- **Esophageal motility study** will confirm nonperistaltic contractions, incomplete LES relaxation, and increased LES tone.
- **Esophagoscopy** is indicated to rule out mass lesions or strictures, and to obtain specimens for biopsy.

TREATMENT

- Medical management: Drugs that relax the LES such as nitrates or calcium channel blockers
- Surgical management: Endoscopic dilatation or esophagomyotomy with fundoplication
  - Esophagomyotomy: Esophagus is exposed via transthoracic (left thoracotomy), transabdominal, thorascopic, or laparoscopic technique. The tunica muscularis of the esophagus is incised distally, with extension to the LES. Complete division of the LES necessitates the addition of an antireflux procedure such as Nissen 360° fundoplication or partial fundoplication.

- Endoscopic dilatation:
  - Lower success rate and a higher complication rate
  - Involves inserting a balloon or progressively larger sized dilators through the narrowed lumen, which causes tearing of the esophageal smooth muscle and decreases the competency of the LES.

COMPLICATIONS

- Risk of squamous cell carcinoma is as high as 10% in patients with long-standing achalasia (15 to 25 years).
- Patients may also develop pulmonary complications such as aspiration pneumonia, bronchiectasis, and asthma, due to reflux and aspiration.

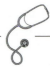

Esophageal perforation is four times more likely following dilatation compared to esophagomyotomy.

DIFFUSE ESOPHAGEAL SPASM (DES)

DEFINITION

DES is a disorder of unknown etiology that, like achalasia, involves a dysfunction of the myenteric plexus. It may be a primary disease process, or it may occur in association with reflux esophagitis, esophageal obstruction, collagen vascular disease, and diabetic neuropathy. Spasm occurs in the distal two thirds of the esophagus and is caused by uncoordinated large-amplitude contractions of smooth muscle.

SIGNS AND SYMPTOMS

- Dysphagia for both solids and liquids.
- Chest pain similar to that seen in myocardial infarction (MI): Acute onset of severe retrosternal pain that may radiate to the arms, jaw, or back. The chest pain may occur at rest, or it may follow swallowing. The degree of chest pain depends on the duration and severity of the contractions.
- No regurgitation (unlike achalasia).

DIAGNOSIS

- Barium swallow may reveal the characteristic "corkscrew" appearance of the esophagus. This appearance is due to the ripples and sacculations that are visible due to uncoordinated esophageal contraction. Barium swallow may be entirely normal, however, because the esophagus may not be in spasm at the time of the study. In contrast to achalasia, the LES appears its normal diameter.
- Esophageal manometry studies will reveal the presence of large, uncoordinated, and repetitive contractions in the lower esophagus. Alternatively, manometry may appear normal when the patient is asymptomatic.
- Esophagoscopy should be performed to rule out mass lesions, strictures, or esophagitis.

TREATMENT

- Nitrates or calcium channel blockers to decrease LES pressure.
- Surgical treatment via esophagomyotomy is not as successful in relieving symptoms as it is for achalasia and is therefore not recommended unless pain or dysphagia are severe and incapacitating (see Table 11-1).

Due to the fact that DES produces cardiac-like complaints, the diagnosis is often delayed until an extensive cardiologic workup is performed. Nutcracker esophagus is another hypermotility disorder, but involves more focal segments of the esophagus.

Patients with DES often have other functional intestinal disorders such as irritable bowel syndrome and spastic colon.

	Achalasia	Diffuse Esophageal Spasm
TABLE 11-1. Achalasia vs. diffuse esophageal spasm.		
Signs and symptoms	Weight loss, cough, diffuse chest pain	Dysphagia, diffuse chest pain
Pattern of contraction	Failure of LES to relax on swallowing Classic: Simultaneous small wave Vigorous: Simultaneous large wave	Swallow-induced large wave
Relieved by	Nitroglycerin	Nitroglycerin
X-ray findings	Absence of gastric bubble, narrowing of terminal esophagus that looks like a beak	Corkscrew appearance
Treatment	Nitroglycerin, local botulinum toxin, balloon dilatation, sphincter myotomy	Nitroglycerin, nifedipine

ESOPHAGEAL VARICES

PATHOPHYSIOLOGY

- Occur as a result of portal hypertension, which is most commonly due to alcoholic cirrhosis.
- As elevated portal system pressure impedes the flow of blood through the liver, and ultimately to the right atrium, various sites of venous anastomosis become dilated secondary to retrograde flow from the portal to systemic circulations.
- Most clinically significant portal-systemic sites:
  - Cardio-esophageal junction—dilation leads to esophageal varices.
  - Periumbilical region—dilation leads to caput medusae.
  - Rectum—dilation leads to hemorrhoids.

SIGNS AND SYMPTOMS

- Painless
- Massive hemorrhage
- Unprovoked (i.e., not post-emetic).
- Can progress to hypovolemic shock

Endoscopic sclerotherapy or band ligation for control of ruptured esophageal varices have a 90% success rate. Patients are usually intubated prior to the procedure to prevent aspiration.

TREATMENT

- Variceal bleeding ceases spontaneously in ~50% of cases.
- Risk for rebleeding is quite high.
- Medical management includes drugs that decrease portal blood flow such as vasopressin, octreotide, or somatostatin. Beta blockers such as propranolol are used to decrease portal pressure.
- Options for ruptured varices:
  1. Volume replacement with normal saline (NS) and packed red blood cells (RBCs)

2. Nasogastric (NG) suction
3. Endoscopic sclerotherapy (injection of the bleeding vessel(s) with a sclerosing agent via a catheter that is passed through the endoscope)
4. Endoscopic band ligation (small elastic band is placed around the bleeding varix resulting in hemostasis)
5. Balloon tamponade (Sengstaken–Blakemore tube)
6. TIPS (transjugular intrahepatic portocaval shunt) (see chapter on transplants)
7. Intraoperative placement of a portocaval shunt
8. Liver transplant

The most serious complication of balloon tamponade for esophageal varices is esophageal perforation.

ESOPHAGEAL PERFORATION OR RUPTURE

DEFINITION

Iatrogenic or pathologic trauma to the esophagus, which may result in leakage of air and esophageal contents into the mediastinum. Carries a 50% mortality.

ETIOLOGY

Iatrogenic: Often occurs in an already diseased esophagus. Comprises 50–75% of cases of esophageal rupture.
- Endoscopy
- Dilatation
- Blakemore tubes
- Intubation of the esophagus
- NG tube placement

Boerhaave syndrome: A *full-thickness* tear. Generally occurs in the relatively weak left posterolateral wall of distal esophagus. Due to:
- Forceful vomiting
- Cough
- Labor
- Lifting
- Trauma

Mallory–Weiss syndrome: A *partial-thickness* tear. Usually occurs in the right posterolateral wall of the distal esophagus and results in bleeding that generally resolves spontaneously. Due to forceful vomiting.

Foreign body ingestion: Objects usually lodge near anatomic narrowings:
- Above the upper esophageal sphincter
- Near the aortic arch
- Above LES

SIGNS AND SYMPTOMS

- Severe, constant pain in chest, abdomen, and back
- Dysphagia
- Dyspnea
- Subcutaneous emphysema
- Mediastinal emphysema heard as a "crunching" sound with heartbeat (Hammon's crunch)

Typical scenario: An alcoholic man presents after severe retching, complaining of retrosternal and upper abdominal pain. *Think:* Boerhaave syndrome (full thickness) or Mallory–Weiss syndrome (partial thickness).

Differential diagnosis of esophageal rupture includes aortic dissection, MI, spontaneous pneumothorax, pancreatitis, and perforated peptic ulcer.

Subcutaneous and mediastinal emphysema require a full-thickness tear.

There is no role for endoscopy in esophageal perforation.

In Boerhaave syndrome the most common site of rupture is the left lateral wall of the esophagus, just above the esophageal hiatus. Iatrogenic perforation occurs most commonly in the pharynx and distal esophagus.

Dysphagia does not usually develop until > 60% of the esophageal lumen is obstructed by tumor.

DIAGNOSIS

- **CXR:** Left-sided pleural effusion, mediastinal or subcutaneous emphysema
- **Esophagogram with water-soluble contrast:** Shows extravasation of contrast
- **Other studies:** Endoscopy, computed tomography (CT), and thoracentesis (check fluid for low pH and high amylase)

TREATMENT

- Surgical repair of full-thickness tears.
- Ninety percent of partial-thickness tears resolve with NG decompression and gastric lavage. The remaining 10% require surgical repair (gastrotomy). Hemostasis is achieved following primary closure of the esophageal mucosa with sutures.

ESOPHAGEAL CARCINOMA

EPIDEMIOLOGY

- Esophageal cancer causes roughly 1–2% of all cancer-related deaths.
- In the United States, each year there are roughly six new cases per 100,000 population; in other regions of the world such as Asia, the incidence of esophageal carcinoma is much higher.
- Most cases occur in patients over the age of 50.
- Males are affected three times more frequently than females.

RISK FACTORS

- Alcohol
- Tobacco
- Diets high in nitrites or nitrosamines
- Esophageal disorders such as achalasia, chronic esophagitis, and Plummer–Vinson syndrome.

SIGNS AND SYMPTOMS

- Gradual development of dysphagia, first for solids and later for both solids and liquids (mechanical dysphagia).
- Anorexia develops as swallowing becomes more painful.
- Decreased PO intake results in profound weight loss, easy fatigability, and weakness.
- Physical exam early in the disease course may be entirely normal.
- With advanced disease, the patient will appear cachectic, and supraclavicular lymphadenopathy may be present.

DIAGNOSIS

- Barium swallow may reveal the presence of a mass.
- Chest x-ray may reveal hilar lymphadenopathy.
- Esophageal duodenoscopy (EGD) is useful to both visualize the mass and to retrieve specimens for biopsy.
- CT scan of the thorax is useful to define the extent of disease and thereby determine appropriate treatment.

TREATMENT

- Most patients who are symptomatic at the time of diagnosis have advanced, widespread disease, with multiple metastases present to the liver, lungs, pleura, and lymph nodes. As a result of this, < 40% of patients will be candidates for "curative" surgery.
- Even when surgery is an option, response is poor; therefore, treatment for esophageal carcinoma is mostly palliative.
- Postoperative complications are common; > 20% of patients will develop fistulae or abscesses and respiratory complications.
- Radiation therapy can shrink the tumor, resulting in at least temporary relief from obstructive symptoms.
- Other options include endoscopic laser therapy, endoscopic dilatation and stent placement, or placement of a gastrostomy or jejunostomy tube.

The 5-year survival rate for esophageal carcinoma is ~5%.

ESOPHAGEAL DIVERTICULA

DEFINITION

- Outpouching of the esophageal mucosa that protrudes through a defect in the tunica muscularis.
- May be either a true diverticulum, involving all three layers of the esophagus, or a false diverticulum, involving only the mucosa and submucosa.
- Characterized by its location: Pharyngoesophageal (Zenker's diverticulum), midesophageal, or epiphrenic.
- Pharyngoesophageal and epiphrenic diverticula are called pulsion diverticula, since they are caused by increased esophageal pressure; they are false diverticula.
- Midesophageal diverticula are traction diverticula and are true diverticula.

Epiphrenic and Pharyngoesophageal = caused by Elevated Pressure (Pulsion) and are Pseudo (false)

SIGNS AND SYMPTOMS

- Pharyngoesophageal type is the most likely to be symptomatic. Typical symptoms include dysphagia, halitosis, regurgitation of food eaten hours to days earlier, choking, and aspiration.
- Midesophageal diverticula are usually asymptomatic.
- Epiphrenic diverticula may cause dysphagia and regurgitation or may be entirely asymptomatic.

DIAGNOSIS

Barium swallow will reveal the presence of all types of diverticula.

TREATMENT

- Treatment of Zenker's diverticulum is recommended to relieve symptoms and to prevent complications such as aspiration pneumonia or esophageal perforation. The most common procedure is a cervical esophagomyotomy with resection of the diverticulum.
- Midesophageal diverticula are resected in the occasional incidence of a fistulous connection between the diverticulum and tracheobronchial tree.

Zenker's causes Zymptoms and requires Zurgery.

- Epiphrenic diverticula may be treated via resection and esophagomyotomy via a left thoracotomy approach.

PATHOPHYSIOLOGY

- Impairment in the functioning of LES will cause the reflux of acidic gastric contents into the esophagus.
- Prolonged exposure to such a low lumenal pH will cause irritation of the esophageal mucosa and the development of reflux esophagitis.
- There are several types of reflux esophagitis, ranging from mild to severe; the type present depends on many factors, including the duration and frequency of reflux episodes.

SIGNS AND SYMPTOMS

- Patients with GERD may report a range of symptoms from heartburn to angina-like chest pain.
- Degree of pain depends on the severity of esophagitis.
- Minimal reflux may cause only minimal, asymptomatic esophagitis, while severe reflux may cause severe esophagitis accompanied by laryngitis, aspiration pneumonitis, or asthma.
- Symptoms are often exacerbated when the patient lies supine and relieved by elevating the head above the level of the stomach.
- Antacids often provide prompt symptomatic relief.
- Presence of dysphagia may indicate peptic stricture formation.

DIAGNOSIS

- Patients presenting with vague symptoms of chest pain must be evaluated for cardiac disease (electrocardiogram [ECG], cardiac enzymes, and admission as appropriate).
- A barium study is useful to assess the severity of reflux, to look for an anatomical cause for the reflux such as a hiatal hernia, and to elucidate pathology resulting from long-standing reflux such as a stricture or ulcer.
- Continuous pH monitoring of the esophagus: A probe that contains pH electrodes is inserted into the patient's esophagus for 24 hours. The probe will continuously record the esophageal pH, thereby enabling the physician to determine the severity of reflux.
- Esophageal motility study is useful in evaluating the competence of the LES.
- Esophagoscopy should be performed to evaluate the esophageal mucosa for the presence of ulcerations, to rule out Barrett's esophagus, and to obtain specimens for biopsy.

TREATMENT

- Initial treatment of GERD involves giving medications that decrease gastric acid production such as:
  - H_2 antagonists (e.g., ranitidine)
  - Antacids
  - Proton pump blockers (e.g., omeprazole)
- Smoking cessation: Nicotine decreases LES tone, thereby increasing reflux.

- Instruct the patient to sleep with the head of the bed elevated.
- For severe cases, agents that increase LES tone such as metoclopramide may be required for symptomatic relief.
- If medical management fails, and the patient develops complications such as chronic esophagitis or stricture, surgical intervention should be considered.
- Esophageal reflux surgery consists of fundoplication. The goal of esophageal reflux surgery is to increase the competency of the LES. This is accomplished by wrapping the gastric fundus around the esophagus either completely or partially.
- Strictures may be treated via forceful dilatation.
- Treatment of GERD is important in order to prevent the development of Barrett's esophagus and secondary esophageal carcinoma. In addition, chronic reflux predisposes the patient to pulmonary complications such as aspiration pneumonia and asthma.

ESOPHAGEAL STRICTURE

DEFINITION

Local, stenotic regions within the lumen of the esophagus resulting from inflammation or neoplasm.

RISK FACTORS AND CAUSES

- Long-standing GERD
- Radiation esophagitis
- Infectious esophagitis
- Corrosive esophagitis
- Subsequent to sclerotherapy for bleeding varices

SIGNS AND SYMPTOMS

- While small strictures may remain asymptomatic, those that obstruct the esophageal lumen significantly will induce progressive dysphagia for solids.
- Odynophagia may or may not be present.

DIAGNOSIS

- Initial evaluation via barium swallow may reveal the presence of stricture.
- Esophagoscopy is necessary in all cases, however, as the stricture must be evaluated for malignancy.
- Esophagoscopy is also necessary to determine appropriate treatment.

TREATMENT

- The esophagus is visualized via endoscopy, and dilators of increasing size are carefully passed through the stricture.
- Dysphagia is relieved in most cases following adequate dilatation of the esophageal lumen.
- The most feared complication of dilatation is esophageal rupture.

The Stomach

See Figure 12-1.

Blood Supply

- Greater curvature: Right and left gastroepiploic arteries
- Lesser curvature: Right and left gastric arteries
- Pylorus: Gastroduodenal artery
- Fundus: Short gastric arteries

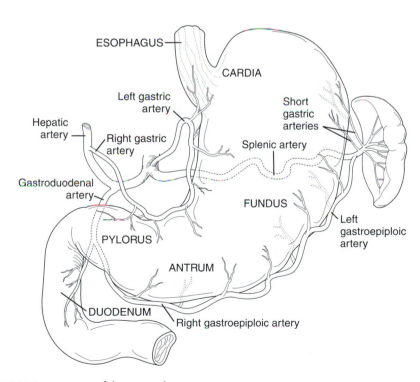

FIGURE 12-1. Anatomy of the stomach.

Innervation

- Anterior gastric wall: Left vagus nerve
- Posterior gastric wall: Right vagus nerve
- Sympathetic afferents from level T5 (below nipple line) to T10 (umbilicus) are responsible for sensation of gastroduodenal pain.

Physiology

- Parietal cells:
  - Secrete intrinsic factor for absorption of vitamin B_{12} in the terminal ileum
  - Secrete hydrochloride (HCl), accounting for highly acidic pH of stomach
  - Located in fundus and body
- Chief cells:
  - Secrete pepsinogen, which digests protein
  - Located in fundus and body
- G cells:
  - Secrete gastrin
  - Located in antrum

PEPTIC ULCER DISEASE (PUD)

PUD consists of duodenal ulcers (DUs) and gastric ulcers (GUs).

EPIDEMIOLOGY

- Two times more common in men.
- Incidence increases with age.
- Smoking and EtOH increase risk.

PATHOPHYSIOLOGY

- Parietal cells secrete HCl into the gastric lumen and bicarbonate into the gastric venous circulation (alkaline tide) and into the protective gastric mucous gel.
- A proton pump exchanges potassium in the gastric lumen for protons.
- The parietal cells are stimulated by gastrin, the vagus nerve, and histamine.
- Gastrin release is stimulated by gastrin-releasing peptide and is inhibited by somatostatin.
- Histamine receptors on parietal cells also stimulate HCl secretion.
- Gastric bicarbonate secretion into the mucous gel is inhibited by non-steroidal anti-inflammatory drugs (NSAIDs), acetazolamide, alpha blockers, and alcohol.
- Gel thickness is increased by prostaglandin E (PGE) and reduced by steroids and NSAIDs.

COMPLICATIONS

- Bleeding: 20% incidence
- Perforation:
  - Incidence: 7%.

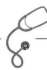

Typical scenario: A patient with known PUD presents with sudden onset of severe epigastric pain. Physical exam reveals guarding and rebound tenderness. *Think:* Perforation.

- Posterior perforation of a duodenal ulcer will cause pain that radiates to the back and can cause pancreatitis or cause GI bleeding. A chest or abdominal film will not show free air because the posterior duodenum is retroperitoneal.
- Anterior perforation will show free air under the diaphragm in 70% of cases. (See Figure 10-1 in acute abdomen chapter.)
- **Gastric outlet obstruction,** due to scarring and edema.

DUODENAL ULCER (DU)

PATHOPHYSIOLOGY

Increased acid production.

ETIOLOGY

- *Helicobacter pylori:* A bacterium that produces urease, which breaks down the protective mucous lining of the stomach. Ten to 20% of persons with *H. pylori* develop PUD.
- NSAIDs/steroids: Inhibit production of PGE, which stimulates mucosal barrier production.
- Zollinger–Ellison (ZE) syndrome:
  - A gastrin-secreting tumor in or near the pancreas.
  - 0.1–1% of patients with ulcer.
  - 20% of ZE patients have associated multiple endocrine neoplasia 1 (MEN-1).
  - Two thirds are malignant.
  - Diarrhea is common.
  - Can see jejunal ulcers

CLINICAL FEATURES

- Burning gnawing epigastric pain that occurs with an empty stomach: Pain is relieved within 30 minutes by food.
- Nighttime awakening (when stomach empties)
- Nausea, vomiting.
- Associated with blood type O.

DIAGNOSIS

- DU: Via endoscopy; however, most symptomatic cases of DU are easily diagnosed clinically. If patient responds to DU therapy, there is no need to do the biopsy.
- *H. pylori:*
  - Endoscopy with biopsy—allows C&S for *H. pylori* (organism is notoriously hard to culture—multiple specimens required during biopsy).
  - Serology: Anti-*H. pylori* immunoglobulin G (IgG) indicates current or prior infection.
  - Urease breath test: $C^{13/14}$ labeled urea is ingested. If gastric urease is present, the carbon isotope can be detected as CO_2 isotopes in the breath.
- ZE: A fasting serum gastrin level > 1,000 pg/mL is pathognomonic for gastrinoma. Secretin stimulation test: Secretin, a gastrin inhibitor, is delivered parenterally (usually with Ca^{2+}) and its effect on gastrin secretion is measured. In ZE syndrome, there is a paradoxical astronomic rise in serum gastrin.

Typical scenario: A 52-year-old woman presents due to 3 months of early satiety, weight loss, and non-bilious vomiting. *Think:* Gastric outlet obstruction.

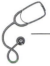

Over 90% of patients with ZE have PUD.

H. pylori may colonize 90% of the population—infection does not necessitate disease.

Typical scenario: A 33-year-old female smoker presents with burning epigastric pain that is improved after eating a meal. *Think:* Duodenal ulcer.

Most common location for DU: Posterior duodenal wall within 2 cm of pylorus

Medical

- Discontinue NSAIDs, steroids, smoking.
- **Proton pump inhibitors** (omeprazole, lansoprazole, pantoprazole): 90% cure rate after 4 weeks.
- **Eradication of H. *pylori*:**
  - Proton pump inhibitor, clarithromycin, and amoxicillin/metronidazole × 14 days: ~90% cure rate
  - Bismuth, metronidazole, tetracycline × 14 days: ~85% cure rate
- **H^2 blockers** (cimetidine, ranitidine, famotidine, nizatidine): 85–95% cure rate after 8 weeks.
- Prostaglandin analogues (e.g., misoprostol) work because of their anti-secretory effect. Not as efficacious as H$_2$ blockers, so no longer recommended.
- Antacids: Over the counter, good for occasional use for all causes of dyspepsia, but better drugs are available for active ulcer disease.

Surgical

- Since the advent of highly effective medical therapy, elective surgery for PUD is quite rare.
- Surgery is indicated when ulcer is refractory to 12 weeks of medical treatment or if hemorrhage, obstruction, or perforation is present.
- Truncal vagotomy and selective vagotomy are not commonly performed anymore due to associated morbidity (high rate of dumping syndrome) despite good protection against recurrence.
- Procedure of choice is **highly selective vagotomy** (parietal cell vagotomy, proximal gastric vagotomy) (see Figure 12-2).
  - Individual branches of the anterior and posterior nerves of Latarjet in the gastrohepatic ligament going to the lesser curvature of the stom-

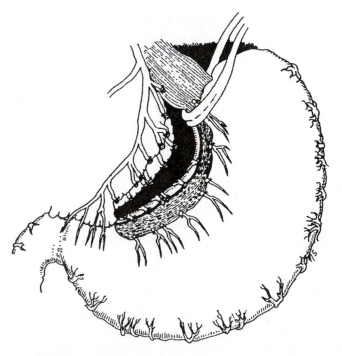

FIGURE 12-2. Highly selective vagotomy. (Reproduced, with permission, from Yamada et al., *Textbook of Gastroenterology.* Lippincott Williams & Wilkins.)

ach are divided from a point 6 cm proximal from the pylorus to a point 6 cm proximal to the esophagogastric junction. The terminal branches to the pylorus and antrum are spared, preserving pyloroantral function and thus obviating the need for gastric drainage.

- Preferred due to its lowest rate of dumping; however, it does have the highest rate of recurrence.
- Recurrence depends on site of ulcer preop: Prepyloric ulcers have the highest recurrence rate at 30%.

■ Laparoscopic option: A posterior truncal vagotomy coupled with an anterior seromyotomy is being done laparoscopically in select centers. Hasn't been around long enough to comment on long-term outcomes.

■ For ZE: The tumor is resected. Occasionally, when focus of tumor cannot be found, a total gastrectomy may be considered in severe cases.

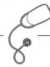

Complications of surgery for peptic ulcer disease:
- Dumping syndrome
- Afferent loop syndrome
- Postvagotomy diarrhea
- Duodenal stump leak
- Efferent loop obstruction
- Marginal ulcer
- Alkaline reflux gastritis
- Chronic gastroparesis
- Postgastrectomy stump cancer

GASTRIC ULCER (GU)

PATHOPHYSIOLOGY

- Decreased protection against acid: Normal or low acid production
- Can be caused by reflux of duodenal contents (pyloric sphincter dysfunction) and decreased mucus and bicarbonate production

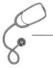

Gastric ulcers can even occur with achlorhydria.

CAUSES

- NSAIDs and steroids inhibit production of PGE.
- PGE stimulates production of the gastric mucosal barrier.
- H. pylori produces urease, which breaks down the gastric mucosal barrier.

CLASSIFICATION

- Type I: Ulcer in lesser curvature at incisura angularis
- Type II: Simultaneous gastric and duodenal ulcer
- Type III: Prepyloric ulcer
- Type IV: Ulcer in gastric cardia

Smoking is a risk factor for GU.

SIGNS AND SYMPTOMS

- Burning, gnawing epigastric pain that occurs with anything in the stomach: Pain is worst 30 minutes after food.
- Anorexia/weight loss
- Vomiting
- Associated with blood type A

Most common location for GU: Lesser curvature

DIAGNOSIS

- Via endoscopy.
- Three percent of GUs are associated with gastric cancer so all GU are biopsied.

TREATMENT

- Medical options same as for duodenal ulcers
- Surgical options:
  - Antrectomy for types I and II

Typical scenario: A 45-year-old Japanese male smoker presents with weight loss and epigastric pain exacerbated by eating. *Think:* Gastric ulcer.

- Burnt paper CURLS
- CUSHING'S ulcer

- Highly selective vagotomy for type III
- Subtotal gastrectomy followed by Roux-en-Y esophagogastrojejunostomy for type IV

Special Gastric Ulcers

- Curling's ulcers: Gastric stress ulcers in patients with severe burns
- Cushing's ulcers: Gastric stress ulcer related to severe central nervous system (CNS) damage

POSTGASTRECTOMY SYNDROMES

Dumping Syndrome

DEFINITION

Complication of gastric surgery thought to result from unregulated movement of gastric contents from stomach to small intestine.

SIGNS AND SYMPTOMS

Typically occur 5 to 15 minutes (early dumping syndrome) or 2 to 4 hours (late dumping syndrome) after eating:
- Nausea, vomiting
- Diarrhea
- Belching
- Tachycardia, palpitations
- Diaphoresis, flushing
- Dizziness, syncope

TREATMENT

Avoid high-sugar food or excessive water intake. Severe cases (1%) that do not respond to dietary modifications can be treated with octreotide.

Postvagotomy Diarrhea

- Seen mostly after truncal vagotomy.
- Usually self-limited.
- Treated symptomatically with kaolin–pectin, loperamide, or diphenoxylate as needed.
- Refractory cases may respond to cholestyramine.

Alkaline Reflux Gastritis

- Diagnosis of exclusion after recurrent ulcer has been ruled out.
- Presents with chronic abdominal pain and bilous vomiting.
- Medical treatment is difficult.
- Surgical management: Roux-en-Y gastrojejunostomy with Roux limb at least 45 to 50 cm long. Recurrence still reported with this procedure.

Afferent Loop Syndrome

DEFINITION

- Obstruction of afferent limb following gastrojejunostomy (Bilroth II)
- Two thirds present in first postoperative week

SIGNS AND SYMPTOMS

- Right upper quadrant (RUQ) pain following a meal
- Bilous vomiting
- Steatorrhea
- Anemia

DIAGNOSIS

Afferent loop will be devoid of contrast on the upper gastrointestinal (UGI) series.

TREATMENT

- Endoscopic balloon dilatation
- Surgical revision

Gastritis

DEFINITION

Acute or chronic inflammation of the stomach lining.

ETIOLOGY

- Increased acid: Smoking, alcohol, stress
- Decreased mucosal barrier: NSAIDs, steroids
- Direct irritant: Pancreatic and biliary reflux, infection

SIGNS AND SYMPTOMS

- Burning or gnawing pain.
- Pain usually worsened with food and relieved by antacids.
- Vomiting may relieve the pain after eating.

DIAGNOSIS

Diagnosis is made by endoscopy.

TREATMENT

- Halt NSAIDs.
- Triple therapy to eradicate *H. pylori* if present.
- Halt cigarettes and alcohol.
- H$_2$ blockers (e.g., cimetidine, ranitidine), sucralfate, or misoprostol.
- Over-the-counter antacids.

COMPLICATIONS

Chronic gastritis leads to:
- Gastric atrophy
- Gastric metaplasia

Typical scenario: A 58-year-old woman who is 6 days postop from a gastrojejunostomy for PUD presents with postprandial RUQ pain and nausea. She reports that vomiting relieves her suffering. *Think:* Afferent loop syndrome.

Etiologies of gastritis: **GNASHING**
- **G**astric reflux (bile or pancreatic secretions)
- **N**icotine
- **A**lcohol
- **S**tress
- ***H**elicobacter pylori* and other infections
- **I**schemia
- **N**SAIDs
- **G**lucocorticoids (long-term use)

Cimetidine is a p450 inhibitor, and therefore prolongs the action of drugs cleared by this system.

- Pernicious anemia (decreased production of intrinsic factor from gastric parietal cells due to idiopathic atrophy of the gastric mucosa and subsequent malabsorption of vitamin B_{12})

GASTRIC OUTLET OBSTRUCTION

COMMON CAUSES

- Malignant tumors of stomach and head of pancreas.
- Obstructing gastric or duodenal ulcers.
- Usually with duodenal ulcer.
- Chronic ulcer causes secondary edema or scarring, which occludes lumen.

SYMPTOMS

Early
- Early satiety
- Gastric reflux
- Weight loss
- Abdominal distention

Late
- Vomiting
- Dehydration
- Metabolic alkalosis

DIAGNOSIS

Endsocopy or barium swallow x-ray.

TREATMENT

- Endoscopic balloon dilatation
- Surgical resection: Truncal vagotomy and pyloroplasty after 7 days of nasogastric decompression and antisecretory treatment

GASTROINTESTINAL HEMORRHAGE

Mallory's Vices Gave (her) An Ulcer.

Upper GI Hemorrhage

ETIOLOGY

- **M**allory–Weiss tear
- **V**arices
- **G**astritis
- **A**rteriovenous malformation
- **U**lcer (peptic)

SIGNS AND SYMPTOMS

- Hematemesis (bright red or coffee grounds).
- Hypotension.
- Tachycardia.

Coffee grounds is the term used to describe old, brown digested blood found on gastric lavage. It usually indicates a source of bleeding proximal to the ligament of Treitz.

- Bleeding that produces 60 cc of blood or more will produce black, tarry stool.
- Very brisk upper GI bleeds can be associated with bright red blood per rectum and hypotension.

DIAGNOSIS

- Gastric lavage with normal saline or free water to assess severity of bleeding (old versus new blood)
- Rectal exam
- Complete blood count (CBC)
- Endoscopy
- Bleeding scan
- Arteriography

TREATMENT

- Depends on etiology and severity
- Bleeding varices are ligated, tamponaded, or sclerosed via endoscopy (see hepatobiliary system chapter).
- Most Mallory–Weiss tears resolve spontaneously.
- For severe bleeds:
  - Intravenous fluids and blood products as needed.
  - Somatostatin (inhibits gastric, intestinal, and biliary motility, decreases visceral blood flow).
  - Consider balloon tamponade for esophageal varices.
- Surgery:
  - Some 5% of the time, UGI bleeding cannot be controlled via endoscopic or other methods and emergent laparotomy will be necessary.
  - For duodenal ulcers, a longitudinal incision is made across the pylorus and proximal duodenum. Bleeding is controlled by undersewing the vessel on either side of the hemorrhage.

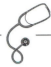

A bleeding scan detects active bleeding by infusing a radioactive colloid or radiolabeled autologous red blood cells (RBCs) and watching for their collection in the GI tract.

Risk of ulcers rebleeding:
- In-hospital: One third.
- GUs are 3 times more likely to rebleed than DUs.

BARIATRIC SURGERY

INDICATION

For morbid obesity, defined as 100 lb above ideal body weight or body mass index > 40 (weight per body surface area in kg/m²) with medical complications, associated with the excess weight

CRITERIA

Participation in supervised dietary program without success *and* morbid obesity.

TYPES

Vertical Banded Gastroplasty (VBG)
- Partitioning of the stomach into a small proximal pouch (< 20 mL) and a more distal one (see Figure 12-3).
- As soon as proximal pouch becomes distended, signal is sent to hypothalamus that satiety has occurred, so patient feels full and stops eating.
- Results in smaller quantity of food consumed in one sitting and delayed gastric emptying.

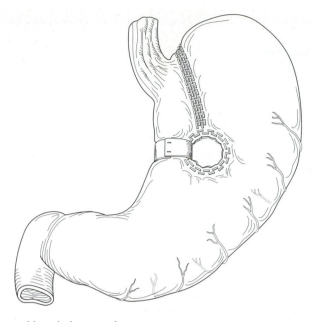

FIGURE 12-3. Vertical banded gastroplasty.

- Advantage of this procedure is that it does not alter anatomy or physiology of GI tract, as pyloric control of stomach emptying is not disturbed.
- Disadvantage—higher recurrence rate

Roux-en-Y Gastric Bypass

- Bypass surgery of stomach, duodenum, and first part of jejunum (100 cm of bowel bypassed) (see Figure 12-4)
- Advantage: Produces greater weight loss
- Disadvantage: Associated with more complications than VBG, including dumping syndrome, stomal ulcer or stenosis, pernicious and iron deficiency anemia

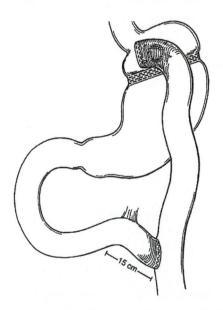

FIGURE 12-4. Roux-en-Y gastric bypass. Jejunum is transected 15 cm past ligament of Treitz. (Reproduced, with permission, from Strauss, Gastric bypass of adolescents with morbid obesity. *J. Pediatr* (138):4; April 2001.)

Adenocarcinoma

EPIDEMIOLOGY

- Highest incidence in age > 60 years.
- Adenocarcinoma comprises 95% of malignant gastric cancer.
- Male predominance.
- Leading cause of cancer-related death in Japan.

RISK FACTORS

- Familial adenomatous polyposis
- Chronic atrophic gastritis
- *H. pylori* infection (6× increased risk)
- Post-partial gastrectomy (15+ years)
- Pernicious anemia
- Diet (foods high in nitrites—preserved, smoked, cured)
- Cigarette smoking

Duodenal ulcer disease may be protective against gastric cancer.

PATHOLOGY

- Polyploid: 25–50%, no substantial necrosis or ulceration
- Ulcerative: 25–50%, sharp margins
- Superficial spreading: 3–10%, involves mucosa and submucosa only, best prognosis
- Linitis plastica: 7–10%, involves all layers, extremely poor prognosis

SIGNS AND SYMPTOMS

- Early: Mostly asymptomatic.
- Late: Anorexia/weight loss, nausea, vomiting, dysphagia, melena, hematemesis; pain is constant, nonradiating, exacerbated by food.
  - Anemia—from blood loss, pernicious
  - **Krukenberg's tumor**—metastasis to ovaries
  - **Blumer's shelf**—metastasis to pelvic cul-de-sac, felt on digital rectal exam
  - **Virchow's node**—metastasis to lymph node palpable in left supraclavicular fossa
  - **Sister Mary Joseph's nodule**—metastasis to the umbilical lymph nodes

DIAGNOSIS

- Upper GI endoscopy: Best method, allows for biopsy, definitive >95% sensitivity and specificity
- Upper GI series: With double contrast; 80–96% sensitivity, 90% specificity (operator dependent); excellent method in skilled hands
- Abdominal CT: Good for detecting distant metastases; also used for preop staging, but suboptimal
- Endoscopic ultrasound: Good for detecting depth of invasion

STAGING

See Table 12-1.

TABLE 12-1. Staging of colorectal cancer by the American Joint Committee on Cancer (TNM classification).[a]

Stage 0	Carcinoma in situ Tis N0 M0
Stage I	Tumor invades submucosa T1 N0 M0
Stage II	Tumor invades through muscularis propria into subserosa, or into nonperitonealized pericolic or perirectal tissues T3 N0 M0 Tumor perforates the visceral peritoneum or directly invades other organs or structures T4 N0 M0
Stage III	Any degree of bowel wall perforation with regional lymph node metastasis N1 1–3 pericolic or perirectal lymph nodes involved N2 4 or more pericolic or perirectal lymph nodes involved N3 Metastasis in any lymph node along a named vascular trunk Any T N1 M0 Any T N2, N3 M0
Stage IV	Any invasion of bowel wall with or without lymph node metastasis, but with evidence of distant metastasis Any T Any N M1

[a]Based on *American Joint Committee on Cancer Staging for Colorectal Cancer* (5th ed.). Lippincott, 1997. Dukes B (corresponds to stage II) is a composite of better (T3, N0, M0) and worse (T4, N0, M0) prognostic groups, as is Dukes C (corresponds to stage III) (any T, N1, M0) and (any T, N2, N3, M0).
T, tumor; N, node; M, metastasis.
Reproduced, with permission, from Friedman SL, McQuaid KR, Grendell JH, eds. *Current Diagnosis and Treatment in Gastroenterology*, 2nd ed. New York: McGraw-Hill, 2002: 424.

TREATMENT

- Radical subtotal gastrectomy can be curative in early disease confined to the superficial layers of the stomach (less than one third of all patients due to typical late presentation)
- Chemotherapy: Sometimes used palliatively for nonsurgical candidates; no role for adjuvant chemotherapy

PROGNOSIS

Prognosis depends on stage of disease. Overall 5-year survival is still only 5–15%.

Gastric Lymphoma

- Second most common malignant gastric cancer
- Comprise only 5% of all gastric tumors
- 5× risk with human immunodeficiency virus (HIV)
- Male predominance 1.7:1

SIGNS AND SYMPTOMS

Nonspecific; include abdominal discomfort, nausea, vomiting, anorexia, weight loss, and hemorrhage.

DIAGNOSIS

- Made by endoscopic biopsy, not readily distinguishable from adenocarcinoma by simple inspection.

- Bone marrow aspiration and gallium bone scans can diagnose metastases.

STAGING (ANN ARBOR CLASSIFICATION)

- Stage I: Disease limited to stomach
- Stage II: Spread to abdominal lymph nodes
- Stage III: Spread to lymph nodes above and below the diaphragm
- Stage IV: Disseminated lymphoma

TREATMENT

- MALT (low grade)—Treat *H. pylori*.
- MALT (high grade) or non-MALT—Radiation/chemo
- Resection reserved for patients with bleeding or perforation

PROGNOSIS

Poor prognostic factors include:
- Involvement of the lesser curvature of the stomach
- Large tumor size
- Advanced stage

Gastric Sarcoma

EPIDEMIOLOGY

- Equal incidence in men and women (unlike gastric adenocarcinoma or gastric lymphoma)
- Usual age at diagnosis is 65 to 70 years

HISTOLOGY

- Most are leiomyosarcomas.
- Spread is hematogenous treatment.
- Surgical resection.

PROGNOSIS

- Low-grade tumors: Five-year survival rate is ~80%
- High-grade tumors: Five-year survival rate is ~30%.

Carney triad:
- **Gastric leiomyosarcoma**
- **Pulmonary chondromas**
- **Extra-adrenal paraganglioma**
Syndrome seen in women under 40

BENIGN TUMORS (10%)

Adenomatous Polyps

- Account for 10–20% of all gastric polyps.
- Are the only ones with any real malignant potential, others are mostly asymptomatic and uncommon.
- Biopsy lesions > 5 mm to check for neoplasia.

Lipoma

- Majority found in antrum
- Most found incidentally on endoscopy
- No need to biopsy or excise unless enlarging—have very low malignant potential

The **"cushion sign"** on endoscopy: A lipoma will feel like a cushion or pillow when pressed with the forceps.

Ectopic Pancreas

- Rare.
- Often presents as "umbilicated dimple."
- Excise to exclude malignancy.

Ménètrier's Disease

DEFINITION

- Autoimmune disease causing a hypertrophic gastritis
- Protein-losing enteropathy
- Enlarged, tortuous gastric rugae
- Mucosal thickening secondary to hyperplasia of glandular cells replacing chief and parietal cells
- Low-grade inflammatory infiltrate—*not* a form of gastritis

SIGNS AND SYMPTOMS

Ménètrier's can look like gastric cancer on barium study.

- Epigastric pain
- Symptoms of protein-losing enteropathy
- Decreased gastric acid secretion
- Less commonly:
  - Nausea, vomiting
  - Anorexia, weight loss
  - Occult GI bleed

DIAGNOSIS

- Endoscopy with deep mucosal biopsy is definitive.
- Barium swallow will reveal large gastric folds and thickened rugae.

COMPLICATIONS

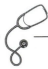

Monitor closely as there may be increased incidence of gastric cancer.

- Gastric ulcer
- Gastric cancer

TREATMENT

- Anticholinergics, H_2 blockers to reduce protein loss
- High-protein diet
- Treatment of ulcers/cancer if present
- Severe disease may require gastrectomy

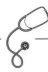

Anticholinergics are thought to reduce the width of tight junctions between gastric mucosal cells.

Bezoars

DEFINITION

- Concretions of nondigestible matter that accumulate in stomach.
- May consist of hair, vegetable matter (especially in patients who may have eaten persimmon), or charcoal (used in management of toxic ingestions)
- May develop after gastric surgery.

- Similar to gastric outlet obstruction
- Occasionally causes ulceration and bleeding

DIAGNOSIS

Upper GI endoscopy.

TREATMENT

- Proteolytic enzymes—papain
- Mechanical fragmentation with endoscope
- Surgical removal

Dieulafoy's Lesion

DEFINITION

Mucosal end artery that causes pressure necrosis and erodes into stomach and ruptures.

SYMPTOMS

Massive, recurrent painless hematemesis.

DIAGNOSIS

Upper GI endoscopy.

TREATMENT

- Endoscopic sclerosing therapy or electrocoagulation
- Wedge resection

GASTRIC DIVERTICULA

DEFINITION

Saccular outpouching through all three stomach layers.

SYMPTOMS

Majority are asymptomatic.

DIAGNOSIS

Upper GI contrast study.

TREATMENT

Diverticulectomy only if there are complications (hemorrhage, diverticulitis).

DEFINITION

Torsion/twisting of stomach typically along long axis. Often associated with paraesophageal hernia. May be acute, but most often chronic.

SYMPTOMS

- Intermittent severe epigastric pain and distention
- Inability to vomit
- Difficult passage of nasogastric (NG) tube

DIAGNOSIS

Upper GI contrast study.

TREATMENT

- Surgical repair of accompanying hernia
- Gastropexy—fixes stomach to anterior abdominal wall
- Gastric resection if there is necrosis

HIGH-YIELD FACTS

The Stomach

Small Bowel

GASTROINTESTINAL (GI) EMBRYOLOGY

Fourth Week

- Primitive gut begins to develop.
  - Endoderm becomes intestinal epithelium and glands.
  - Mesoderm becomes connective tissue, muscle, and wall of intestine.

Fifth Week

- Intestine elongates and midgut loop herniates through umbilicus.
- Midgut loop has cranial and caudal limbs:
  - *Cranial* limb becomes distal duodenum to proximal ileum.
  - *Caudal* limb becomes distal ileum to proximal two thirds transverse colon.

Tenth Week

Midgut loop returns to the abdominal cavity after rotating a total of 270 degrees.

GROSS ANATOMY

General

- Total length: 5 to 10 m (approximately 25 cm duodenum, 100 to 110 cm jejunum, 150 to 160 cm ileum); longest organ in GI tract.
- Duodenum has 4 parts:
  - First part—duodenal bulb: 5 cm long, site of most ulcers
  - Second part—descending duodenum: 10 cm long, associated with head of pancreas, becomes retroperitoneal
  - Third part—transverse duodenum
  - Fourth part—ascending duodenum to the ligament of Treitz
- Jejunum begins and duodenum ends at the *ligament of Treitz*.

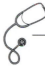

All of small intestine is derived from the midgut except for the proximal duodenum, which is derived from the foregut.

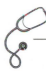

The vitelline duct joins the yolk sac at the junction of the cranial and caudal limbs of the midgut loop. It persists as *Meckel's diverticulum* in 2% of the population.

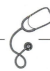

The midgut loop rotates a total of 270 degrees around the axis of the superior mesenteric artery before it reaches its final fixed position in the abdomen.

All of the small bowel is supplied by branches of the SMA except the proximal duodenum (which is supplied by branches from the celiac trunk).

The small bowel has an abundant collateral circulation via the vascular arcades that course through the mesentery.

One way to distinguish between the jejunum and ileum is by their arcades. The jejunum has few (1 to 2) arcades with long vasa recta, and the ileum has many arcades with short vasa recta.

- Duodenum is retroperitoneal and thus tethered to the posterior abdominal wall; it has no serosa at its posterior aspect.
- Prominent plicae circulares (transverse mucosal folds in the lumen of the small bowel) present throughout the distal duodenum and jejunum.

Vasculature

Small bowel consists of three sequential sections: Duodenum, jejunum, and ileum.

- Duodenum: Begins at pylorus and ends at the ligament of Treitz
  - Proximal: *Gastroduodenal artery* (first branch of proper hepatic artery); bifurcates caudally into the anterior superior and posterior superior pancreaticoduodenal arteries.
  - Distal: *Inferior pancreaticoduodenal artery* (branch of superior mesenteric artery [SMA]); bifurcates cranially into the anterior inferior and posterior inferior pancreaticoduodenal arteries.
  - Venous drainage:
    - Anterior and posterior pancreaticoduodenal veins drain into the superior mesenteric vein (SMV), which joins the splenic vein behind the neck of the pancreas to form the portal vein.
- Prepyloric vein is landmark for pylorus.
- Jejunum and ileum:
  - Jejunum is proximal 40% of small intestine distal to ligament of Treitz.
  - Ileum is remaining 60% of small intestine.
  - No clear boundaries between the two.
  - Combined length is 5 to 10 m.
  - Both supplied by branches of SMA.

Lymphatics

- Drainage: Bowel wall → mesenteric nodes → lymph node channels parallel to SMV → cisterna chyli (a retroperitoneal structure between the aorta and inferior vena cava [IVC])→ thoracic duct (also between the aorta and IVC) → left subclavian vein
- Participate in absorption of fat

Innervation

PARASYMPATHETIC SYSTEM

- Source: Fibers originate from vagus and celiac ganglia.
- Function: Enhances bowel secretion, motility, and other digestive processes.

SYMPATHETIC SYSTEM

- Source: Fibers originate from ganglion cells that reside in a plexus at the base of the SMA.
- Function: Opposes effects of parasympathetic system on bowel.

ENTERIC NERVOUS SYSTEM

- Source: Myenteric plexus, which consists of Meissner plexus at base of submucosa and Auerbach plexus between the inner circumferential and outer longitudinal layers of the muscle wall

- Function: Neural control of all GI function including motility, blood flow, secretion, and absorption. Facilitates digestion along with parasympathetic and sympathetic nervous systems.

GI MOTILITY

Peristalsis

- Intestinal contractions at a rate of 1 to 2 cm/sec.
- Main function is to move chyme through the intestine.
- Migrating myoelectric complexes (MMCs)
- Individual phasic contractions
- Migrating clustered complexes
- Giant migrating contractions
- Retrograde giant contractions

GI HORMONES

See Table 13-1.

DIGESTION

Major Stages of Digestion

Three major stages: Intraluminal, intestinal (mucosal), and transport.

INTRALUMINAL STAGE

- Prepares ingested nutrients for absorption.
- Hydrolysis of food by salivary, pancreatic, and gastric enzymes.
- Fats and fat-soluble enzymes hydrolyzed by bile salts.
- Fatty acids and monoglycerides form micelles, facilitating uptake at brush border.

INTESTINAL (MUCOSAL) STAGE

- Includes final digestion of carbohydrates and protein and absorption of nutrients by epithelial cells.
- Carbohydrates hydrolyzed by brush border oligosaccharidases and disaccharidases.
- Peptides hydrolyzed by brush border and intracellular peptidases.
- Enterokinase, a brush border enzyme, activates trypsinogen (secreted by the pancreas) to trypsin, which in turn converts many other pancreatic enzymes to their active form within intestinal lumen.

TRANSPORT STAGE

Involves lymphatic transport of fats via the lacteals and portal system and transport of protein and carbohydrate breakdown products.

Typical scenario: A 70-year-old male with a history of peripheral vascular disease and hyperlipidemia presents to the emergency department with severe, diffuse abdominal pain. His blood pressure is 170/100 and his pulse is 90 bpm. Supine abdominal radiograph shows air within the wall of the small intestine. What is the most likely diagnosis? *Think:* Small bowel infarction.

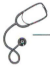

Sympathetic nerves inhibit GI motility by decreasing acetylcholine release.

Since > 93% of ingested fat is normally absorbed, > 6 g of fecal fat collected over a 24-hour time period in a diet with 100 g of lipid ingested per day would be defined as *steatorrhea*.

TABLE 13-1. Hormones of the GI tract.

Hormone	Site of Release	Action	Stimulated By	Inhibited By
Gastrin	Antrum	■ Gastric acid secretion ■ Cell growth	■ Vagus ■ Food in antrum ■ Gastric distention ■ Calcium	■ Antral pH < 2.0 ■ Somatostatin
Cholecystokinin (CCK)	Duodenum	■ Gallbladder contraction stimulates pancreatic acinar cell growth ■ Inhibits gastric emptying	■ Polypeptides ■ Amino acids ■ Fat ■ Hydrochloride (HCl)	■ Chymotrypsin ■ Trypsin
Secretin	Duodenum	■ Stimulates pancreatic secretion of H_2O and HCO_3 ■ Bile secretion of HCO_3 ■ Pepsin secretion ■ Inhibits gastric acid secretion	■ Low pH (acid) ■ Intraluminal duodenal fat	■ High duodenal pH
Somatostatin	Pancreas	■ Increases small bowel reabsorption of H_2O and electrolytes ■ Inhibits cell growth; GI motility; gallbladder contraction; pancreatic, biliary, and enteric secretion of gastric acid; and secretion/action of all GI hormones	■ Intraluminal fat ■ Gastric and duodenal mucosa ■ Catecholamines	■ Acetylcholine release
Pancreatic polypeptide	Pancreas	■ Clinical usefulness of pancreatic polypeptide is limited to being a marker for other endocrine tumors of the pancreas	■ Cephalic—vagus ■ Gastric—reflexes ■ Intestinal—food in small bowel	
Neurotensin	Small bowel/colon	■ Pancreatic secretion ■ Vasodilation ■ Inhibits gastric acid secretion	■ Fat	
Peptide YY	Small bowel/colon	■ Inhibits gastric acid secretion, pancreatic exocrine secretion, and migrating myoelectric complexes (MMCs)		
Glucagon	Small bowel/colon	■ Increases glycogenolysis, lipolysis, gluconeogenesis	■ Low serum glucose	■ Somatostatin
Motilin		■ Inhibits MMCs ■ Increases gastric emptying ■ Increases pepsin secretion	■ Vagus ■ Fat ■ Intraduodenal alkaline environment	■ Pancreatic polypeptide

Absorption Overview

See Table 13-2.

Intestinal Immune Function

- Gut is largest immune organ in human body.
- Immunoglobulin A (IgA) is most prevalent type of immunoglobulin in lumen of GI tract, part of initial immune defense.
- Lymphoid nodules, mucosal lymphocytes, and isolated lymphoid follicles in appendix and mesenteric lymph nodes together constitute the mucosa-associated lymphoid tissue (MALT).
- Lymphoid tissue throughout small intestine and colon lies within mucosa and submucosa, producing broad dome-like projections into intestinal lumen.

Short-chain fatty acids, unlike carbohydrates, are absorbed in the large intestine and can be used as an alternative energy source for persons who suffer from carbohydrate malabsorption.

TABLE 13-2. Absorption in the small intestine.

	Duodenum	Jejunum	Ileum
Water	+	+++	++
Sodium	+	+++	++
Potassium	+	+++	+
Chloride	+	++	+++
Fats	++	+++	+
Proteins	++	+++	+
Carbohydrates	++	+++	+
Bile salts	0	0	+++
Fat-soluble vitamins[a]	+	+++	+
Water-soluble vitamins			
Vitamin B$_{12}$	0	0	+++
Folic acid	+	+++	++
Ascorbic acid	?	+	+++
Minerals	+++	++	0
Iron	+++	++	0
Calcium	++	+++	+
Magnesium	+	++	++
Zinc[b]	0	+	++

[a] Vitamin K (endogenously produced fraction) absorbed in colon.
[b] Based on animal studies.
Reproduced, with permission, from Wilson JAP, Owyang C. Physiology of digestion and absorption. In: Nelson RL, Nyhus LM (eds.): *Surgery of the Small Intestine*. Appleton & Lange, 1987: 22.

Small Bowel

DEFINITION

Transmural inflammation of any part of the GI tract from mouth to anus, with affected areas neighboring unaffected ones, characterized by periods of clinical remission and progression. Unknown etiology but postulated to be caused by infection, genetic defect, or autoimmune process.

EPIDEMIOLOGY

- Most common surgical disease of small bowel
- Occurs in 3 to 6/100,000 people
- Incidence highest in northern climates and developed nations and lowest in southern climates and developing nations
- Approximately 500,000 persons with the disease in the United States

RISK FACTORS

- Jewish descent
- Urban dwelling
- Onset most common between 15 and 40 or 50 and 80 years of age (bimodal age distribution)
- Positive family history
- Smoking
- Diet high in refined sugar, nonsteroidal anti-inflammatory drug (NSAID) use, or oral contraceptive use (all are controversial)

SIGNS AND SYMPTOMS

- Diarrhea, weight loss, and fever
- Crampy abdominal pain
- Bleeding (hemoccult + stools common, but gross lower GI bleeding less common than in ulcerative colitis)(see Table 14-2)
- Perianal disease in up to one third of patients
- Signs and symptoms of intestinal perforation and/or fistula formation (e.g., combination of localized peritonitis, fever, abdominal pain, tenderness, and palpable mass on physical exam)

DIAGNOSIS

- Typical history of prolonged diarrhea with abdominal pain, weight loss, and fever with or without gross bleeding.
- Physical exam can be normal, nonspecific, or suggestive of Crohn's disease with perianal skin tags, sinus tracts, and a palpable abdominal mass.
- Clinch diagnosis by colonoscopy, esophagogastroduodenoscopy (EGD), and/or air-contrast barium enema, depending on suspected site of involvement.
- Radiographic evidence: Nodular contour of bowel; narrowed lumen, sinuses, and clefts; linear ulcers; asymmetrical involvement of bowel wall; string sign

TREATMENT

- Medical: Corticosteroids, aminosalicylates (sulfasalazine, 5-ASA), immune modulators (azathioprine, mercaptopurine, cyclosporine), metronidazole.

- Surgical: Most patients ultimately require surgical therapy, though physicians tend to avoid it as long as possible since Crohn's disease is not curable, and surgical resection of an affected area does not preclude future development in adjacent or distant parts of the bowel.
  - Indications: Complication such as obstruction, abscess, fistula, perforation, perianal disease, or cancer.
  - For strictures, stricturoplasty.
  - For fistulas, fistula resection; if patient is septic, excise grossly involved portion only followed by intraoperative open debridement.
  - For cancer, operate just as if the patient did not have Crohn's.

PROGNOSIS

- Typical course is one of intermittent exacerbations followed by periods of remission.
- Ten to 20% of patients experience prolonged remission after initial presentation.
- Approximately 80% of patients ultimately require surgical intervention.
  - Resection with anastomosis has 10–15% clinical recurrence rate per year.
  - Total colectomy with ileostomy has 10% recurrence rate over 10 years in remaining small bowel.

BENIGN NEOPLASMS OF SMALL INTESTINE

INCIDENCE

- Adenomas > leiomyomas > lipomas (but leiomyomas most likely to cause symptoms).
- Most common cause of adult intussusception.
- See Table 13-3 for individual small bowel tumor types.

RISK FACTORS

- Consumption of red meat and salt-cured foods
- Specific disease states:
  - Peutz–Jeghers syndrome (hamartomatous polyps)
  - Crohn's disease (adenocarcinoma)
  - Gardner syndrome (adenoma)
  - Familial adenomatous polyposis (adenoma)
  - Celiac disease (lymphoma, carcinoma)
  - Immunodeficiency states, autoimmune disorders (lymphoma)

SIGNS AND SYMPTOMS

- Intermittent obstruction
- Intussusception
- Occult bleeding
- Palpable abdominal mass
- Abdominal pain

DIAGNOSIS

- Majority of patients: Small bowel series with follow-through followed by enteroclysis or extended enteroscopy if negative
- High-risk patients: Enteroclysis

Typical scenario: A patient presents with pigmented spots on his lips and a history of recurrent colicky abdominal pain. What is the cause of his abdominal pain? *Think:* Peutz–Jeghers syndrome. The hamartomatous polyps are likely causing intermittent intussusception.

Enteroclysis is a double-contrast study that involves passing a tube into the proximal small intestine and injecting barium and methylcellulose. It can detect tumors missed on conventional small bowel follow-through. Extended small bowel enteroscopy (Sonde enteroscopy) is much like enteroclysis but involves advancement of the enteroscope by peristalsis. It visualizes up to 70% of the small bowel mucosa and detects tumors missed by enteroclysis.

TABLE 13-3. Benign neoplasms of the small intestine.

Type	Risk Factors	Signs and Symptoms	Location
Hamartoma		Recurrent colicky abdominal pain (from intermittent intussusception	
Adenoma (35% of benign small bowel tumors)	Gardner's syndrome Familial adenomatous polyposis	Obstruction Bleeding	Duodenum (20%) Jejunum (30%) Ileum (50%)
Hemangioma (3–4% of benign small bowel tumors)		Bleeding	
Fibroma		Obstruction Asymptomatic mass	
Lipoma		Obstruction Bleeding	Ileum
Leiomyoma		Obstruction Bleeding	Jejunum

- Other diagnostic modalities: Computed tomography (CT) scan, upper GI series, upper endoscopy (visualizes to duodenum), push endoscopy (extends visualization to proximal jejunum)

TREATMENT

Surgical, with segmental resection and primary anastomosis.

MALIGNANT NEOPLASMS OF SMALL INTESTINE

DESCRIPTION

Risk factors, signs and symptoms, and diagnosis essentially the same as benign neoplasms of small intestine (see Table 13-4).

TREATMENT

- Wide *en bloc* resection, including lymph nodes.
- Patients with duodenal lesions may require Whipple procedure.
- Bypass may be required for palliation.

PROGNOSIS

- Overall 5-year: ≤ 20%
- Survival by tumor type:
  - Periampullary carcinoma: 30–40%
  - Leiomyosarcoma: 30–40%
  - Non-Hodgkin's lymphoma: 30%

TABLE 13-4. Malignant neoplasms of the small intestine.

Type	Risk Factors	Signs and Symptoms	Location
Adenocarcinoma (25–50% of primary small bowel malignancies)	Crohn's disease	Obstruction Bleeding Mass	Duodenum; ileum
Carcinoid (up to 40% of primary small bowel malignancies)		Often asymptomatic Obstruction Carcinoid syndrome	Ileum
Lymphoma	Celiac disease Immunosuppression Autoimmune disease	Fatigue Weight loss Pain Obstruction Mass Bleeding	Ileum
Sarcoma		Obstruction Pain Bleeding	Jejunum; ileum; Meckel's diverticulum
Neuroendocrine		Mass Hormone-specific symptoms	Proximal small intestine
Metastatic	History of melanoma, breast, lung, ovarian, colon, or cervical cancer		Obstruction; bleeding

CARCINOID

DEFINITION

- Malignant tumor of enterochromaffin cell origin, part of APUD (amine precursor uptake and decarboxylation) system.

INCIDENCE

- Peak incidence between 50 and 70 years of age
- Occurs with same frequency as adenocarcinoma but has variable malignant potential:
  - > 90% diagnosed in GI system
  - 46% in appendix (but 3% metastasize)
  - 28% in ileum (but 35% metastasize)
  - 17% in rectum
  - 30–40% present with multiple lesions

SIGNS AND SYMPTOMS

- Frequently asymptomatic.
- Slow growing.
- Most common symptom is abdominal pain.

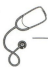

The carcinoid syndrome develops when the tumor produces amines and peptides outside of the portovenous circulation. Classically, appendiceal and small intestinal carcinoids cause the carcinoid syndrome only after they have metastasized to the liver.

Typical scenario: A 60-year-old male presents with a history of cutaneous flushing, diarrhea, wheezing, and an unintentional 15-lb weight loss. *Think:* Carcinoid syndrome; the wheezing is a clue that the lesion may be endobronchial. Order a 24-hour urine 5-HIAA level to confirm the diagnosis.

- Obstruction; rectal bleeding (from rectal carcinoid), pain, weight loss.
- Carcinoid syndrome: 10% of cases:
  - Due to production of serotonin, bradykinin, or tryptrophan by tumor and exposure of products to systemic circulation prior to breakdown by the liver
  - Characterized by cutaneous flushing, diarrhea, valvular lesions (right > left), and bronchoconstriction

DIAGNOSIS

- Most found incidentally during appendectomy or surgery for intestinal obstruction
- If patient has carcinoid syndrome, increased 5-HIAA (hydroxyindolacetic acid) or 5-HTP (hydroxytryptophan; indicates bronchial location) in 24-hour urine collection clinches diagnosis
- Otherwise diagnosed as any other small bowel neoplasm

TREATMENT

- Medical: Serotonin antagonists (e.g., cyproheptadine) or somatostatin analogues (e.g., octreotide) for symptoms of carcinoid syndrome.
- Surgical:
  - Appendiceal carcinoid < 2 cm: Appendectomy
  - Appendiceal carcinoid > 2 cm: Right hemicolectomy
- Small intestinal carcinoid: Resect tumor with mesenteric lymph nodes.
- Otherwise, resect tumor and any solitary liver metastasis considered resectable.

PROGNOSIS

- Overall survival roughly 54%.
- Five-year survival after palliative resection is 25%; after curative resection is 70%.

FISTULA

DEFINITION

A communication between two epithelialized cavities.

RISK FACTORS

- Previous abdominal surgery (most common)
- Diverticular disease
- Crohn's disease
- Colorectal cancer

SIGNS AND SYMPTOMS

- If associated with an abscess, can be accompanied by fever and leukocytosis
- Drainage of succus entericus (bowel contents) from skin (enterocutaneous)
- Diarrhea (entero-enteric; especially if between proximal and distal small bowel or colon)
- Pneumaturia and symptoms of urinary tract infection (UTI) (enterovesicular)

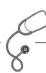

Proximal fistulas cause more problems than distal fistulas because the draining contents are more acidic, more fluids and electrolytes are lost, and more absorptive material is lost.

DIAGNOSIS

- CT
- Cystoscopy
- Colonoscopy
- Gastrograffin enema
- Small bowel follow-through

TREATMENT

- Localize site and extent of fistula and determine whether distal obstruction present.
- Consider percutaneous drainage to help protect skin.
- Consider somatostatin for high-output fistulas (does not change rate of closure of fistula but does decrease loss of volume and electrolytes).
- Bowel rest.
- IV antibiotics until clinical improvement.
- If 6 weeks pass without improvement, resect tract and consider proximal ostomy if abscess found.

PROGNOSIS

Mortality at least 20%.

Factors that can keep a fistula tract open: **FRIEND**
Foreign body
Radiation
Inflammation
Epithelialization
Neoplasm
Distal obstruction

SMALL BOWEL OBSTRUCTION (SBO)

DEFINITION

Cessation, impairment, or reversal of the physiologic transit of intestinal contents secondary to a mechanical or functional cause.

TYPES

- Open loop obstruction: Flow is blocked but proximal decompression is possible.
- Closed loop obstruction:
  - Inflow and outflow both blocked
  - Seen with incarcerated hernia, torsion, adhesions, volvulus
  - Requires emergent surgery

ETIOLOGY

Mechanical

- Intraluminal (gallstone ileus, foreign body, intussusception)
- Intramural (Crohn's disease, lymphoma, radiation enteritis)
- Extrinsic (adhesion, hernia, cancer, abscess, congenital)

Functional (Paralytic Ileus)

- Hypokalemia
- Peritonitis
- Ischemia
- Medications (opiates, anticholinergics)
- Hemoperitoneum
- Retroperitoneal hematoma
- Postoperative

The most common causes of small bowel obstruction are extrinsic: **ABC**
Adhesions
Bulge (hernias)
Cancer

RISK FACTORS

- Previous abdominal surgery (most common risk factor in United States)
- Hernia
- Inflammatory bowel disease
- Diverticular disease
- Cholelithiasis
- Ingested foreign body

SIGNS AND SYMPTOMS

- Colicky abdominal pain
- Abdominal distention
- High-pitched bowel sounds
- Nausea
- Vomiting

DIAGNOSIS

- Usually clear from history and physical examination.
- Confirm by supine and upright abdominal x-rays: Dilated loops of small intestine without evidence of colonic distention on supine x-ray; multiple air–fluid levels in a "stepladder" arrangement on upright films (Figure 13-1).
- CT scan sometimes helpful when x-rays are nondiagnostic (Figure 13-2).
- Strangulated bowel (in which the vascular supply to a segment of intestine is compromised) can lead to intestinal infarction and requires im-

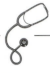

"Never let the sun rise or set on an SBO" (unless the patient is postop, has carcinomatosis, known Crohn's disease, or partial small bowel obstruction).

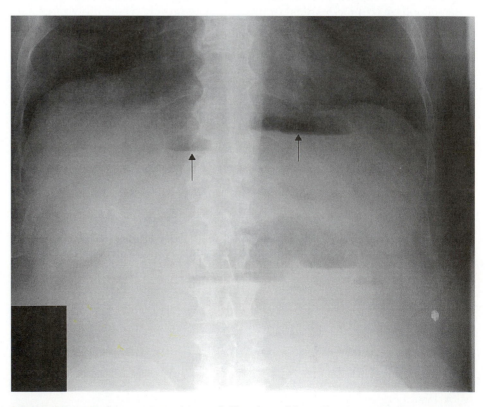

FIGURE 13-1. AXR demonstrating loops of dilated small bowel in the midabdomen, suggestive of small bowel obstruction.

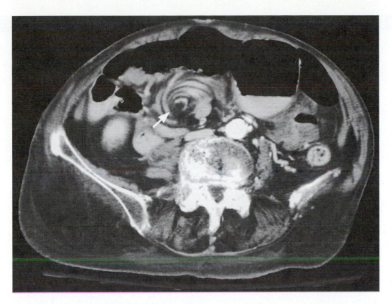

FIGURE 13-2. Contrast abdominal CT scan demonstrating midgut volvulus as a cause of small bowel obstruction.

mediate laparotomy. Classic signs include fever, tachycardia, leukocytosis, and constant, noncramping abdominal pain.

- Upright chest radiograph: A sensitive way to detect free air under the diaphragm and thus detect bowel perforation.

TREATMENT

If the patient is stable or has partial small bowel obstruction, give a trial of nonoperative management:

- IV hydration.
- NPO.
- Nasogastric tube (NGT) decompression.
- Check upright abdominal x-ray (AXR) for dilated loops of small bowel, air–fluid levels, gas in colon and rectum.
- Check electrolytes, especially for hypokalemic, hypochloremic metabolic alkalosis.

If the patient fails conservative management (a day passes, fever develops, or abdomen becomes increasingly tender), perform an exploratory laparotomy.

- Adhesions call for LOA (lysis of adhesions).
- Hernias should be repaired or, if contents of sac are strangulated, resected.
- Cancer requires en bloc resection with lymph node sampling.
- Crohn's disease requires resection or stricturoplasty of affected area only.

There are no clinical or laboratory parameters that can reliably differentiate between simple small bowel obstruction and strangulated bowel.

Typical scenario: A 5-year-old child presents with increasing irritability, colicky abdominal pain, and rectal bleeding with stools that have a currant jelly appearance. A tubular mass is palpated in the right lower quadrant. Upright abdominal x-ray shows air–fluid levels with a stepladder pattern. *Think:* Intussusception. Barium enema is both diagnostic and therapeutic.

Large Bowel

Embryology

- Origin: Embryonic midgut (up to mid-transverse colon) and hindgut (rest of colon, proximal anus, and lower genitourinary [GU] tract). Distal anus derives from ectoderm.
- Development of midgut: Discussed in small bowel chapter.
- Development of hindgut: Cloaca divided in the sixth week into ventral UG sinus and dorsal rectum by the anorectal septum.
- Development of anus: Formed by the eighth week from ectoderm. The *dentate line* marks the transition between hindgut and ectoderm.

Gross Anatomy

See Figure 14-1.

COLON

- Extends from the ileocecal valve to the rectum and consists of: right colon, transverse colon, left colon, sigmoid colon.
- Three to five feet in length.
- Cecum is widest; the colon progressively narrows distally.
- Unlike the small intestine, the colon has taenia coli, haustra, and appendices epiploicae (fat appendages that hang off antimesenteric side of colon).
- The taenia coli—three distinct bands of longitudinal muscle—converge at the appendix and spread out to form a longitudinal muscle layer at the proximal rectum.
- Retroperitoneal attachments of ascending and descending colon fix it to the posterior abdominal wall.
- Retroperitoneal: Ascending colon, descending colon, posterior hepatic and splenic flexures.
- Intraperitoneal: Cecum, transverse colon, sigmoid colon.
- Long mesentery of transverse colon enables it to hang in dependent position in abdomen.
- One end of omentum attaches to anterior–superior aspect of transverse colon; other end attaches to stomach.

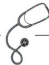

In development, the midgut loop rotates 270° counterclockwise around the axis of the superior mesenteric artery (SMA). Developmental anomalies may include malrotation or failure of right colon to elongate.

The blood supply is based on embryology:
- Midgut: SMA
- Hindgut: Inferior mesenteric artery (IMA)
- Distal anus: Internal pudendal artery branches

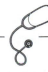

The ileocecal valve functions to prevent reflux of bowel contents from the cecum back to the ileum.

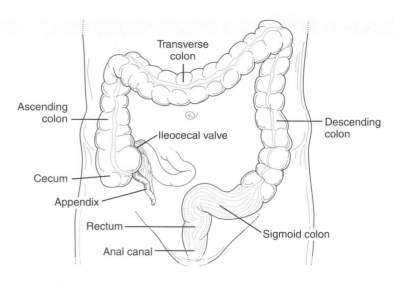

FIGURE 14-1. Bowel anatomy.

Large Bowel

The anatomy and physiology of the colon affect how colon cancers typically present. Because the colon progressively narrows distally and functions physiologically to absorb water, left-sided colon cancers tend to present with a change in bowel habits (e.g., small-caliber stools), obstruction, and hematochezia (gross blood). To the contrary, right-sided colon cancers tend to present in a more indolent fashion with microcytic anemia, fatigue, and melena (dark, tarry stools) because the proximal colon has a larger circumference and the stool is less solid.

RECTUM

- 12 to 15 cm in length
- Rectum has distinct peritoneal covering:
  - Anterior peritoneal reflection 5 to 9 cm above anus
  - Posterior peritoneal reflection 12 to 15 cm above anus
  - Upper third of rectum: Covered anteriorly and laterally by peritoneum
  - Middle third of rectum: Covered anteriorly by peritoneum
  - Lower third of rectum: No peritoneum
- Fascia:
  - Waldeyer's fascia: Rectosacral fascia that extends from S4 vertebral body to rectum
  - Denonvilliers' fascia: Anterior to lower third of rectum
- Pelvic floor: Levator ani (composed of pubococcygeus, iliococcygeus, and puborectalis muscles); innervated by S4 nerve

ANUS

- Anal canal runs from pelvic diaphragm to anal verge (junction of anoderm and perianal skin).
- Dentate line: A mucocutaneous line that separates proximal, pleated mucosa from distal, smooth anoderm (1 to 1.5 cm above anal verge).
- Anal mucosa proximal to dentate line lined by columnar epithelium; mucosa distal to dentate line (anoderm) lined by squamous epithelium and lacks glands and hair.
- Columns of Morgagni: 12 to 14 columns of pleated mucosa superior to the dentate line separated by crypts.
- Anal sphincter:
  - Internal: Consists of specialized rectal smooth muscle (from inner circular layer); involuntary, contracted at rest, responsible for 80% of resting pressure
  - External: Consists of 3 loops of voluntary striated muscle; a continuation of puborectalis muscle; responsible for 20% of resting pressure and 100% of voluntary pressure.

Blood Supply

ARTERIAL

- **Superior mesenteric artery (SMA):** Supplies the cecum, ascending colon, and proximal two thirds of the transverse colon via the ileocolic, right colic, and middle colic arteries, respectively
- **Inferior mesenteric artery (IMA):** Supplies the distal two thirds of the transverse colon, sigmoid colon, and superior rectum via the left colic, sigmoidal, and superior rectal (hemorrhoidal) arteries, respectively
- **Internal iliac artery:** Supplies the middle and distal rectum via the middle rectal and inferior rectal arteries, respectively (the inferior rectal artery is a branch of the internal pudendal artery)
- **Internal pudendal artery:** Supplies the anus; is a branch of the internal iliac artery

VENOUS

- **Superior mesenteric vein (SMV):** Drains the cecum and ascending and transverse colon before joining the splenic vein
- **Interior mesenteric vein (IMV):** Drains the descending colon, sigmoid colon, and proximal rectum before joining the splenic vein
- **Internal iliac vein:** Drains the middle and distal rectum
- **Middle rectal vein:** A branch of the internal iliac vein; drains upper anus
- **Inferior rectal vein:** A branch of the internal pudendal vein; drains lower anus
- **Hemorrhoidal complexes:** Three complexes within the anus that drain into the superior rectal veins and one external complex that drains into the pudendal veins

Lymphatic Drainage

- Lymphatics of the colon, rectum, and anus generally follow the arterial supply, with several levels of nodes as one moves centrally toward the aorta (e.g., ileocolic nodes, superior mesenteric nodes, etc.).
- Tumor metastases generally move from one lymph node group to another in a centripetal fashion.
- Lymph node groups of colon (from lateral to medial):
  - Epicolic
  - Paracolic
  - Intermediate (named according to the artery they follow)
  - Main (around SMA and IMA)

Innervation

- Derives primarily from autonomic nervous system
- Sympathetic nerves:
  - T7–T12 for right colon, L1–L3 for left colon and rectum
  - Inhibit peristalsis
- Parasympathetic nerves:
  - Vagus nerve for proximal colon, sacral nerves (S2–S4) for distal colon
  - Stimulate peristalsis

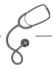

The rectum has two major angles that play a significant role in continence. The first angle is formed at the origin of the rectum at the sacral promontory as it bends posteriorly and inferiorly, following the curve of the sacrum. The second angle, the anorectal angle, is formed by the puborectalis muscle as it joins the anus, pulling the rectum forward. A Valsalva maneuver enhances these angles, closing off the rectum.

Anal canal above dentate line drains to IM nodes or to internal iliac nodes. Lower anal canal drains to inguinal nodes.

Histology

From inner lumen to outer wall:
- Colon: Mucosa, submucosa, inner circular muscle layer, outer longitudinal muscle (taenia coli)
- Rectum: Mucosa, submucosa, inner circular muscle, outer longitudinal muscle (confluent)
- Anus: Anoderm (epithelium that is richly innervated, but without secondary skin appendages)

Microbiology

- Colon sterile at birth; normal flora established shortly thereafter
- Normal flora: 99% anaerobic (predominantly *Bacteroides fragilis*); 1% aerobic (predominantly *Escherichia coli*)

PHYSIOLOGY

The rectum can store approximately 500 cc of feces.

General

- The colon and rectum have two primary physiologic functions:
  1. Absorption of water and electrolytes from stool
  2. Storage of feces

Motility

Auerbach's plexus primarily inhibits colonic activity.

- Characterized by three types of contractions:
  1. Retrograde movements: From transverse colon to cecum, these movements slow the transit of luminal contents, thereby prolonging their exposure to absorptive epithelium.
  2. Segmental contractions: The most common variety, these are localized simultaneous contractions of the longitudinal and circular muscles of the colon.
  3. Mass movements:
     - Contractions of long segments of colon that are 30 seconds in duration and result in antegrade propulsion of luminal contents at a rate of 0.5 to 1 cm/sec.
     - Occur 3 to 4 times each day, especially after waking up or after eating, and may result in bowel movements.
- Neuronal control of colon:
  1. Extrinsic: Parasympathetic and sympathetic (as described above)
  2. Intrinsic (from mucosa to bowel wall): Mucosa, *submucosal (Meissner's) plexus*, circular muscle layer, *myenteric (Auerbach's) plexus*, longitudinal muscle layer, *subserosal plexus*, serosa

Constipation consists of the ability to pass flatus but the inability to pass stool, whereas *obstipation* refers to the inability to pass flatus or stool.

Defecation

1. Mass movement causes feces to move into rectal vault.
2. Sampling reflex: Rectal distention leads to involuntary relaxation of internal sphincter, allowing descent of rectal contents and sensation of feces at transitional zone.

3. Voluntary relaxation of external sphincter pushes contents down anal canal.
4. Voluntary increase in intra-abdominal pressure assists in propelling rectal contents out of anus.

Flatus

- Voluntary contraction of pelvic floor muscles (puborectalis and external sphincter) causes selective passage of gas with retention of stool.
- Gas:
  - Components are N_2, O_2, CO_2, H^+, CH_4; these gases are odorless.
  - Odor due to trace substances (dimethyl sulfide and methanethiol).
  - Approximately 600 cc/day normally produced.

DISORDERS OF MOTILITY

Irritable Bowel Syndrome (IBS)

DEFINITION

Abnormal state of intestinal motility modified by psychosocial factors for which no anatomic cause can be found.

INCIDENCE

Affects up to 17% of U.S. population, 2 females:1 male, young adults.

SIGNS AND SYMPTOMS

Episodes of altered bowel function (constipation, diarrhea, or both) occurring intermittently over a prolonged period of time with or without abdominal pain.

DIAGNOSIS

History with symptoms exacerbated by physical or emotional stress; must first exclude organic disease.

TREATMENT

- Not a surgical disease
- Reassurance, education, and medical treatment for refractory symptoms of anxiety and/or depression

Constipation

- Definition < 3 stools/week while consuming high-fiber diet.
- Diagnosis: By history; differentiate between acute constipation (persistent change in bowel habits for < 3 months), and chronic constipation (persistent change in bowel habits > 3 months).

CAUSES

- Diet-related (fluid, fiber)
- Lack of physical activity

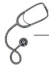

IBS is often regarded as a wastebasket diagnosis for a change in bowel habits along with complaints of abdominal pain after other causes have been excluded.

- Medications (especially opiates and anticholinergics)
- Medical illness (irritable bowel syndrome, diabetes, hypothyroidism)
- Depression
- Neurologic disease (Parkinson's disease, multiple sclerosis)
- Many other causes

TREATMENT

- Short-term: Stool softeners; Fleet's enema if suppository fails.
- Long-term: After ruling out a treatable cause, encourage dietary changes such as increasing fiber and fluid consumption.
- If dietary changes fail, assess colonic transit time. Defecography or anometry may prove helpful.

Surgical consultation is frequently obtained for **fecal impaction:**
- Typically older, often institutionalized adults, with history of chronic constipation, and no bowel movements reported for several days.
- On exam, abdomen is distended and rectal vault is filled with hard stool.

TREATMENT

- Manual disimpaction.
  - Complications: When disimpaction is not successful or the patient presents too late, perforation may occur (stercoral ulcer), causing fecal peritonitis and sepsis. Urgent laparotomy is required.
- Followed by enemas, stool softeners.
- Recommend increasing dietary fiber.

Diarrhea

DEFINITION

- Passage of >three loose stools/day.
- Surgeons are likely to encounter diarrhea in post-op patients. In the hospitalized patient, a workup may be indicated to rule out infectious or ischemic etiologies. In the outpatient follow-up setting, diarrhea may occur due to extensive small bowel resection (short bowel syndrome), due to disruption of innervation, or even as an expected outcome (gastric bypass).

DIAGNOSIS

- Stool sample for enteric pathogens and *Clostridium difficile* toxin.
- Check stool for white blood cells (WBCs) (IBD or infectious colitis), red blood cells (RBCs) without WBCs (ischemia, invasive infectious diarrhea, cancer).

TREATMENT

Individualized based on the treatable cause, and is addressed with the specific problems that may cause diarrhea (colitis, ischemia).

Postvagotomy diarrhea occurs in 20% of patients after truncal vagotomy. Denervation of the extrahepatic biliary tree and small intestine leads to rapid transit of unconjugated bile salts into the colon, impeding water absorption and causing diarrhea. Cholestyramine is the medical treatment. If that fails, surgical reversal of a segment of the small intestine to prolong transit time and increase absorptive capacity may be considered.

Fecal Incontinence

DEFINITION

- True incontinence: Complete loss of solid stools
- Minor incontinence: Flatus or occasional soilage of undergarments from seepage or urgency

SIGNS AND SYMPTOMS

Decreased resting tone and squeeze pressure on rectal examination; rule out other anorectal pathology such as hemorrhoids or rectal prolapse.

ETIOLOGY

- Mechanical: Anal sphincter trauma (i.e., secondary to childbirth or iatrogenic, s/p fistulotomy for abscess or perianal fistula)
- Systemic disease (scleroderma)
- Fecal impaction
- Neurogenic: Pudendal nerve injury

DIAGNOSIS

- Anal manometry: Detects resting and squeeze pressures of internal and external sphincters
- Endoanal ultrasound: More accurate; detects occult lesions
- Pelvic floor electromyography: Differentiates between anatomic and neurogenic incompetence
- Pudendal nerve terminal motor latency testing: Predicts likely success of surgical repair

COLITIS

Infectious

PSEUDOMEMBRANOUS COLITIS

- Definition: An acute colitis characterized by formation of an adherent inflammatory exudate (pseudomembrane) overlying the site of mucosal injury.
- Typically occurs after antibiotics, especially clindamycin, ampicillin, or cephalosporins.
- Due to overgrowth of *Clostridium difficile*.
- Signs and symptoms: Vary from a self-limited diarrheal illness to invasive colitis with megacolon or perforation as possible complications.
- Diagnosis: Detection of *C. difficile* toxin in stool; proctoscopy or colonoscopy if diagnosis uncertain.
- Treatment: Stop offending antibiotic; give flagyl or vancomycin PO (if patient unable to take PO, give flagyl IV).
- Prognosis: High rate of recurrence (20%) despite high response rate to treatment.

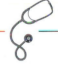

Patients with *C. difficile* colitis should be placed on contact isolation, as infection is contagious.

ACTINOMYCOSIS (*ACTINOMYCES ISRAELII*)

- Definition: Infection of the gastrointestinal (GI) tract (usually the ileocecal region) with *A. israelii* classically after appendectomy

- Signs and symptoms: Weight loss, night sweats, draining fistulas, and an abdominal mass
- Diagnosis: Characteristic "sunburst" pattern of sulfur granules on histopathologic evaluation; culture
- Treatment: Surgical drainage and antibiotics (tetracycline or penicillin)

NEUTROPENIC

- Definition: A syndrome characterized by diffuse mucosal ulceration, invasive infection with enteric organisms, and sepsis
- Incidence: Occurs in cancer patients receiving chemotherapy, particularly those with acute myelogenous leukemia (AML) or aplastic anemia
- Signs and symptoms: Fever, abdominal pain (and/or PSBO), and diarrhea in a patient with < 100 neutrophils/mL; patients frequently septic
- Diagnosis: Diarrhea in appropriate clinical setting; cecal edema sometimes noted on computed tomography (CT) scan
- Treatment: Bowel rest, IV fluids, and broad-spectrum antibiotics; surgery only if complications (e.g., perforation) arise

Radiation Induced

See Table 14-1.

- Associated with external radiation therapy (XRT) to pelvis usually for endometrial, cervical, prostate, bladder, and rectal cancer
- Risk factors: Atherosclerosis, diabetes, hypertension, old age, adhesions from previous abdominal operation
- Chance of developing disease is dose dependent:

< 4,000 cGy	0 patients
5,000–6,000 cGy	Some patients
> 6,000 cGy	Most patients

TABLE 14-1. Radiation-induced colitis.

	Early (During Course of XRT)	Late (Weeks to Years Later)
Signs and symptoms	Nausea, vomiting, cramps, diarrhea, tenesmus, rectal bleeding	Tenesmus, bleeding, abscess, fistula involving rectum (rectal pain, stool per vagina)
Diagnosis	Plain abdominal films, barium enema	Barium enema, CT scan
Etiology	Mucosal edema, hyperemia, acute ulceration	Submucosal arteriolar vasculitis, microvascular thrombosis, wall thickening, mucosal ulceration, strictures, perforation
Treatment	Treat symptoms. If no improvement, decrease dose of XRT or discontinue treatment	Treat with stool softener, topical 5-ASA, corticosteroid enema ■ Strictures: Gentle dilatation or diverting colostomy after excluding cancer ■ Rectovaginal fistula: Proximal colostomy and low colorectal anatomosis or coloanal temporary colostomy

Ischemic

DEFINITION

Acute or chronic intestinal ischemia secondary to decreased intestinal perfusion or thromboembolism:

- Embolus or thrombus of the inferior mesenteric artery
- Poor perfusion of mucosal vessels from arteriole shunting or spasm

INCIDENCE

Ninety percent of cases occur in patients > 60 years of age.

RISK FACTORS

- Old age
- s/p Abdominal aortic aneurysm (AAA) repair
- Hypertension
- Coronary artery disease
- Diabetes
- Adhesions from previous abdominal surgery
- Underlying obstructive lesion of colon

SIGNS AND SYMPTOMS

- Mild lower abdominal pain and rectal bleeding, classically after AAA repair
- Pain more insidious in onset than small bowel ischemia

DIAGNOSIS

Clinical history; characteristically shows "thumbprinting" on barium enema (but contrast enema is contraindicated in the setting of suspected bowel gangrene).

TREATMENT

If symptoms mild, observe; if moderate (with fever and increased WBC), give IV antibiotics; if severe (with peritoneal signs), exploratory laparatomy with colostomy.

Ischemic colitis often affects the splenic flexure.

A 70-year-old white male with a history of hypertension develops cramping lower abdominal pain 2 days s/p AAA repair. A few hours later he develops bloody diarrhea. What's the diagnosis? *Think:* Ischemic colitis should be suspected in any elderly patient who develops acute abdominal pain followed by rectal bleeding. Furthermore, the most common setting for ischemic colitis is the early postoperative period after AAA repair when impaired blood flow through the inferior mesenteric may put the colon at risk.

INFLAMMATORY BOWEL DISEASE: ULCERATIVE COLITIS

DEFINITION

Inflammation confined to mucosal layer of colon that extends from the rectum proximally in a continuous fashion.

INCIDENCE

Highest in third and fourth decades of life; whites 4× > nonwhites; industrialized nations >> developing nations

RISK FACTORS

- Jewish descent
- White race
- Urban dwelling
- Age between 15 and 40 or 50 and 80 (bimodal age distribution)
- Positive family history

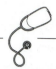

Both ulcerative colitis (UC) and Crohn's disease can present with bloody diarrhea, but bloody diarrhea is more common in UC.

- Diet high in refined sugar, NSAID use, or oral contraceptive use (all are controversial)
- Nicotine *decreases risk* (unlike Crohn's disease)

SIGNS AND SYMPTOMS

Two characteristic presentations:
- Insidious, recurrent abdominal pain, anorexia, weight loss, and mild diarrhea
- Acute onset of *bloody diarrhea*, abdominal pain ± tenesmus, vomiting, and fever

DIAGNOSIS

- Endoscopy with histolopathologic evaluation of biopsies
- Barium enema: "Lead pipe" appearance of colon classic but no longer test of choice

TREATMENT

- Medical: Similar to Crohn's (see Table 14-2):
  - Mild/moderate disease: 5-ASA, corticosteroids PO or per rectum
  - Severe disease: IV steroids
  - Proctitis: Topical steroids
  - Refractory disease: Immunosuppression
- Surgical:
  - Indications: Failure of medical therapy, increasing risk of cancer in long-standing disease, bleeding, perforation
  - Procedure: Proctocolectomy (curative)
  - If patient is acutely ill and unstable, due to perforation, a diverting loop colostomy is indicated. Once stabilized, the patient may undergo a more definitive operation.

TABLE 14-2. Ulcerative colitis vs. Crohn's disease.

	Ulcerative Colitis	Crohn's Disease
Pathology	■ Inflammation of the **mucosa only** (exudate of pus, blood, and mucus from the "crypt abscess") ■ Always **starts in rectum** (up to one third don't progress)	■ Inflammation involves **all bowel wall layers,** which is what may lead to fistulas and abscess ■ Rectal sparing in 50%
Diagnosis	■ Continuous lesions ■ Rare ■ **Lead pipe colon** appearance due to chronic scarring and subsequent retraction and loss of haustra	■ **Skip lesions:** Interspersed normal and diseased bowel ■ **Aphthous ulcers** ■ **Cobblestone** appearance. From submucosal thickening interspersed with mucosal ulceration
Complications	■ Perforation ■ Stricture ■ Megacolon	■ Abscess ■ Fistulas ■ Obstruction ■ Perianal disease

PROGNOSIS

Approximately 10% risk of cancer at 10 years, and 2%/year thereafter.

DIVERTICULAR DISEASE

DEFINITION

- Herniation of the mucosa and submucosa through the muscular layers of the bowel wall at sites where arterioles penetrate, forming small outpouchings or diverticula.
- Diverticula occur on the mesenteric side of the colon.
- Are generally numerous and collectively referred to as diverticulosis.

INCIDENCE

- > 50% of Americans over 70 years of age
- Men and women equally affected
- Sigmoid colon most commonly involved with progressively decreasing frequency of involvement as one proceeds proximally

RISK FACTORS

- Old age
- Low-fiber diet

SIGNS AND SYMPTOMS

Diverticulosis
- 80% of patients asymptomatic.
- May cause recurrent, intermittent left lower quadrant (LLQ) pain and tenderness that often follows a meal and is relieved by flatus or defecation.
- LLQ rope-like mass sometimes palpable on exam.
- **Massive lower GI bleeding is classic** (notably absent in diverticulitis).

Diverticulitis
- Persistent abdominal pain initially diffuse in nature that often becomes localized to the LLQ with development of peritoneal signs
- LLQ and/or pelvic tenderness
- Ileus
- Fever, anorexia, nausea, vomiting, and change in bowel habits (usually constipation)
- Elevated WBC

DIAGNOSIS

Diverticulosis
- Characteristic history and physical exam confirmed by diverticula identified on barium enema and/or colonoscopy.
- See section on lower GI bleed (LGIB) for management of patients with this presentation.

Diverticulitis
- Characteristic history and physical exam with elevated WBCs
- Abdominal x-ray: Ileus, distention, and/or free intraperitoneal air

Unless all the colonic and rectal mucosa is removed, the patient is still at risk for cancer.

Recommend colonscopy after 7 years of pancolitis, after 10 years of left-sided colitis, then scope and biopsy every 1 to 2 years.

The diverticula of common diverticulosis are *false* diverticula, because only the mucosa and submucosa herniated rather than all the layers of the bowel wall.

Pathology of diverticulitis: A peridiverticular inflammation caused by (usually tiny) perforation of the diverticulum secondary to increased pressure or obstruction by inspissated feces. Feces extravasate onto the serosal surface but infection is usually well contained in a patient with normal immune function.

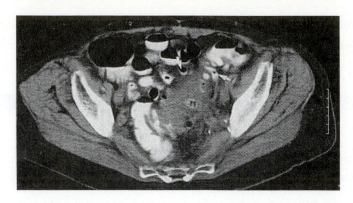

FIGURE 14-2. CT scan demonstrating multiple small sigmoid diverticuli (arrows). (Reproduced, with permission, from Gupta H & Dupuy DE: *Surg Clin North Am* 6(77); December 1997.)

- CT scan: Pericolonic inflammation with or without abscess formation (barium enema and colonoscopy may induce perforation and are contraindicated in the acute setting but should be obtained in follow-up) (see Figure 14-2)

TREATMENT

- Diverticulosis:
  - High-fiber diet, stool softeners.
- Mild diverticulitis:
  - Outpatient management: Clear liquid diet, PO antibiotics, and non-opioid analgesics with close follow-up.
  - Follow-up includes colonoscopy and dietary recommendations once acute infection has subsided.
- If outpatient therapy fails, admit for IV antibiotics and IV hydration with bowel rest. Nasogastric tube (NGT) is placed when there is evidence of ileus or small bowel obstruction (SBO), with nausea and vomiting.
- Severe diverticulitis with peritonitis and/or perforation: Two-stage procedure with initial surgical drainage and diverting colostomy followed by colonic reanastomosis 2 to 3 months later.
- Elective resection of affected bowel may be considered in the patient who has recurrent episodes of diverticulitis requiring treatment.

PROGNOSIS

- Seventy percent of patients have no recurrence after one episode of uncomplicated diverticulitis.
- After a second episode, 50% recur.

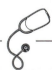

Ten to 25% of LGIBs eventually require surgery despite the fact that 85% of bleeds initially stop spontaneously.

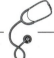

An extensive operation is indicated when no site is identified in an unstable patient because although < 10% will rebleed, the mortality for those 10% is approximately 30%.

LOWER GI BLEED (LGIB)

DEFINITION

- Bleeding of an origin distal to the ligament of Treitz. LGIB is considered massive when the patient requires 3 or more units of blood within 24 hours.

- Most common causes are diverticulosis and angiodysplasia. Other causes include IBD, ischemic colitis, cancer, and anticoagulation treatment.

MANAGEMENT

See Table 14-3.

TABLE 14-3. Management of lower GI bleeding (LGIB).

	Diverticulosis	Angiodysplasia
Incidence	50% of patients are > 60	25% of patients are > 60 Adult men > adult women
Character	Painless 75% of bleeding from right colon	Cecum and ascending colon
Quantity and rate	Massive and rapid	Slow
Signs and symptoms	Melena and/or hematochezia often with symptoms of orthostasis	
Diagnosis	<ul><li>First rule out upper GI bleeding with nasogastric lavage</li><li>To identify site of bleed:</li></ul>1. Colonoscopy 2. ≥ 0.5 mL/min: Bleeding scan with Tc-sulfur colloid identifies bleeding; label lasts for up to 24 hours so a patient can be easily rescanned when rebleeding occurs after a negative initial scan 3. ≥ 1 mL/min: Angiography (selective mesenteric angiography best method to diagnose angiodysplasia) Colonoscopy	
Treatment	1. Resuscitation 2. Therapeutic options if site identified: Octreotide, embolization, vasoconstriction with epinephrine, vasodestruction with alcohol or sodium compounds, or coagulation/cautery with heat 3. If site identified but bleeding massive or refractory, segmental colectomy 4. Without identification of bleeding site and persistent bleeding in an unstable patient, total abdominal colectomy with ileostomy	
Cause	Disruption of arteriole at either dome or antimesenteric neck of diverticulum (almost always on mucosal side, so bleed occurs into lumen rather than into peritoneal cavity)	Chronic intermittent obstruction of submucosal veins secondary to repeated muscular contractions results in dilated venules with incompetent precapillary sphincters and thus arteriovenous communication
Prognosis	10% overall mortality	

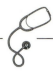

The three most common causes of obstruction of the large bowel are adenocarcinoma (65%), scarring secondary to diverticulitis (20%), and volvulus (5%).

Ogilvie syndrome is associated with any severe acute illness, neuroleptics, opiates, malignancy, and certain metabolic disturbances.

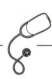

In Ogilvie syndrome, pharmacologic decompression of the bowel with neostigmine is particularly useful because diagnosis with contrast enema or colonoscopy can be exceedingly difficult without bowel decontamination.

LARGE BOWEL OBSTRUCTION

INCIDENCE

Most commonly occurs in elderly patients; much less common than small bowel obstruction.

SIGNS AND SYMPTOMS

- Abdominal distention
- Cramping abdominal pain
- Nausea, vomiting
- Obstipation
- High-pitched bowel sounds

DIAGNOSIS

- Supine and upright abdominal films: Distended proximal colon, air–fluid levels, and no distal rectal air.
- Establish 8- to 12-hour history of obstipation; passage of some gas or stool indicates partial small bowel obstruction, a nonoperative condition.
- Barium enema: May be necessary to distinguish between ileus and pseudo-obstruction

TREATMENT

1. Correction of fluid and electrolyte abnormalities.
2. NGT for intestinal decompression.
3. Broad-spectrum IV antibiotics (e.g., cefoxitin).
4. Relieve obstruction surgically (colonic obstruction is a surgical emergency since a nasogastric tube will not decompress the colon)

PSEUDO-OBSTRUCTION (OGILVIE SYNDROME)

DEFINITION

Massive colonic dilation without evidence of mechanical obstruction thought to result from an imbalance between parasympathetic and sympathetic control of intestinal motility.

INCIDENCE

More common in older, institutionalized patients.

RISK FACTORS

Severe infection, recent surgery or trauma.

SIGNS AND SYMPTOMS

Marked abdominal distention with mild abdominal pain and decreased or absent bowel sounds.

DIAGNOSIS

- Abdominal radiograph with massive colonic distention.
- Check for free air under diaphragm with upright chest x-ray (CXR).

- Exclude mechanical cause for obstruction with water-soluble contrast enema and/or colonoscopy.

TREATMENT

1. NGT and rectal tube for proximal and distal decompression, respectively.
2. Correction of electrolyte abnormalities.
3. Discontinue narcotics, anticholinergics, or other offending medications.
4. Turn patient frequently and mobilize from bed.
5. Consider pharmacologic decompression with neostigmine (a cholinesterase inhibitor).
6. If the cecal diameter is > 11 cm or if peritoneal signs develop, the patient should undergo prompt exploratory laparotomy with cecostomy or loop colostomy.

VOLVULUS

DEFINITION

Rotation of a segment of intestine about its mesenteric axis; characteristically occurs in the sigmoid colon (70% of cases) or cecum (30%).

INCIDENCE

> 50% of cases occur in patients over 65.

RISK FACTORS

- Elderly (especially institutionalized patients)
- Hypermobile cecum secondary to incomplete fixation during intrauterine development (cecal volvulus)

SIGNS AND SYMPTOMS

Same as other causes of large bowel obstruction.

DIAGNOSIS

- Abdominal films: Markedly dilated sigmoid colon or cecum with a "kidney bean" appearance
- Barium enema: Characteristic "bird's beak" at areas of colonic narrowing

TREATMENT

- Cecal volvulus: Right hemicolectomy if vascular compromise; cecopexy otherwise adequate (suturing the right colon to the parietal peritoneum)
- Sigmoid volvulus (see Figure 14-3):
  1. Sigmoidoscopy with rectal tube insertion to decompress the volvulus.
  2. Emergent laparotomy if sigmoidoscopy fails or if strangulation or perforation is suspected.
  3. Elective resection at a later date to prevent recurrence (40% of cases recur after nonoperative reduction).

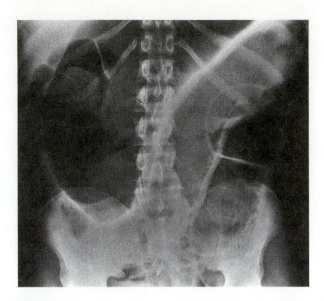

FIGURE 14-3. Abdominal x-ray shows a grossly distended coffee bean–shaped loop of bowel in the right upper quadrant, findings that are typical of a sigmoid volvulus. (Reproduced, with permission, from Rozycki GS et al. *Annals of Surgery* 5(235); May 2002. Lippincott Williams & Wilkins.)

BENIGN TUMORS OF THE LARGE BOWEL

Colorectal Polyps

MORPHOLOGY

Broadly divided into sessile (flat) and pedunculated (on a stalk).

HISTOLOGIC TYPES

1. Inflammatory (pseudopolyp): Seen in UC
2. Lymphoid: Mucosal bumps containing intramucosal lymphoid tissue; no malignant potential
3. Hyperplastic: Overgrowth of normal tissue; no malignant potential
4. Adenomatous: Premalignant; are classified (in order of increasing malignant potential) as tubular (75%), tubulovillous (15%), and villous (10%)
5. Hamartomatous: Normal tissue arranged in abnormal configuration; juvenile polyps, Peutz–Jeghers polyps

INCIDENCE

Thirty to 40% of individuals over 60 in the United States.

SIGNS AND SYMPTOMS

- Asymptomatic (most common)
- Melena
- Hematochezia
- Mucus
- Change in bowel habits

Malignant potential of a polyp is determined by: size, histologic type, and epithelial dysplasia.

SIZE	RISK of CA
< 1 cm	1–3%
1–2 cm	10%
>2 cm	40%

HISTOLOGY	RISK
Tubular	5%
Tubulovillous	20%
Villous	40%

ATYPIA	RISK
Mild	5%
Moderate	20%
Severe	35%

DIAGNOSIS

Flexible endoscopy (sigmoidoscopy or colonoscopy)

TREATMENT

- Attempt colonoscopic resection if: Pedunculated, well or moderately well differentiated, no venous or lymphatic invasion, invades only into stalk, margins negative.
- Otherwise, a segmental colon resection is indicated.

POLYPOSIS SYNDROMES

See Table 14-4.

COLORECTAL CARCINOMA (CRC)

INCIDENCE

- Second most common cause of cancer deaths overall (behind lung cancer).
- 130,000 new cases and 55,000 deaths each year.
- Incidence increases with increasing age starting at age 40 and peaks at 60 to 79 years of age.
- See Table 14-5 for screening recommendations from the U.S. Preventative Services Task Force.

RISK FACTORS

- Age > 50
- Personal history of resected colon cancer or adenomas
- Family history of colon cancer or adenomas
- Low-fiber, high-fat diet
- Inherited colorectal cancer syndrome (familial adenomatous polyposis [FAP], hereditary nonpolyposis colon cancer [HNPCC])
- Long-standing UC or Crohn's disease

ADENOMA–CARCINOMA SEQUENCE

Normal → hyperproliferative → early adenoma → intermediate adenoma → late adenoma → carcinoma (→ metastatic disease)

1. APC loss or mutation
2. Loss of DNA methylation
3. Ras mutation
4. Loss of DCC gene
5. Loss of p53

SIGNS AND SYMPTOMS

- Typically asymptomatic for a long period of time; symptoms, if present, depend on location and size
- Right-sided cancers: Occult bleeding with melena, anemia, and weakness

At diagnosis of CRC:
10% in situ disease
One third local disease
One third regional disease
20% metastatic disease

Microcytic anemia in an elderly male or postmenopausal woman is colon cancer until proven otherwise.

TABLE 14-4. Polyposis syndromes of the bowel.

Syndrome	Inheritance Pattern	Risks/Associated Findings

Familial polyposis coli (FAP)	Autosomal dominant	■ Polyps develop between the second and fourth decades; colon cancer inevitable without prophylactic colectomy
		■ Caused by abnormal gene on chromosome 5
		■ Indication for operation: Polyps
		■ Operations
		  1. Proctocolectomy with Brooke's ileostomy
		  2. Proctocolectomy with continent ileostomy
		  3. Colectomy with ileorectal anastomosis
		  4. Proctocolectomy with ileal pouch—anal anastomosis

Gardner's syndrome	Autosomal dominant	Innumerable polyps with associated osteomas, epidermal cysts, and fibromatosis; colon cancer inevitable without surgery
Turcot's syndrome	Autosomal recessive	Multiple adenomatous colonic polyps with central nervous system (CNS) tumors (especially gliomas)
Cronkite–Canada syndrome	None	GI polyposis with alopecia, nail dystrophy, and hyperpigmentation; minimal malignant potential
Peutz–Jeghers syndrome	Autosomal dominant	Hamartomatous polyps of the entire GI tract with melanotic pigmentation of face, lips, oral mucosa, and palms; increased risk for cancer of the pancreas, breast, lung, ovary, and uterus
Hereditary nonpolyposis colon cancer syndrome (HNPCC or Lynch syndrome)	Autosomal dominant	Lynch syndrome I: Patients without multiple polyps who develop predominantly right-sided colon cancer Lynch syndrome II: Same as Lynch I but additional risk for extracolonic adenocarcinomas of the uterus, ovary, cervix, and breast

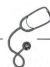

Rule out metastases from colorectal cancer with CXR, CT of abdomen and pelvis, and liver function tests. Measure carcioembryonic antigen (CEA) to establish a baseline level.

- Left-sided cancers: Rectal bleeding, obstructive symptoms, change in bowel habits and/or stool caliber
- Both: Weight loss, anorexia

DIAGNOSIS

- Colon cancer: Flexible sigmoidoscopy or colonoscopy (need to evaluate entire colon and rectum to look for synchronous lesions), barium enema

TABLE 14-5. Screening recommendations from U.S. Preventative Services Task Force, March 2000.

Screening Measure/Condition	Recommended Cancer Screening Measure(s)/Treatment
Digital rectal examination	Every year after 40
Fecal occult blood test	Every year after 50
Flexible sigmoidoscopy	Every 5 years after 50, with fecal occult blood test (FOBT)
Colonoscopy	Every 10 years
Persons at high risk for colon cancer (FAP, HNPCC, UC, high-risk adenomatous polyps)	Regular endoscopic screening by a specialist
Follow-up after resection of colorectal carcinoma (CRC)	▪ Perioperative colonoscopy to remove any synchronous cancer ▪ Colonoscopy 1 year postop and yearly thereafter to look for metachronous lesions ▪ Colonoscopy 3 years after one negative test ▪ Colonoscopy every 5 years once a 3-year test is negative

- Rectal cancer: Digital rectal exam, proctoscopy/colonoscopy, barium enema, also consider transrectal ultrasound (TRUS), CT, or magnetic resonance imaging (MRI) to assess depth of local tumor invasion and local lymph node status.

TREATMENT

- Surgical resection (see Table 14-6):
    - Goal is to remove primary tumor along with lymphatics draining involved bowel.
    - Involves at least a 2-cm margin both proximally and distally (traditionally requires a 5-cm margin).
    - In rectal cancer, the circumferential radial margin (CRM) is crucial to local recurrence. A recent study found local recurrence to be 55% in patients with a positive CRM, 28% with a margin < 1 mm, and 10% with a margin > 1 mm. (Birbeck et al. *Annals of Surgery* 235(4): 449–457, 2002)

    Adjuvant treatment:
    - Dukes C colon cancer: 5-FU and levamisol or 5-FU and leucovorin
    - Fixed rectal cancer: Preop XRT
    - Rectal cancer that is transmural or has positive nodes: Pelvic radiation, using 5-FU as a radiosensitizer

STAGING AND PROGNOSIS

Dukes System
A: Limited to wall
B: Through wall of bowel but not to lymph nodes
C: Metastatic to regional lymph nodes
D: Distant mets

Typical scenario: A 65-year-old male presents complaining of rectal bleeding and increasing constipation with thinning of stool caliber. A barium enema is performed (see Figure 14-4). What is the most likely diagnosis? *Think:* This elderly individual is at risk for colon cancer, and his obstructive symptoms likely indicate that it is left-sided. The "apple core" filling defect in the descending colon on barium enema is classic for left-sided colon cancer.

CRC 5-year survival by stage:
Stage I: T1N0M0/T2N0M1 (74%)
Stage II: T3N0M0/T4N0M0 (63%)
Stage III: anyTN1M0/anyTN2-3M0 (46%)
Stage IV: anyT anyN M1 (5%)

Rectal cancer: 5-year survival
I: 72%
II: 54%
III: 39%
IV: Rare

Local recurrence after resection with intent to cure is 5–30%, with total mesorectal excision, 3.5%. Recurrence may require pelvic exenteration.

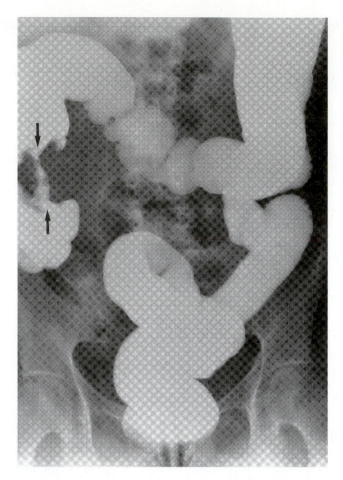

FIGURE 14-4. Apple core filling defect of colon cancer seen on barium enema. (Reproduced, with permission, from Schwartz, *Principles of Surgery*, 7th ed., Fig. 26–72, New York: McGraw Hill, p. 1347.)

TNM system
T1: Invasion of submucosa
T2: Invasion of muscularis propria
T3: Invasion of subserosa, or nonperitonealized pericolic or perirectal tissues
T4: Invasion of visceral peritoneum or direct invasion of other organs
N0: No nodal disease
N1: 1 to 3 pericolic or perirectal lymph nodes
N2: 4 or more pericolic or perirectal lymph nodes
N3: Involvement of any lymph node along the course of a named vessel
M0: No evidence of distant mets
M1: Distant mets

TABLE 14-6. Operative management of CRC based on tumor location.

Tumor Location	Operation
Cecum	Right hemicolectomy: ■ Resection of terminal ileum, cecum, ascending and proximal transverse colon ■ Ligation of ileocolic, right colic, and right branch of middle colic arteries
Right colon	Right hemicolectomy
Proximal/mid-transverse colon	Extended right hemicolectomy: ■ Resection as above plus remainder of transverse colon and splenic flexure ■ Ligation of ileocolic, right colic, and middle colic artery
Splenic flexure and left colon	Left hemicolectomy: ■ Resection through descending colon ■ Ligation of left colic artery
Sigmoid or rectosigmoid colon	Sigmoid colectomy: ■ Ligation of inferior mesenteric artery (IMA) distal to takeoff of left colic artery including sigmoidal and superior rectal arteries
Proximal rectum	**Low anterior resection (LAR):** ■ Tumors > 4 cm from anal verge (with distal intramural spread < 2 cm) ■ Must be able to get 2-cm margin ■ Includes total mesorectum excision ■ Involves complete mobilization of rectum, with division of lateral ligaments, posterior mobilization through Waldeyer's fascia to tip of coccyx, dissection between rectum and vagina or prostate ■ Complications: Incontinence, urinary dysfunction, sexual dysfunction, anastomotic leak (5–10%), stricture (5–20%)
Distal rectum	**Abdominal–perineal resection (APR):** ■ Tumors not fitting criteria for LAR ■ Involves creation of end ostomy, with resection of rectum, total mesorectal excision (TME), and closure of anus ■ Complications: Stenosis, retraction or prolapse of ostomy, perineal wound infection
Other situations	■ Obstructing cancer: Attempt to decompress ■ Perforated cancer: Remove disease and perforated segments ■ Synchronous or metachronous lesions, or proximal perforation with distal ca: Subtotal colectomy with ileosigmoid or ileorectal anastomosis ■ Very distal rectal tumor and/or patient not stable for big operation: Transanal excision of tumor, endoscopic microsurgery, or endocavitary radiation

HIGH-YIELD FACTS

Large Bowel

Hemorrhoids

See Table 14-7.

- Prolapse of the submucosal veins located in the left lateral, right anterior, and right posterior quadrants of the anal canal
- Classified by type of epithelium: **Internal** if covered by columnar mucosa (above dentate line), **external** if covered by squamous mucosa (below dentate line), and **mixed** if both types of epithelia are involved
- Incidence: Male = female
- Risk factors: Constipation, excessive diarrhea, pregnancy, increased pelvic pressure (ascites, tumors), portal hypertension
- Diagnosis: Visualize with anoscope

Anal Fissure

DEFINITION

Painful linear tears in the anal mucosa below the dentate line induced by constipation or excessive diarrhea.

SIGNS AND SYMPTOMS

- Pain with defecation
- Bright red blood on toilet tissue
- Markedly increased sphincter tone and extreme pain on digital examination
- Visible tear upon gentle lateral retraction of anal tissue

TABLE 14-7. Grade description, syptoms, and treatments of hemorrhoids.

	Grade Description	Symptoms	Treatment
I	Protrudes into lumen, no prolapse	Bleeding	Nonresectional measures[1]
II	Prolapse with straining, spontaneous return	Bleeding, perception of prolapse	Nonresectional measures
III	Prolapse, requires manual reduction	Bleeding, prolapse, mucous soilage, pruritus	Consider trial of nonresectional measures; many require excision
IV	Prolapse cannot be reduced	Bleeding, prolapse, mucous soilage, pruritus, pain[2]	Excision

[1] Nonresectional methods (rubber-band ligation, infrared coagulation, or injection sclerotherapy) can be used in insensate tissue only (above the dentate line).
[2] Pain if thrombosed or ischemic.
Reproduced, with permission, from Niederhuber JE. *Fundamentals of Surgery*. Stamford, CT: Appleton & Lange, 1998: 317.

DIAGNOSIS

History and physical exam.

TREATMENT

- Sitz baths.
- Fiber supplements.
- Increased fluid intake.
- If nonsurgical therapy fails, options include lateral internal sphincterotomy or forceful anal dilation (Lord procedure).

Anorectal Abscess

DEFINITION

Obstruction of anal crypts with resultant bacterial overgrowth and abscess formation within the intersphincteric space.

RISK FACTORS

- Constipation
- Diarrhea
- IBD
- Immunocompromise
- History of recent surgery or trauma
- History of colorectal carcinoma
- History of previous anorectal abscess

SIGNS AND SYMPTOMS

Rectal pain, often of sudden onset, with associated fever, chills, malaise, leukocytosis, and a tender perianal swelling with erythema and warmth of overlying skin.

TREATMENT

Surgical drainage.

Fistula In Ano

DEFINITION

Tissue tracts originating in the glands of the anal canal at the dentate line that are usually the chronic sequelae of anorectal infections, particularly abscesses.

CLASSIFICATION OF ANORECTAL FISTULAS

1. **Intersphincteric (70%):** Fistula tract stays within intersphincteric plane.
2. **Transsphincteric (25%):** Fistula connects the intersphincteric plane with the ischiorectal fossa by perforating the external sphincter.
3. **Suprasphincteric (4%):** Similar to transsphincteric, but the fistula loops above the external sphincter to penetrate the levator ani muscles.
4. **Extrasphincteric (1%):** Fistula passes from rectum to perineal skin without penetrating sphincteric complex.

Typical scenario: A 24-year-old male with chronic constipation complains of intense anal pain. He has a tender, swollen, bluish lump at the anal orifice. What is the treatment? *Think:* This young man's history of constipation and physical exam findings are classic for a thrombosed external hemorrhoid. The treatment is surgical excision if the pain has been present for less than 48 hours or is persistent. Pain typically subsides after 48 hours, and treatment is symptomatic.

Goodsall's rule can be used to clinically predict the course of an anorectal fistula tract. Imagine a line that bisects the anus in the coronal plane. Any fistula that originates anterior to the line will course anteriorly in a direct route. Fistulae that originate posterior to the line will have a curved path. Fistula tracts that diverge from this rule should increase one's suspicion for IBD.

RISK FACTORS

- History of ischiorectal abscess
- Crohn's disease
- Trauma
- Foreign body
- Tuberculosis (TB)
- Colorectal carcinoma

SIGNS AND SYMPTOMS

Recurrent or persistent perianal drainage that becomes painful when one of the tracts becomes occluded.

DIAGNOSIS

- Bidigital rectal exam
- Intrarectal ultrasound

TREATMENT

Intraoperative unroofing of the entire fistula tract with or without placement of setons (heavy suture looped through the tract to keep it patent for drainage and to stimulate fibrosis; subsequent opening of the tract after adequate fibrosis decreases risk of incontinence).

Pilonidal Disease

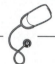

The terms *pilo* and *nidus* are Latin terms for "hair" and "origin," respectively, indicating that the lesion is associated with hair follicles. Pilonidal disease results from trauma to hair follicles in the gluteal region with resultant infection.

DEFINITION

A cystic inflammatory process generally occurring at or near the cranial edge of the gluteal cleft.

INCIDENCE

Most commonly seen in young men in their late teens to the third decade.

SIGNS AND SYMPTOMS

Can present acutely as an abscess (fluctuant mass) or chronically as a draining sinus with pain at the top of the gluteal cleft.

TREATMENT

- Acute abscess: Incision and drainage under local anesthesia with removal of involved hairs
- Chronic pilonidal sinuses overlying a cyst: Various surgical techniques that, when possible, keep the incision off of the midline

Anal Cancer

DEFINITION

Neoplasms of the anorectal region that are classified into tumors of the perianal skin (anal margin carcinomas) and tumors of the anal canal.

INCIDENCE

Rare (1–2% of all colon cancers); more common in women than men; average age 50 to 70.

RISK FACTORS

- Human papillomavirus (HPV)
- Human immunodeficiency virus (HIV)
- Cigarette smoking
- Multiple sexual partners
- Anal intercourse
- Immunosuppressed state

SIGNS AND SYMPTOMS

Often asymptomatic; can present with anal bleeding, a lump, or itching; an irregular nodule that is palpable or visible externally (anal margin tumor) or a hard, ulcerating mass that occupies a portion of the anal canal (anal canal tumor).

DIAGNOSIS

- Surgical biopsy with histopathologic evaluation.
- Histology: Anal margin tumors include squamous and basal cell carcinomas, Paget's disease, and Bowen's disease. Anal canal tumors are usually epidermoid (squamous cell carcinoma or transitional cell/cloacogenic carcinoma) or malignant melanoma.
- Clinical staging: Involves history, physical exam, proctocolonoscopy, abdominal or pelvic CT or MRI, CXR, and liver function tests.

TREATMENT

- Squamous cell carcinoma—nigro protocol—radiation and chemo; surgery is reserved for recurrence.
- Other anal margin tumors: Wide local excision alone or in combination with radiation and/or chemotherapy is successful in 80% of cases without abdominal–perineal resection (APR) if tumor is small and not deeply invasive.
- Anal canal tumors: Local excision not an option; combined chemotherapy (5-FU and mitomycin C) with radiation often successful; APR only if follow-up biopsy indicates residual tumor.

PROGNOSIS

- Anal margin tumors: 80% overall 5-year survival
- Anal canal tumors:
  - Epidermoid carcinoma: 50% overall 5-year survival
  - Malignant melanoma: 10–15% 5-year survival

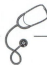

Two unique in situ tumors of the perianal skin are Paget's disease and Bowen's disease. Paget's disease of the anus is adenocarcinoma in situ, and anal Bowen's disease is squamous carcinoma in situ.

The Appendix

EMBRYOLOGY AND DEVELOPMENT

- The appendix buds off from the cecum beginning at about the sixth week of life. During ante- and postnatal development, the growth rate of cecum exceeds that of the appendix. Appendix is displaced medially/proximally toward ileocecal valve
- Whereas the base of the appendix is constant in position, the tip can be in varioius locations with differing clinical implications (see acute appendicitis below).

Lymphoid Tissue

- First appears 2 weeks after birth.
- Grows through puberty.
- Remains constant for 1 decade postpuberty.
- Decreases steadily with age.
- By 60 years of age it's gone, and complete obliteration of lumen is common.

LAYERS OF COLON WALL

- Mucosa, submucosa, inner circular muscle, outer longitudinal muscle, serosa
- Longitudinal muscle: Separated into three distinct bands called teniae coli
- Positioned 120° apart about the circumference of the colon
- **Appendices epiploicae:** Fatty appendages attached to the teniae

BLOOD SUPPLY

Superior mesenteric artery (SMA) to the ileocolic artery to appendicular artery.

LANDMARKS

- Three teniae coli converge at the junction of the cecum and appendix (they disappear at the rectum and sacral promontory).
- **Fold of Treves:** Ileal fold just proximal to the ileocecal valve, contains the only antimesenteric fatty appendage on the small bowel.

SIZE

- Length ranges from 2 to 20 cm, averages 6 to 9 cm
- Luminal capacity is approximately 0.1 mL (*Note:* There is no real lumen.)

ANATOMIC VARIANCES

- Absence
- Duplication
- Diverticula

FUNCTION

- Immunologic organ that secretes immunoglobulins (especially IgA).
- Integral part of gut-associated lymphoid tissue (GALT) system.
- Not an essential organ (vestigial).
- Appendectomy isn't associated with predisposition to sepsis or any other immunological compromise.
- In children, prophylactic appendectomy should be considered when undergoing abdominal surgery during which the appendix will be incidentally exposed.

ACUTE APPENDICITIS

INCIDENCE

- One of the most common acute surgical diseases.
- Incidence parallels lymphoid development with the peak in early adulthood.
- More frequent in males 1.3:1 (especially during puberty).
- There is a second peak in the incidence of appendicitis in the elderly.
- Eighty-four percent of all appendectomies are performed for acute pathology.

CAUSES OF LUMINAL OBSTRUCTION

- Lymphoid hyperplasia
- Fecalith (30%)

- Foreign objects (e.g., inspissated Ba^{2+} from previous x-ray study, vegetable and fruit seeds)
- Stricture (tumor)
- Parasites (especially *Ascaris* spp.)

PROBABLE SEQUENCE OF EVENTS WITH CLOSED LOOP OBSTRUCTION OF LUMEN

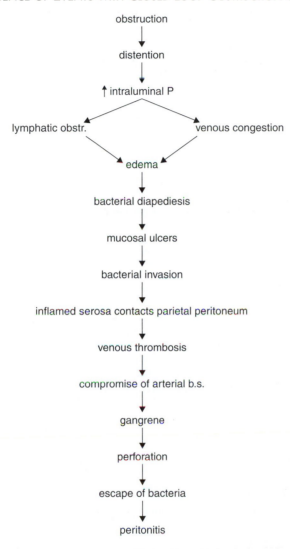

obstruction

↓

distention

↓

↑ intraluminal P

lymphatic obstr.   venous congestion

edema

↓

bacterial diapediesis

↓

mucosal ulcers

↓

bacterial invasion

↓

inflamed serosa contacts parietal peritoneum

↓

venous thrombosis

↓

compromise of arterial b.s.

↓

gangrene

↓

perforation

↓

escape of bacteria

↓

peritonitis

SYMPTOMS

- Abdominal pain that precedes vomiting (opposite of gastroenteritis)
- Pain intially diffuse, over epigastrium or umbilicus (periumbilical) then localizes to right lower quadrant (RLQ)
- Fever
- Leukocytosis

SIGNS

See Table 15-1.
- Direct rebound tenderness, maximal at or near McBurney's point
- Rovsing's sign: Pain in RLQ when palpation pressure is exerted in LLQ
- Iliopsoas sign: Pelvic pain upon extension of the right thigh (presence signifies retrocecal appendicitis)

Just 0.5 mL raises the appendiceal intraluminal pressure by ~60 cm H_2O.

The anatomic site of the tip of the appendix is responsible for the corresponding principal locus of somatic phase of pain:
- Long tip: Left lower quadrant (LLQ) pain
- Retrocecal: Flank or back pain
- Pelvic: Suprapubic pain
- Retroileal: Testicular pain (from irritation of spermatic art and ureter)
- Malrotation: Perplexing pattern of pain

McBurney's point: One third the distance along a line from the anterior superior iliac spine to the umbilicus

TABLE 15-1. Likelihood ratios (LRs) for signs and symptoms of appendicitis.

Sign/Symptom	Positive LR	Negative LR
Right lower quadrant (RLQ) pain	8.0	0.0–0.28
Rigidity	3.76	
Migration of pain (periumbilical→ RLQ)	3.2	0.5
Pain that precedes vomiting	2.8	
Psoas sign	2.38	
Fever	1.9	
Rebound tenderness	1.1–6.3	0.0–0.86
No similar pain previously		0.3

NOTE: LR is the amount by which the odds of a disease change with new information, as follows:

Likelihood ratio	Degree of change in probability
> 10 or < 0.1	Large (often conclusive)
5–10 or 0.1–0.2	Moderate
2–5 or 0.2–0.5	Small (but sometimes important)
– or 0.5–1	Small (rarely important)

Source: Hardin DM Jr: Acute Appendicitis: Review and Update, *American Family Physician* 1999;60: 2027–2034.

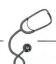

Things that lower the odds for appendicitis (low likelihood ratio [LR]–):
- Absence of RLQ pain
- History of similar pain in the past

Things that raise the odds for appendicitis (high LR+):
- Presence of RLQ pain

- Obturator sign: Pelvic pain upon internal rotation of the right thigh (presence signifies pelvic appendicitis)
- Dunphy's sign: Increased pain with coughing

DIFFERENTIAL DIAGNOSIS

- Gastroenteritis
- Ectopic pregnancy
- Mesenteric adenitis
- Meckel's diverticulum (see pediatric surgery chapter)
- Intussusception (see pediatric surgery chapter)
- Typhoid fever
- Regional enteritis
- Torsion and infarction of epiploic appendages
- Urinary tract infection
- Ureteral stone
- Pyelonephritis
- Primary peritonitis
- Henoch–Schönlein purpura

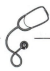

Yersinia enterocolitis is the great mimicker of appendicitis.

DIAGNOSIS: LABS

Complete Blood Count (CBC)
- Will demonstrate mild leukocytosis (10,000 to 18,000/mm³) with moderate polymorphonuclear (PMN) predominance.
- If white blood count (WBC) > 18,000/mm³, consider perforation with or without abscess.

Urinalysis

- Several WBCs or red blood cells (RBCs) may be found in appendicitis secondary to ureter or bladder irritation from inflamed appendix.
- Bacteriuria from catherized specimen is not seen in appendicitis.

DIAGNOSTIC IMAGING

Abdominal X-Ray (AXR)

- Will reveal an appendicolith/fecalith < 15% of the time (see Figure 15-1)

Abdominal Computed Tomography (CT) with Contrast

- Sensitivity of 95–98%
- Specificity of 83–90%
- Positive findings include:
  - > 6 mm dilatation of the appendix
  - Appendiceal thickening
  - Periappendiceal streaking (densities within perimesenteric fat)
  - Presence of appendicolith (see Figure 15-2)

Graded Compression Ultrasonography

- Sensitivity of 85%.
- Specificity of 92%.
- Very much operator dependent.
- Main positive finding is an enlarged (> 6 mm) noncompressible appendix (see Figure 15-3).
- Primary role is to exclude gynecologic pathology for which it is an excellent modality.

With mesenteric adenitis, there is usually a concurrent or antecedent history of respiratory tract infection.

HIGH-YIELD FACTS

The Appendix

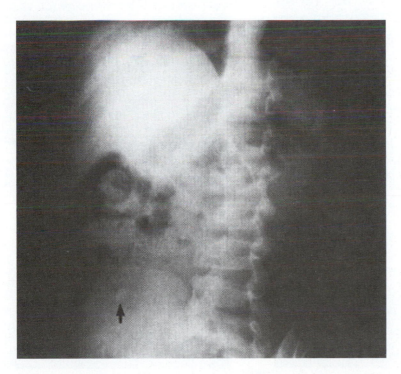

FIGURE 15-1. AXR demonstrating appendicolith. (Reproduced, with permission, from Heller. *J Pediatr* 135(5); November 1999, pp. 632–639.)

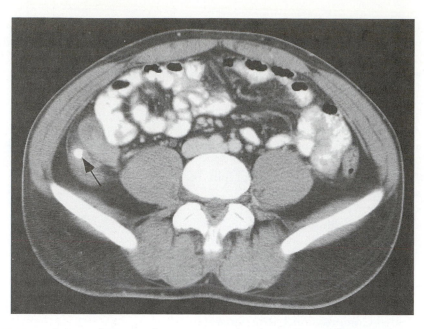

FIGURE 15-2. Abdominal CT scan demonstrating appendicolith and acute appendicitis.

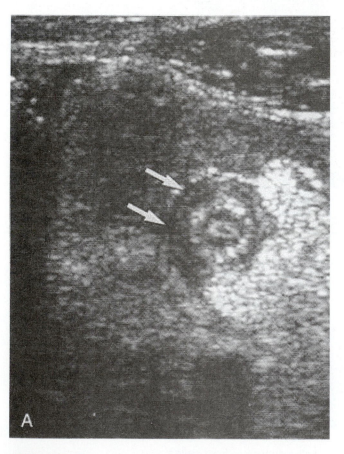
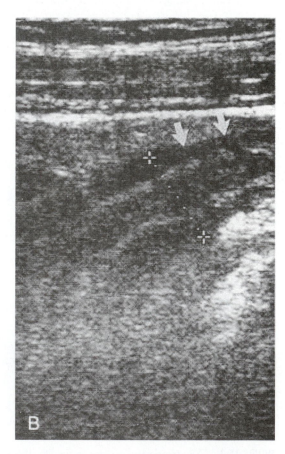

FIGURE 15-3. Transverse (A) and saggital (B) ultrasonographic views of the appendix demonstrate an inflamed, noncompressible, blind-ending tubular structure (arrows) with a diameter of 13 cm. Findings consistent with an acute appendicitis. (Reproduced, with permission, from *Surg Clin North Am* 77(6): December 1997. Copyright © 1997. WB Saunders Company.)

- False positive seen with:
  - Periappendix from surrounding inflammation.
  - Dilated fallopian tube.
  - Insipissated stool: Looks like appendicolith.
  - Obese patients: Appendix is noncompressible secondary to overlying fat.
- False negatives seen with:
  - Inflammation that is confined to the tip of the appendix.
  - Retrocecal cecum.
  - Large appendix: Mistaken for small bowel.
  - Perforation: Appendix now becomes compressible.

TREATMENT

- The definitive treatment of appendicitis is appendectomy.
- Peritoneal washout and parenteral antibiotics for perforation.

Approximately one third of appendixes rupture prior to appendectomy.

APPENDICITIS IN SPECIAL POPULATIONS

Pregnant Patients

- Appendicitis is the most common surgical emergency in the pregnant patient. Incidence: 1:2,000 pregnancies.
- Most frequent in first trimester.
- Fetal mortality increases 3–8% with early appendicitis to 30% with perforation.
- Surgery during pregnancy carries a risk of premature labor of 10–15% but is standard treatment.

Elderly Patients

- Present late in the course.
- Perforation rate is higher (> 50%).
- Tend to present with atypical findings (report less pain, have less peritonitis).
- Delayed leukocytosis.

Immunocompromised Patients

Examples: Patients with acquired immune deficiency syndrome (AIDS), those receiving high-dose chemotherapy

- Are susceptible to cytomegalovirus (CMV)-related bowel perforation and neutropenic colitis

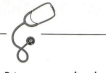

Primary appendiceal neoplasms are rare.

APPENDICEAL NEOPLASMS

Carcinoid

See small bowel chapter for further discussion.
- Most common type of appendiceal tumor.
- Comprise two thirds of all appendiceal tumors.
- Tumors < 2 cm treated with appendectomy.
- Tumors > 2 cm require right hemicolectomy.
- Medical treatment consists of serotonin antagonists (e.g., cyproheptadine) or somatostatin analogues (e.g., octreotide) for symptoms of carcinoid syndrome.

Mucinous Tumors

- Rupture of the tumor leads to mucin in the peritoneum (pseudomyxoma peritonei). Secondary complications include bowel obstruction and perforation.
- Sometimes associated with migratory thrombophlebitis.

Adenocarcinoma

Quite rare; see description of colon adenocarcinoma.

APPENDICEAL ABSCESS

SIGNS AND SYMPTOMS

Can present with symptoms similar to appendicitis including:
- Increasing RLQ pain
- Anorexia
- Fever
- A tender, fluctuant RLQ mass that is palpable on rectal examination
- Localizing peritonitis

DIAGNOSIS

- Leukocytosis on CBC.
- CT scan confirms the diagnosis.

TREATMENT

- Percutaneous drainage
- Operative drainage

The Hepatobiliary System

HEPATIC ANATOMY

See Figure 16-1.
- Arterial supply:
  - Celiac trunk comes off the aorta, giving off the left gastric, splenic, and common hepatic arteries.
  - Common hepatic artery divides into the proper hepatic artery and the supraduodenal artery.
  - Proper hepatic artery divides into the right and left hepatic arteries.
- Venous drainage:
  - The left, middle, and right hepatic veins drain into the inferior vena cava (IVC).
- Ligaments of the liver:
  - *Falciform ligament:* Connects the anterior abdominal wall to the liver; contains the ligamentum teres (obliterated umbilical vein)
  - *Coronary ligament:* Peritoneal reflection on the cranial aspect of the liver that attaches it to the diaphragm

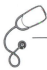

The right and left hepatic arteries supply 50% of the liver's oxygen. The portal vein supplies the remaining 50%. However, the liver receives 75% of its blood supply from the portal vein and only 25% from the hepatic arteries. The different degrees of oxygen saturation within the arterial and venous systems account for this fact.

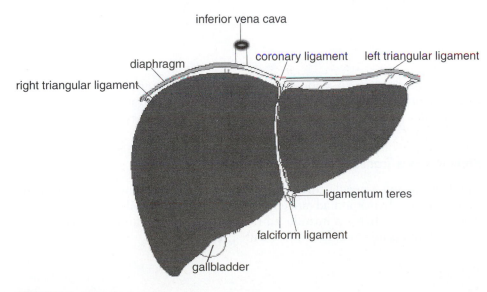

FIGURE 16-1. Hepatic anatomy.

The hepatoduodenal ligament contains the common bile duct, portal vein, and proper hepatic artery. It forms the anterior boundary of the epiploic foramen of Winslow and connects the greater and the lesser peritoneal cavities.

- *Triangular ligaments:* The right and left lateral extensions of the coronary ligament
- *Bare area:* The posterior section of the liver against the diaphragm; has no peritoneal covering.
- **Glisson's capsule:** The peritoneal membrane that covers the liver.
- *Cantlie's line* (portal fissure): A line that passes from the left side of the gallbladder to the left side of the IVC, dividing the liver into right and left lobes. It is based on blood supply and is the basis of the four classic types of hepatic resection.
- Liver enzymes: Aspartate transaminase (AST) and alanine transaminase (ALT) are made by hepatocytes; alkaline phosphatase (alk phos) is made by ductal epithelium.

COMMON PROCEDURES OF THE HEPATOBILIARY SYSTEM

Pringle Maneuver

Compression of the hepatoduodenal ligament. It is performed to control bleeding from the liver.

Liver Resection

Up to 80% of the liver can be removed and still retain adequate function.

Sphincterotomy (Papillotomy)

A cut through the sphincter of Oddi to allow the passage of stones from the common bile duct (CBD) into the duodenum. It is often performed during endoscopic retrograde cholangiopancreatography (ERCP).

Kocher Incision

An incision at the right subcostal margin performed during open cholecystectomy.

ERCP

Involves passage of an endoscope into the duodenum, introduction of a catheter into the ampulla of Vater, and injection of contrast medium into the CBD and/or pancreatic duct; conscious sedation is necessary.

Percutaneous Transhepatic Cholangiography (PTCA)

Involves passing a needle through the skin and subcutaneous tissues into the hepatic parenchyma and advancement into a peripheral bile duct. When bile is aspirated, a catheter is introduced through the needle, and radiopaque contrast medium is injected. It complements ERCP.

- Constituents: Cholesterol, lecithin, bile acids, and bilirubin.
- Function: Emulsifies fats.
- Enterohepatic circulation: Bile acids are released from the liver into the duodenum, reabsorbed at the terminal ileum, and transported back to the liver via the portal vein.
- Cholecystokinin:
  - Released by duodenal mucosal cells.
  - Stimulates gallbladder contraction and release of bile (along with vagal stimulation).
  - Causes opening of the ampulla of Vater and slows gastric emptying.
  - Is stimulated by fat, protein, amino acids, and hydrochloride (HCl).
  - Trypsin and chymotrypsin inhibit its release.

JAUNDICE

DEFINITION

- Yellowing of the skin and sclera due to an elevation in total bilirubin > 2.5. Categorized into prehepatic, hepatic, or posthepatic causes (see Table 16-1).

SIGNS AND SYMPTOMS

- Yellow skin and sclera.
- Pruritus.
- Can have hepatomegaly, tenderness of the right upper quadrant (RUQ), or signs of cirrhosis.
- Dark urine, clay-colored stools, anorexia, and nausea indicate obstructive jaundice.

DIAGNOSIS

See Table 16-1.

TREATMENT

Treat the underlying disorder.

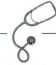

In obstructive jaundice, the alkaline phosphatase (ALP) level rises more quickly than the bilirubin level. Also, when the obstruction is relieved, the ALP level falls more quickly than the bilirubin level.

TABLE 16-1. Causes of increased bilirubin.

Classification	Causes	Direct Bilirubin	Indirect Bilirubin
Prehepatic	Hemolysis Gilbert's disease Crigler–Najjar syndrome	Normal	High
Hepatic	Alcoholic cirrhosis Acute hepatitis Primary biliary cirrhosis	High	High
Posthepatic	Gallstones Tumor	High	Normal

HEPATIC ABSCESSES

DEFINITION

A collection of pus in the liver of bacterial, fungal, or parasitic origin that most commonly involves the right lobe. The two main subtypes are pyogenic (bacterial) and amebic.

INCIDENCE

- Pyogenic: 8 to 15/100,000
- Amebic: 1.3/100,000

RISK FACTORS

- Pyogenic: Usually secondary to bacterial sepsis or biliary or portal vein infection; can also occur from a perforated infected gallbladder, cholangitis, diverticulitis, liver cancer, or liver metastases
- Amebic: Patients from Central America, homosexual men, institutionalized patients, and alcoholics

SIGNS AND SYMPTOMS

Fever, chills, RUQ pain, jaundice, sepsis, and weight loss; amebic abscesses tend to have a more protracted course.

DIAGNOSIS

- Leukocytosis
- Elevated liver function tests (LFTs)
- Ultrasound or computed tomography (CT) of the liver
- Serology for amebic abscesses

TREATMENT

- Pyogenic: Ultrasound or CT-guided percutaneous drainage with IV antibiotics; operative drainage indicated if percutaneous attempts fail or cysts are multiple or loculated
- Amebic: Operative drainage not indicated unless abscesses do not resolve with IV metronidazole or are superinfected with bacteria

PROGNOSIS

Mortality is low for uncomplicated abscesses, but complicated abscesses carry a 40% mortality risk.

HEPATIC CYSTS

Hydatid Cyst

DEFINITION

A hepatic cyst caused by *Echinococcus multilocularis* or *Echinococcus granulosus* that is usually solitary and involves the right lobe of the liver.

RISK FACTORS

Exposure to dogs, sheep, cattle, foxes, wolves, domestic cats, or foreign travel.

SIGNS AND SYMPTOMS

Most commonly asymptomatic; can cause hepatomegaly.

DIAGNOSIS

Often picked up incidentally on ultrasound, CT, or abdominal films, which may show calcifications outlining the cyst; eosinophilia, serology.

TREATMENT

Never aspirate these cysts or they will spill their contents. Treat with albendazole or mebendazole followed by resection.

Nonparasitic Cysts

DEFINITION

Benign cysts within the liver parenchyma that most commonly involve the right lobe; are thought to be of congenital origin.

INCIDENCE

Rare; 4:1 female:male ratio.

SIGNS AND SYMPTOMS

Most cysts are small and asymptomatic; large cysts (rare) can present with increasing abdominal pain and girth and can bleed or become infected.

DIAGNOSIS

Usually incidental; ultrasound or CT.

TREATMENT

Small asymptomatic cysts require no treatment; large, symptomatic cysts should be surgically excised.

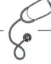

Nonparasitic cysts of the liver are associated with polycystic kidney disease.

BENIGN LIVER TUMORS

Cavernous Hemangioma

DEFINITION

A benign vascular tumor resulting from abnormal differentiation of angioblastic tissue during fetal life; usually located in the right posterior segment of the liver.

INCIDENCE

Most common benign tumor of the liver; occurs at all ages.

SIGNS AND SYMPTOMS

Usually asymptomatic; rarely presents with pain, a mass, or hepatomegaly.

DIAGNOSIS

Usually discovered incidentally; can be detected by ultrasound, CT, magnetic resonance imaging (MRI), radionuclide scan, or arteriography; **do not** biopsy, as hemorrhage can occur.

TREATMENT

Surgical resection if symptomatic or in danger of rupture; otherwise, observe.

Hamartoma

DEFINITION

A benign focal lesion of the liver that consists of normal tissue that has differentiated in an abnormal fashion; are multiple subtypes, depending on the types of cells involved (e.g., bile duct hamartoma, mesenchymal hamartoma, etc.).

INCIDENCE

Rare.

SIGNS AND SYMPTOMS

Typically asymptomatic; can present with RUQ pain or fullness.

DIAGNOSIS

Usually discovered incidentally during radiologic imaging; may require histopathologic evaluation.

TREATMENT

Surgical excision.

Adenomas

DEFINITION

A mass lesion of the liver characterized by a benign proliferation of hepatocytes.

INCIDENCE

Most common in premenopausal females with a multiyear history of oral contraceptive (OCP) use.

RISK FACTORS

OCP use, long-term anabolic steroid therapy, glycogen storage disease.

SIGNS AND SYMPTOMS

- Abdominal pain
- Abdominal mass
- Bleeding
- Can also be asymptomatic

Hepatocellular adenomas present with abdominal pain secondary to tumor rupture or bleeding in approximately one third of patients.

A 27-year-old female presents to her obstetrician with a history of a hepatocellular adenoma that resolved after discontinuing OCPs. She now wants to get pregnant. Does she have any specific health risks? *Think:* Hepatocellular adenomas treated by cessation of OCPs rather than by resection are at risk for rupture and hemorrhage during future pregnancies.

DIAGNOSIS

Ultrasound with needle biopsy.

TREATMENT

- Cessation of OCPs
- Surgical excision

Focal Nodular Hyperplasia (FNH)

DEFINITION

A benign hepatic tumor thought to arise from hepatocytes and bile ducts that has a characteristic "central scar" on pathologic evaluation.

INCIDENCE

Most common in premenopausal females.

SIGNS AND SYMPTOMS

Usually asymptomatic; 10% of patients present with abdominal pain and/or a RUQ mass.

DIAGNOSIS

Usually incidental on ultrasound or CT; can be differentiated from hepatocellular adenoma by a Tc-99 study.

TREATMENT

Resect if patient is symptomatic.

Like hepatic adenomas, focal nodular hyperplasia is associated with long-term OCP use.

MALIGNANT LIVER TUMORS

Hepatocellular Carcinoma (Hepatoma)

DEFINITION

A malignant tumor derived from hepatocytes frequently found in association with chronic liver disease, particularly cirrhosis.

INCIDENCE

- Accounts for 80% of liver cancers, but < 2% of all cancers
- Much more common in males (3:1)
- Usually diagnosed in the fifth or sixth decade.

RISK FACTORS

- Hepatitis B
- Hepatitis C
- Cirrhosis
- Aflatoxins (found in peanuts)
- Liver flukes

Eighty to 90% of patients with hepatocellular carcinoma have underlying cirrhosis, with alcoholic cirrhosis being the predominant type in Western countries. In the Far East, posthepatic cirrhosis is more common.

- Hemochromatosis
- Alpha-1-antitrypsin deficiency
- Anabolic steroid use

SIGNS AND SYMPTOMS

- Weight loss
- Weakness
- Dull pain in the RUQ or epigastrium
- Nausea, vomiting
- Jaundice
- Nontender hepatomegaly
- Splenomegaly (33%)
- Ascites (50%)

DIAGNOSIS

- Increased ALP, AST, ALT, gamma-glutamyl transferase (GGT), alpha-fetoprotein, and des-gamma-carboxy prothrombin (DCP).
- Contrast CT and ultrasound can visualize the tumor.
- CT or ultrasound-guided needle biopsy will give the definitive diagnosis.

TREATMENT

- Surgical resection is the only cure, consisting of either lobectomy or segmental resection. A 1-cm margin is required.
- Transplant is also a possibility, but there often is a high recurrence rate due to the continued presence of the underlying risk factor (e.g., hepatitis B, hepatitis C, etc.).

PROGNOSIS

Most patients die within the first 4 months if the tumor is not resected. After resection or transplant, the 5-year survival is approximately 25%.

Metastatic Neoplasms

SIGNS AND SYMPTOMS

- Patients are usually asymptomatic until the disease has become advanced and the liver begins to fail.
- Symptoms may include fatigue, weight loss, epigastric fullness, dull RUQ pain, ascites, jaundice, or fever.

DIAGNOSIS

- Increased ALP, GGT, lactic dehydrogenase (LDH), AST, and ALT (nonspecific).
- Metastases will enhance on contrast CT (see Figure 16-2).
- Intraoperative ultrasound with liver palpation is the most sensitive diagnostic tool.

TREATMENT

Resection, if possible, is the treatment of choice.

A bruit can commonly be heard over a hepatocellular carcinoma due to its abundant vascularity.

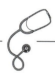

The most common hepatic malignancy is metastases. The primary is usually from colon, breast, or lung, with bronchogenic carcinoma being the most common primary cancer.

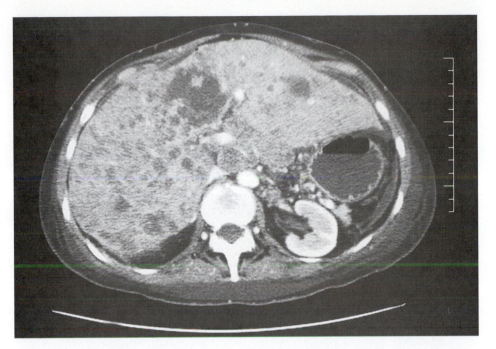

FIGURE 16-2. Abdominal CT in hepatic metastasis. Note slitlike appearance of intrahepatic IVC secondary to compression by mets. Also note presence of ascites and bilateral pleural effusions, left greater than right.

LIVER FAILURE

Child-Pugh Score

Child's classification estimates hepatic reserve in patients with liver failure (see Table 16-2).

TABLE 16-2. Child–Pugh Score for liver failure.

Variable	Number of Points Accorded		
	1	2	3
Bilirubin (mg/dL)	< 2.0	2.0–3.0	> 3.0
Albumin (mg/dL)	> 3.5	2.8–3.5	< 2.8
Ascites (clinical evaluation)	None	Easily controlled	Poorly
Neurologic disorder	None	Minimal	Advanced
Prothrombin time (sec > control)	< 4.0	4.0–6.0	> 6.0

Correlation with Child's class: 5–6 points, Class A; 7–9 points, Class B; 10–15 points, Class C.

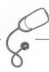

The most common cause of portal hypertension in the in the United States is cirrhosis from alcoholism. The most common cause outside North America is schistosomiasis.

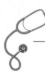

Rule of two thirds for portal hypertension:
Two thirds of patients with cirrhosis develop portal hypertension.
Two thirds of patients with portal hypertension develop esophageal varices.
Two thirds of patients with esophageal varices will bleed from them.
Note: Only 10–15% of alcoholics develop cirrhosis.

Splenomegaly is the most common clinical finding in portal hypertension.

DEFINITION

Portal pressure > 10 mm Hg (measure with indirect hepatic vein wedge pressure).

CAUSES

- *Prehepatic:* Congenital atresia, cyanosis, or portal vein thrombosis
- *Intrahepatic:* Cirrhosis, hepatic fibrosis from hemochromatosis, Wilson's disease, or congenital fibrosis
- *Posthepatic:* Budd–Chiari syndrome (thrombosis of the hepatic veins), hypercoagulable state, lymphoreticular malignancy

SIGNS AND SYMPTOMS

- Jaundice
- Splenomegaly
- Palmar erythema
- Spider angiomata
- Ascites
- Truncal obesity with wasting of the extremities
- Asterixis (a flapping hand tremor)
- Hepatic encephalopathy

Portosystemic Collaterals and Their Clinical Manifestations
- Left gastric vein to the esophageal veins—**esophageal varices**
- Umbilical vein (via the falciform ligament) to the epigastric veins— **caput medusa**
- Superior hemorrhoidal vein to the middle and inferior hemorrhoidal veins—**hemorrhoids**
- Veins of Retzius (posterior abdominal wall veins) to the retroperitoneal lumbar veins—**retroperitoneal varices**

DIAGNOSIS

- Suggestive history and physical examination
- Duplex Doppler ultrasound: Initial procedure of choice
- Venous phase of visceral angiography: Defines portal anatomy more precisely

TREATMENT

- Shunts (see Figure 16-3):
  - **Splenorenal (Warren shunt):** Connects the splenic vein to the left renal vein. Used for patients with esophageal varices and a history of bleeding.
  - **End to side:** Connects the end of the portal vein to the side of the IVC. This is considered a total shunt.
  - **Side to side:** Connects the side of the portal vein to the side of the IVC. This is considered a partial shunt.
  - **Portocaval H graft:** A synthetic graft is attached from the portal vein to the IVC. This is considered a partial graft.
  - **Mesocaval H graft:** A synthetic graft is attached from the superior mesenteric vein (SMV) to the IVC.

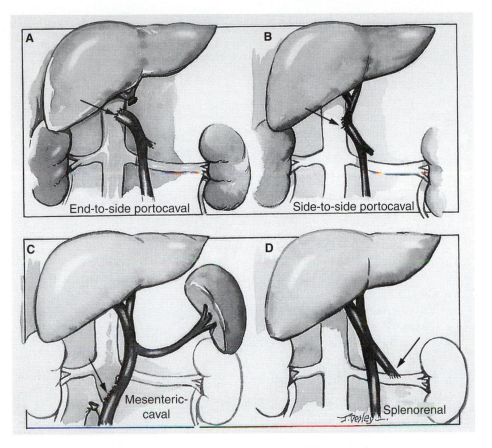

FIGURE 16-3. Types of portocaval shunts. (Copyright 2003 Mayo Foundation.)

- Complications: Increased incidence of hepatic encephalopathy because more toxins are diverted to the systemic circulation (except for the Warren shunt), and death from hepatic failure due to decreased blood flow to the liver.
- *Liver transplant:* Ideal candidate is a young patient with cirrhosis and an episode of bleeding from esophageal varices.

HEPATIC ENCEPHALOPATHY

DEFINITION

- Altered mental status due to hepatic insufficiency.
- Toxins that are normally cleared by the liver are retained in the circulation.
- The exact toxin that causes the central nervous system (CNS) changes is unknown but has been theorized to be ammonia, gamma-aminobutyric acid (GABA), mercaptens, or short-chain fatty acids.

EPIDEMIOLOGY

- Occurs in all cases of fulminant hepatic failure
- Occurs in one half of patients with end-stage liver disease requiring transplantation
- Occurs in one third of cirrhotics

TABLE 16-3. Grading of asterixis.

Grade	Asterixis: Flaps per minute
0	None
1+	Rare (2–4/min)
2+	Occasional (6–8/min)
3+	Frequent (10–60/min)
4+	Continuous

CAUSE

Precipitating factors include:

- Infection (watch for spontaneous bacterial peritonitis [SBP])
- Potassium, magnesium, or other electrolyte depletion
- Use of opiates, sedatives, or other hepatically cleared drugs
- Gastrointestinal (GI) bleed
- Excess dietary protein

SIGNS AND SYMPTOMS

- Change in level of consciousness
- Lethargy, coma
- Normal electroencephalogram (EEG)
- Asterixis (see Table 16-3)

DIAGNOSIS

An elevated serum ammonia level along with signs of altered mental status is diagnostic.

TREATMENT

- Lactulose and neomycin (PO or PR) to reduce intestinal absorption of ammonia
- Liver dialysis

In hepatic encephalopathy, the serum ammonia level **does not** correlate with the degree of encephalopathy.

ASCITES

DEFINITION

- Excess fluid in the peritoneal cavity.
- Sodium and fluid retention by the kidney, low plasma oncotic pressure due to low albumin production by the failing liver, and elevated hydrostatic pressure in the hepatic sinusoids or portal veins cause fluid to be lost into the peritoneal cavity.

SIGNS AND SYMPTOMS

Distended abdomen, fluid wave, shifting dullness

TREATMENT

- Reduce sodium intake.
- Potassium sparing diuretic (e.g., spironolactone).
- Abdominal paracentesis:
  - Removing too much ascitic fluid or removing the fluid too quickly will cause intravascular fluid to be drawn into the peritoneal cavity. This leads to a loss of intravascular volume and can cause hypovolemic shock.

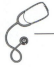

A **LeVeen shunt** is a peritoneal–jugular shunt used to decrease ascites. One drawback is that it may increase hepatic encephalopathy.

ESOPHAGEAL VARICES

DEFINITION

Engorged esophageal or gastric veins.

SIGNS AND SYMPTOMS

- Asymptomatic unless rupture occurs
- With rupture: Upper GI bleeding with hematemesis, melena, and/or hematochezia

DIAGNOSIS

Esophagogastroduodenostomy (EGD).

TREATMENT OF RUPTURED VARICES

Options include:
- Endoscopic sclerotherapy
- Vasopressin or somatostatin injection
- Balloon tamponade (Sengstaken–Blakemore tube)
- TIPS (transjugular intrahepatic portocaval shunt)
- Intraoperative placement of a portocaval shunt
- Liver transplant

Beta blockers can be used to decrease portal pressure and reduce the incidence of rupture.

PROGNOSIS

Poor even with treatment. Ruptured esophageal varices have a 50% death rate.

CAPUT MEDUSA

DEFINITION

Engorged abdominal wall veins.

SIGNS AND SYMPTOMS

Mass of veins extending from around the umbilicus, periumbilical bruit (Cruveilheir–Baumgarten bruit)

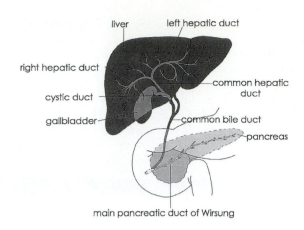

right hepatic duct

common hepatic duct

cystic duct

gallbladder

common bile duct

pancreas

main pancreatic duct of Wirsung

FIGURE 16-4. Anatomy of the biliary tree. (Modified, with permission, from *LifeArt Emergency Medicine Professional Collection.* Lippincott Williams & Wilkins, 2000.)

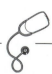

Calot's triangle: Inferior border of the liver, common hepatic duct, and cystic duct. The cystic artery runs through it, and the associated lymph node is called Calot's node. The right hepatic artery is adjacent to the cystic duct in Calot's triangle and, as such, is susceptible to injury during cholecystectomy.

The infundibulum of the gallbladder is also called **Hartman's pouch.**

Only 15% of gallstones have enough calcium to be radiopaque. The majority of kidney stones, on the other hand, have sufficient calcium to be radiopaque on plain films.

ANATOMY OF THE BILIARY TREE

See Figure 16-4.

- Intrahepatic ducts converge to become the right and left hepatic ducts.
- Right and left hepatic ducts converge, forming the common hepatic duct.
- Cystic duct comes off the gallbladder and joins the common hepatic duct to become the common bile duct (CBD).
- CBD empties into the duodenum via the ampulla of Vater.

ANATOMY OF THE GALLBLADDER

- The proximal end of the gallbladder near the cystic duct is called the *infundibulum*, and the larger distal end of the gallbladder is called the *fundus*.
- The valves within the cystic duct are called the *spiral valves of Heister*.
- The gallbladder collects bile directly from the liver via small bile ducts called ducts of Luschka.

CHOLELITHIASIS

DEFINITION

Stones in the gallbladder. Eighty-five percent of stones are composed primarily of cholesterol, while the remaining 15% are pigmented.

INCIDENCE

Approximately 10% of the U.S. population has gallstones; incidence increases with age.

RISK FACTORS

The typical ones are: Female, fat, fertile, and forty; other risk factors include Native American race, pregnancy, oral contraceptives, Western diet, inflammatory bowel disease (IBD), hyperlipidemia, ileal resection, and total parenteral nutrition (TPN).

SIGNS AND SYMPTOMS

- Most patients are asymptomatic.
- Symptomatic patients classically complain of severe RUQ pain that radiates to the back, epigastrium or left upper quadrant (LUQ) that tends to be worse after eating (especially after fatty foods) and may be associated with nausea and vomiting.
- The symptom complex is called *biliary colic* and typically resolves over a few hours.

DIAGNOSIS

- Often incidental, as most patients are asymptomatic.
- Abdominal plain films pick up 15% of gallstones.
- Ultrasound: Procedure of choice; classic findings include an acoustic shadow ("headlight") and gravity-dependent movement of gallstones with patient repositioning (see Figure 16-5).

TREATMENT

Asymptomatic cholelithiasis does not require cholecystectomy unless the patient:

- Has a porcelain gallbladder (which has an increased incidence of carcinoma)
- Has sickle cell anemia
- Has a stone > 2 to 3 cm
- Is a pediatric patient

Symptomatic cholelithiasis requires cholecystectomy. A laparoscopic cholecystectomy can be performed on 95% of patients. Medical treatment of cholelithiasis involves chenodeoxycholic acid or ursodeoxycholic acid, drugs

Risk factors for cholelithiasis:
- Female
- Fat
- Fertile
- Forty
- Flatulent
- Famillal
- Fibrosis, cystic
- F-Hgb (sickle cell disease)

Mirizzi's syndrome is external compression of the common hepatic duct by a gallstone impacted in the cystic duct.

Hydrops of the gallbladder: Complete obstruction of the cystic duct by a gallstone, causing the gallbladder to fill with fluid from the gallbladder mucosa. The fluid is often milky white.

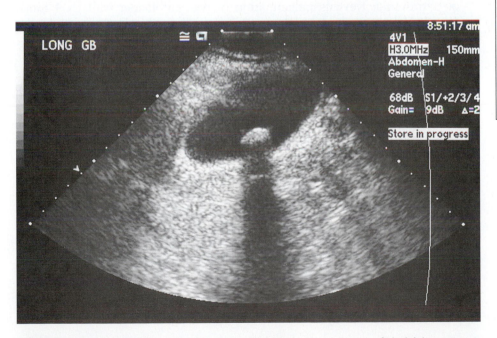

FIGURE 16-5. Sonogram demonstrating classic "headlight" appearance of cholelithiasis.

that can be used to dissolve cholesterol stones. These are not effective as surgical management.

PROGNOSIS

Three to 5% of patients with cholelithiasis develop complications.

CHOLECYSTITIS

Acute Calculous Cholecystitis

DEFINITION

Inflammation of the gallbladder wall, usually due to obstruction of the cystic duct by gallstones.

SIGNS AND SYMPTOMS

- RUQ tenderness and guarding are present, distinguishing it from uncomplicated biliary colic.
- Pain typically lasts > 3 hours.
- Fever, nausea, vomiting, and anorexia are nonspecific and variable.
- Murphy's sign: Pain on deep inspiration resulting in inspiratory arrest (positive in about one third of patients).
- Sonographic Murphy's: Pain over RUQ when palpated with ultrasound probe (87% sensitivity).
- One third of patients develop exquisitely tender RUQ mass late in course.

DIAGNOSIS

- Labs: Leukocytosis, with or without increased ALP, LFTs, amylase, and total bilirubin.
- Ultrasound: Reveals inflammation of the gallbladder wall (> 4 mm), pericholecystic fluid and stones in the gallbladder. Positive predictive value of all three is 90%. Will also see dilation of the CBD if the stone has passed.
- HIDA scan (most sensitive) (see Figures 16-6 and 16-7): A radionucleotide scan in which Technetium-99m labeled iminodiacetic acid is injected intravenously into hepatocytes. A normal gallbladder would be visualized within 1 hour.

TREATMENT

- NPO.
- IV fluids.
- IV antibiotic.
- IV analgesia.
- Cholecystectomy within 24 to 48 hours.
- Often done laparoscopically; if inflammation prevents adequate visualization of important structures, convert to open cholecystectomy.

Emphysematous Cholecystitis

See Figures 16-8 and 16-9.

In acute cholecystitis, the pain is similar in character to cholelithiasis but typically lasts longer (> 3 hours).

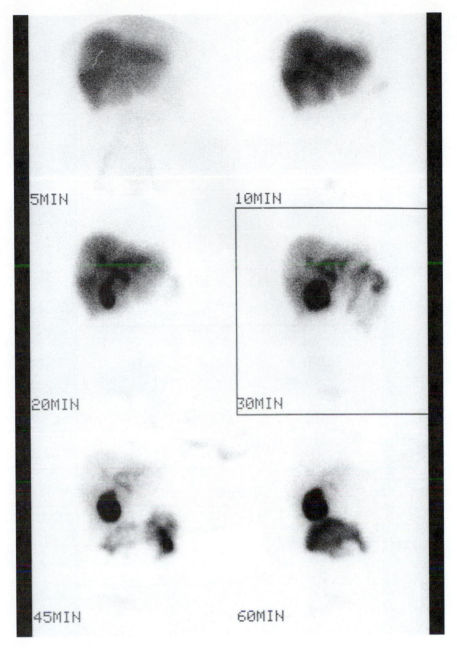

FIGURE 16-6. Normal HIDA scan, demonstrating uptake of contrast in intrahepatic bile ducts and gallbladder at 20 minutes and excretion into small bowel at 30 minutes.

- Severe variant of cholecystitis caused by gas-forming bacteria
- Relatively rare
- Often results in perforation of the gallbladder, high mortality and morbidity
- Typically affects elderly diabetic men

Acalculous Cholecystitis

DEFINITION

Acute cholecystitis without evidence of gallstones; thought to be due to biliary stasis.

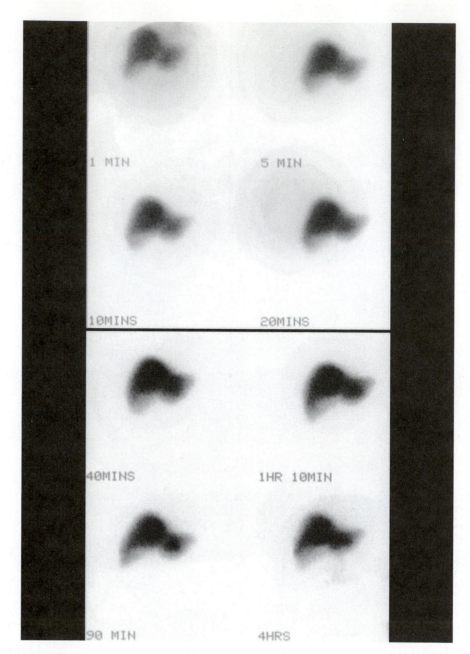

FIGURE 16-7. HIDA scan, consistent with acute cholecystitis. The gallbladder is not visualized even at 4 hours, even though the small bowel is.

INCIDENCE

Ten percent of cases of acute cholecystitis.

RISK FACTORS

Most often seen in intensive care unit (ICU) patients with multiorgan system failure, trauma (especially after major surgery), burns, sepsis, and TPN.

DIAGNOSIS

- Labs: Leukocytosis, with or without increased ALP, LFTs, amylase, and total bilirubin

Ten percent of cases of acute cholecystitis are not associated with gallstones. This is referred to as acalculous cholecystitis.

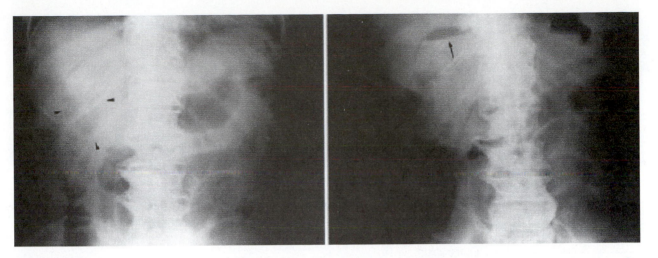

FIGURE 16-8. AXR demonstrating rimlike gas within gallbladder. (Reproduced, with permission, from Ise N et al., *Surg Today* (2002) 32: 183–185.)

- Ultrasound: Biliary sludge and inflammation; can also be used to detect complications (e.g., gangrene, empyema, or perforation of the gallbladder)
- HIDA scan: To confirm diagnosis

TREATMENT

Urgent cholecystectomy; percutaneous cholecystectomy is an option in patients with high surgical risk.

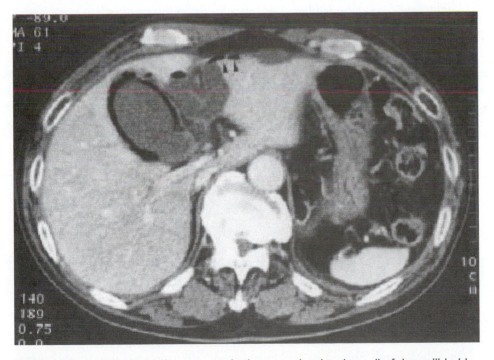

FIGURE 16-9. Abdominal CT shows air in the lumen and within the wall of the gallbladder, surrounding fatty infiltration and intraperitoneal gas. (Reproduced, with permission, from Ise N et al., *Surg Today* (2002) 32: 183–185.)

DEFINITION

Obstruction of the common bile duct by a stone.

INCIDENCE

Found in 6–15% of acute calculous cholecystitis and 1–2% of acalculous cholecystitis at surgery.

SIGNS AND SYMPTOMS

Epigastric or RUQ pain and tenderness, jaundice, cholangitis, or recurrent attacks of acute pancreatitis without other known risk factors.

DIAGNOSIS

- Labs: Increased ALP, LFTs, and total and direct bilirubin
- ERCP: Gold standard for diagnosis of CBD stones; also provides a therapeutic option (see below)
- Endoscopic ultrasound: Less sensitive than ERCP but also less invasive; more sensitive than transabdominal ultrasound
- Transabdominal ultrasound: Highly specific but not very sensitive for CBD stones

TREATMENT

- ERCP: Involves endoscopic sphincterotomy with retrieval of the CBD stone(s) with a basket (85–90% successful).
- If ERCP fails, the CBD can be opened surgically and the stones removed. A T-tube is placed so bile can drain externally. It is removed 2 to 3 weeks later on an outpatient basis.

Acute (Ascending) Cholangitis

DEFINITION

Bacterial infection of the bile ducts usually associated with obstruction of the CBD by a gallstone.

SIGNS AND SYMPTOMS

- Fever, chills
- Nausea, vomiting
- Abdominal pain with or without altered mental status and septic shock

DIAGNOSIS

- Labs: Leukocytosis with increased bilirubin, ALP, and LFTs.
- Ultrasound: Should be the initial study; dilation of common and intrahepatic bile ducts is suggestive.
- ERCP/percutaneous transhepatic cholangiography (PTC): Provides a definitive diagnosis; can also be therapeutic.

HIGH-YIELD FACTS

The Hepatobiliary System

Ascending cholangitis is a life-threatening emergency.

Charcot's triad:
- RUQ pain
- Fever
- Jaundice

Reynold's pentad:
- Charcot's triad plus
- Central nervous system (CNS) symptoms
- Septic shock

Common causes of CBD obstruction: **SINGE**
- **S**tricture
- **I**atrogenic causes (ERCP/PTC or biliary stent placement)
- **N**eoplasm
- **G**allstones
- **E**xtrinsic compression (e.g., pancreatic pseudocyst/pancreatitis)

- Bile cultures: Obtain to facilitate proper antibiotic treatment; offending organisms are usually enteric gram negatives and enterococci.

TREATMENT

- NPO, IV fluids, and IV antibiotics.
- If patient is in shock, decompress bile duct and remove obstruction immediately by ERCP/PTC. If unsuccessful, intraoperative decompression with T-tube placement is indicated.
- If the patient is stable, continue conservative management with definitive treatment later.

Sclerosing Cholangitis

DEFINITION

A chronic, progressive inflammatory process of the biliary tree of unknown etiology that results in strictures and, in most cases, leads to cirrhosis and liver failure.

INCIDENCE

2:1 male predominance with median age of onset at 40 years.

RISK FACTORS

IBD, pancreatitis, diabetes, trauma to the common hepatic duct.

SIGNS AND SYMPTOMS

Many patients are asymptomatic at the time of diagnosis, but symptoms can include fever, weight loss, fatigue, pruritus, jaundice, hepatomegaly, splenomegaly, and hyperpigmentation.

Seventy percent of patients with sclerosing cholangitis have IBD, whereas 3 to 7.5% of patients with IBD have sclerosing cholangitis.

DIAGNOSIS

ERCP/PTC reveal a "beads on a string" appearance of the bile ducts (see Figure 16-10). ALP is almost always elevated.

TREATMENT

- Balloon dilation with stent placement can be performed for palliative purposes, but definitive treatment varies depending on the location of the strictures.
- Extrahepatic strictures: Hepatoenteric anastomosis with removal of the extrahepatic ducts and T-tube placement for external drainage of bile.
- Intrahepatic strictures: Liver transplant.

Complications of sclerosing cholangitis:
- Cirrhosis
- Cholangitis
- Obstructive jaundice
- Cholangiocarcinoma

PROGNOSIS

- Ten percent of patients develop cholangiocarcinoma.
- Ten-year survival is 75%.

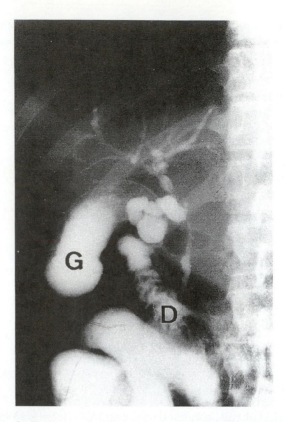

FIGURE 16-10. ERCP demonstrating beads on a string appearance of bile ducts in sclerosing cholangitis. G, gallbladder; D, duodenum. (Reproduced, with permission, from Nakanuma Y et al. Definition and pathology of primary sclerosing cholangitis. *J. Hepatobiliary Pancreat Surg* 1999; 6: 333–342.)

GALLSTONE ILEUS

DEFINITION

- Small bowel obstruction caused by a gallstone; the ileocecal valve is the most common site of obstruction.
- Most often a large stone has eroded a hole through the gallbladder wall to the duodenum, causing a cholecystenteric fistula. A gallstone escapes through this hole into the GI tract and eventually gets stuck in the ileum, causing small bowel obstruction.

INCIDENCE

Most common in women over 70.

SIGNS AND SYMPTOMS

Symptoms of acute cholecystitis followed by signs of small bowel obstruction (nausea, vomiting, abdominal distention, RUQ pain).

DIAGNOSIS

- Abdominal plain films: May show the pathognomonic features of pneumobilia, dilated small bowel, and a large gallstone in the RLQ
- Ultrasound: Useful to confirm cholelithiasis; may also identify the fistula

Typical scenario: A 75-year-old female with a past history of cholelithiasis presents complaining of RUQ pain that radiates to her back, with nausea, vomiting, and abdominal distention. Abdominal plain films show air in the biliary tree and a "'stepladder" appearance of the small bowel. *Think:* The history is consistent with both cholelithiasis and small bowel obstruction, and findings on abdominal radiograph are suggestive of gallstone ileus.

- Upper and lower GI series: Other diagnostic options that are usually unnecessary

TREATMENT

Exploratory laparotomy, removal of the gallstone, and possible small bowel resection with or without cholecystectomy and fistula repair.

CARCINOMA OF THE GALLBLADDER

DEFINITION

Malignant neoplasm of the gallbladder, the majority of which are adenocarcinomas.

INCIDENCE

Extremely rare (< 1% of patients with cholelithiasis); incidence increases with age with a peak at 75 years; female:male ratio 3:1

RISK FACTORS

Include porcelain gallbladder, gallstones, choledochal cysts, gallbladder polyps, and typhoid carriers with chronic inflammation.

SIGNS AND SYMPTOMS

Most patients are asymptomatic until late in the course when findings may include abdominal pain, nausea, vomiting, weight loss, RUQ mass, hepatomegaly, or jaundice.

DIAGNOSIS

Ultrasound, CT, MRI, or ERCP/PTC

TREATMENT

Varies depending on the extent of tumor involvement.
- Tumor confined to gallbladder mucosa: Cholecystectomy
- Tumor involving muscularis or serosa: Radical cholecystectomy, wedge resection of overlying liver, and lymph node dissection
- Tumor involving liver: Consider palliative measures such as decompression of the proximal biliary tree or a bypass procedure of the obstructed duodenum

Courvoisier's sign: A palpable, nontender gallbladder often associated with cancer in the head of the pancreas or the gallbladder.

BENIGN TUMORS OF THE BILE DUCTS

DEFINITION

Tumors that arise from ductal glandular epithelium most commonly found at the ampulla of Vater; most are adenomas, of polypoid morphology, and < 2 cm in size.

SIGNS AND SYMPTOMS

Intermittent jaundice and RUQ pain.

DIAGNOSIS

Intraoperative cholangiogram, ultrasound, ERCP/PTC.

TREATMENT

Resection of the tumor with a margin of duct wall either intraoperatively or endoscopically.

A cholangiocarcinoma that arises at the junction of the right and left hepatic ducts is called a **Klatskin tumor.**

CHOLANGIOCARCINOMA

DEFINITION

An uncommon tumor that may occur anywhere along the intrahepatic or extrahepatic biliary tree but is most commonly located at the bifurcation of the right and left hepatic ducts (60–80% of cases). Nearly all are adenocarcinomas.

INCIDENCE

- Increases with age with peak at 55 to 65 years; 1/100,000 people per year
- No sex predilection

RISK FACTORS

Choledochal cyst, ulcerative colitis, sclerosing cholangitis, liver flukes, toxins, contrast dye.

SIGNS AND SYMPTOMS

- Jaundice
- Clay-colored stools
- Dark urine
- Pruritus
- Pain
- Malaise
- Weight loss

DIAGNOSIS

- Ultrasound: Shows bile duct dilation
- CT: Identifies tumors located near the hilum of the liver
- Biopsy via ERCP/PTC under ultrasound guidance

TREATMENT

- Varies depending on location of the tumor.
- Proximal tumors: Resect with a Roux-en-Y hepaticojejunostomy.
- Distal tumors: Whipple procedure.
- If both hepatic ducts or the main trunk of the portal vein are extensively involved, the tumor may be unresectable.

PROGNOSIS

Five-year survival rate is 15–20%.

The Pancreas

EMBRYOLOGY

- Begins development during fourth week of gestation from endoderm of duodenum.
- Two pouches develop, the ventral and dorsal pancreas, which rotate and fuse by eighth week.
- **Heterotopic pancreas**—wrong location of pancreatic tissue (stomach, duodenum, Meckel's diverticulum).
- **Pancreas divisum**—failure to fuse two duct systems (duct of Santorini becomes main duct); 5% of population. The resulting inadequate drainage results in chronic pain and recurrent bouts of pancreatitis.
- **Annular pancreas**—ventral pancreas malrotates and encircles second portion of duodenum (pancreatitis, upper gastrointestinal [GI] obstruction, peptic ulcer).

ANATOMY

- Location: Lies retroperitoneal, posterior to stomach, transverse mesocolon and lesser omentum, at the level of body of L2.
- Head: Includes uncinate process.
- Neck: Portion anterior to superior mesenteric vein.
- Body: Lies to the left of the neck, forms posterior floor of lesser sac.
- Tail: Enters splenorenal ligament, adjacent to splenic hilum; susceptible to injury during splenectomy.
- Ducts: Duct of Wirsung is the main duct; runs entire length of pancreas. Joins common bile duct to form ampulla within papilla of Vater (40% of time). Duct of Santorini is accessory duct.
- Sphincter of Oddi: Smooth muscle around ampulla.

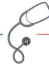

Resection of head of pancreas requires resection of duodenum also.

BLOOD SUPPLY

See Figure 17-1.

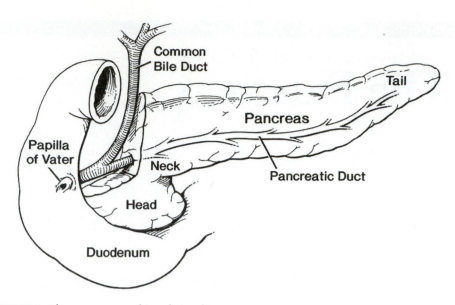

FIGURE 17-1. The pancreas and its relationships.

Splanchnicectomy can be done for pain control in pancreatic disease.

Secretin is the most potent endogenous stimulant of bicarbonate secretion.

The exocrine pancreas makes up 85% of pancreatic volume; the endocrine pancreas accounts for only 2%, with the rest composed of extracellular matrix and vessels or ducts.

- Head is closely associated with duodenum (anterior and posterior pancreaticoduodenal arteries).
- Body and tail are supplied by branches of dorsal pancreatic artery, and splenic artery.
- Sympathetics: From thoracic sympathetic ganglia to the splanchnic nerves to the celiac ganglia (pain).
- Parasympathetics: From vagal nuclei (for islets, acini and ducts).

PHYSIOLOGY

Exocrine

Secretion of 1 to 5 L/day of isosmotic, pH 8 fluid, with Na^+ and K^+ similar to that in plasma.

- **Acinar cells:** Secrete enzymes (e.g., chymotrypsin, trypsin, carboxypeptidase, amylase, lipase).
- **Centroacinar and ductal cells:** Secrete water and electrolytes.
- Phases:
  1. Cephalic phase: Stimuli by sight, smell of food activates vagal fibers. Gastric acid production → duodenal acidification → secretin release → pancreatic bicarbonate (HCO_3) release.
  2. Gastric phase: Antral distention and protein causes release of gastrin → gastric acid secretion → duodenal acidification → secretin release → pancreatic HCO_3 release.
  3. Intestinal phase: Dudodenal acid and bile stimulate secretin, and duodenal fat and protein release cholecystokinin (CCK) → releases pancreatic enzymes.

Endocrine

- Islets of Langerhans make up 1.5% of pancreas by weight.
- Hormones:
  - Insulin: From beta cells in islets of Langerhans
  - Glucagon: From islet alpha cells (glycogenolysis and release of glucose)
- Pancreatic polypeptide
- Somatostatin: From islet delta cells (generally causes inhibitory functions of gastrointestinal tract)

ACUTE PANCREATITIS

DEFINITION

Inflammation of the pancreas due to parenchymal autodigestion by proteolytic enzyme.

ETIOLOGY

- Metabolic:
  - Alcohol: 35–40%
  - Hyperlipidemia: Types I and IV hypertriglyceridemia
  - Hypercalcemia: Seen in hyperparathyroidism
- Mechanical:
  - Gallstones: Biliary disease (40%)
- Trauma and post-op (e.g, endoscopic retrograde cholangiopancreatography [ERCP])
  - Pancreatic duct obstruction (e.g., tumor, pancreatic divisum)
  - Duodenal obstruction
- Vascular:
  - Ischemia
  - Vasculitis
- Infectious:
  - Scorpion venom
  - Viral infection (e.g., mumps, coxsackie B, cytomegalovirus)
- Drugs (e.g., isoniazid, estrogens, azathioprine, hydrochlorothiazide, sulfonamides, pentamidine, didanosine)

SIGNS AND SYMPTOMS

- Severe, constant mid-epigastric or left upper quadrant (LUQ) pain, radiates to the back. Pain sometimes improved when patient sits up and leans forward.
- Nausea, vomiting.
- Low-grade fever.
- Tachypnea.
- Abdomen is usually tender with guarding, but no rebound.
- Fluid sequestration in retroperitoneum can be massive.
- Ninety percent have mild, self-limited disease.
- Cullen and Grey–Turner signs are indicative of severe, hemorrhagic pancreatitis.

GlucAgon = Alpha cells

Somatostatin may be used clinically to:
1. Treat symptoms of neuroendocrine tumors (islet cell, carcinoid, gastrinoma, VIPoma, and acromegaly).
2. To convert high-output fistulae to low-output fistulae (because of its anti-motility and anti-secretory effects).

Causes of pancreatitis: **GET SMASHED**
Posterior perforation of peptic ulcer
Alcohol
Neoplasm
Cholelithiasis (biliary disease)
Renal disease (end stage)
ERCP
Anorexia (malnutrition)
Trauma
Infections
Toxins (drugs)
Incineration (burns)
Surgery, scorpion bite

Be aware of MED VIPS
Methyldopa/metronidazole
Estrogen
Didanosine
Valproate
Isoniazid
Pentamidine
Sulfonamides

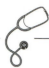

Cullen's sign: Bluish discoloration of periumbilicus (think of **cUL**len and **UmbiLicus**).
Grey–Turner's sign: Bluish discoloration of flank (think of **turn** on your side/flank).

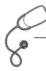

High amylase levels are also seen in intestinal disease, perforated ulcer, ruptured ectopic, salpingitis, and salivary gland disorders.

DIAGNOSIS

- Amylase:
  - Secreted by the pancreas to break down carbohydrates.
  - Also found in salivary glands, small bowel, ovaries, testes, skeletal muscle.
  - May be persistently elevated in renal insufficiency.
  - A level three times the upper limit of normal is 75% specific and 80–90% sensitive for pancreatitis.
  - Still widely used as a marker but has false-negative rate of 10% and is not specific.
  - High amylase associated with acute, not chronic pancreatitis.
- Lipase:
  - Secreted by the pancreas to break down triglycerides.
  - Also found in gastric and intestinal mucosa, and liver.
  - A level two times the upper limit of normal is 90% specific and 80–90% sensitive.
- Elevation in urinary amylase, amylase–creatinine clearance ratio.
- Sentinel loop sign (on abdominal x-ray [AXR]).
- Colon cutoff sign (on AXR).
- Computed tomography (CT) scan: Diagnostic test of choice (90% sensitive and 100% specific) (see Figure 17-2).

TREATMENT

- Hydration: Maintain adequate intravascular volume.
- Monitor electrolytes.
- Nasogastric tube: For severe disease with vomiting.
- Antibiotics: If infection identified.
- NPO.

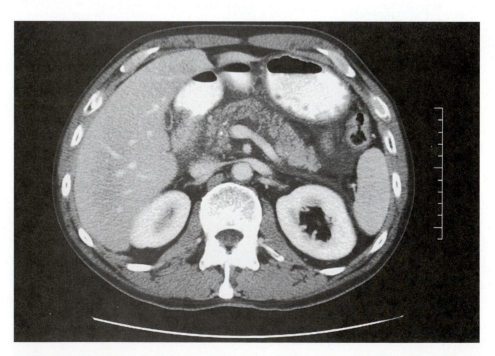

FIGURE 17-2. Abdominal CT demonstrating stranding in the peripancreatic region, consistent with acute pancreatitis.

TABLE 17-1. Ranson's criteria (predicts risk of mortality in pancreatitis).

On Admission	After 48 hours
Age > 55	Drop in hematocrit > 10%
Blood sugar > 200	Increase in blood urea nitrogen (BUN) > 5
White blood count (WBC) > 16,000	Calcium < 8
Serum glutamic oxaloacetic transaminase (SGOT) > 250	PO_2 < 60 mm Hg
Lactic dehydrogenase (LDH) > 700	Base deficit > 4
	Fluid deficit > 6 L

Number of Risk Factors	Mortality
< 3	1%
3 or 4	16%
5 or 6	40%
> 6	70–100%

- Surgery indicated for:
    - Uncertainty of diagnosis
    - Secondary infected necrosis
    - Correction of associated biliary tract disease
    - Progressive deterioration with medical care

PROGNOSIS

- See Table 17-1 for Ranson's criteria.

A sentinel loop is distention and/or air–fluid levels near a site of abdominal distention. In pancreatitis, it is secondary to pancreatitis-associated ileus.

CHRONIC PANCREATITIS

ETIOLOGY

- Most commonly alcohol abuse
- Also hyperparathyroidism, cystic fibrosis, congenital pancreatic anomalies, hemochromatosis
- Associated with chronic liver disease

SIGNS AND SYMPTOMS

- Pain similar to acute pancreatitis
- Malabsorption
- Steatorrhea
- Elevated blood sugars
- Polyuria

Typical scenario: A 32-year-old male who underwent laparotomy for a gunshot wound to the abdomen 2 days ago is found to have a tender belly without rebound and is leaning forward on his stretcher breathing at a rate of 28/min. *Think:* Pancreatitis.

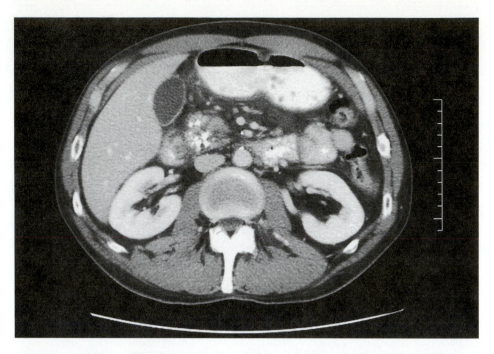

FIGURE 17-3. Abdominal CT demonstrating calcificaton involving the entire head of the pancreas, consistent with chronic pancreatitis.

Gallstones are not a common cause of chronic pancreatitis.

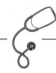

Pancreatic calcifications are associated with chronic pancreatitis.

DIAGNOSIS

- Patient history very important
- **Pancreatic calcifications** on x-ray
- **Chain of lakes** pattern on pancreatography
- **Pseudocysts:** On CT scan (see Figure 17-3) (use ultrasound for follow-up of pseudocysts)

TREATMENT

- Nonoperative management: Includes control of abdominal pain, endocrine and exocrine insufficiency
- Operative management: In general for pain relief:
  - Ampullary procedures
  - Ductal drainage procedures (to decompress the pancreatic duct)
  - Ablative procedures (resection of portions of pancreas)
- For pseudocysts: Thirty percent of pseudocysts resolve on their own with bowel rest (TPN and NPO). Internal drainage can be after 4 weeks (pseudocyst wall needs that time to mature) done via Roux-en-Y cyst-jejunostomy or cyst-gastrostomy.
- Indications for surgery:
  - Persistent pain
  - Gastrointestinal or biliary obstruction
  - Pseudocyst infection, hemorrhage, or rupture
  - Enlarging pseudocysts

ETIOLOGY

- From exocrine pancreas.
- Fourth most common cause of cancer death in the United States.
- Male:female: 2:1.
- Blacks > whites.
- Associated with smoking and older age.
- Most occur in head of pancreas.
- Associated with genetic lesions.

SIGNS AND SYMPTOMS

- Weight loss
- Jaundice (due to obstruction in head)
- Pain radiating to back
- Phlebitis

DIAGNOSIS

- Elevated CA 19-9, alkaline phosphatase, direct bilirubin.
- Initial study is an ultrasound if biliary obstruction suspected.
- CT scan very useful.
- Percutaneous transhepatic cholangiography (PTC) and endoscopic retrograde cholangiopancreatography (ERCP) useful in periampullary lesions.
- Angiography may also be useful.

TREATMENT

- Preoperative nutritional optimization.
- Preoperative internal biliary decompression with stent may be considered.
- Most patients are not candidates for Whipple procedure (pancreaticoduodenectomy).
- If unresectable, palliative procedure considered:
  - **Relieve biliary obstruction.**
  - **Relieve duodenal obstruction.**
  - **Chemical splanchicectomy (pain control).**
- Postoperative chemoradiation therapy controversial.

Courvoisier's sign:
Palpable nontender gallbladder (don't confuse with Murphy's sign).

Whipple procedure:
Removal of gallbladder, common bile duct (CBD), antrum of stomach, duodenum, proximal jejunum and head of pancreas (en bloc); high morbidity and mortality.

HIGH-YIELD FACTS

The Pancreas

- Commonly females age 40 to 60 years
- In body and tail
- Malignant potential
- < 2 % of all pancreatic exocrine tumors
- Present with abdominal/back pain
- Prognosis better than adenocarcinoma
- Treatment: Surgical resection

Pancreatic cystadenoma:
Mucinous = **m**alignant
potential

CYSTADENOMA

- Older and middle-aged women
- Present with vague abdominal symptoms
- Two types:
  - Serous: Benign
  - Mucinous: Generally benign but has potential to be malignant
- Treatment: Surgical

ENDOCRINE TUMORS (ISLET CELL TUMORS)

Note: Islet cell tumor cancer vaccines, which use the patient's own live cancer cells to induce remission or fight relapse, are in clinical trials.

Insulinoma

DEFINITION

Overproduction of insulin.

Typical scenario: A 30-year-old male complains of feeling faint and confused most notably after he exercises. His symptoms improve after he has a soft drink. *Think:* Insulinoma—check fasting serum insulin level.

EPIDEMIOLOGY

- Most common islet cell tumor.
- Eighty-five percent are benign.
- Most are solitary lesions.
- Found with equal frequency in head, body, and tail of pancreas.

SIGNS AND SYMPTOMS

- "Spells" or blackouts due to hypoglycemia
- Aggressiveness, confusion, coma

DIFFERENTIAL DIAGNOSIS

- Obesity
- Surreptitious insulin administration
- Circulating insulin antibodies
- Renal insufficiency

DIAGNOSIS

Fasting serum insulin level > 25 uU/mL (normal: < 15 uU/mL)

Insulinoma is characterized by **Whipple's triad:**
1. Symptoms of hypoglycemia with fasting
2. Glucose < 50
3. Relief of symptoms with glucose

TREATMENT

- Surgical resection is usually curative.
- Diazoxide can improve hypoglycemic symptoms.

Gastrinoma

DEFINITION

- Overproduction of gastrin
- Also known as Zollinger–Ellison syndrome

EPIDEMIOLOGY

- Second most frequent islet cell tumor
- 50% found in tail of pancreas
- Small, slow-growing, multiple, 60% malignant
- Tumor most commonly located in pancreatic head (70%) or duodenal bulb (10%)

SIGNS AND SYMPTOMS

- Signs of peptic ulcer disease
- Epigastric pain most prominent after eating
- Occasionally diarrhea

DIFFERENTIAL DIAGNOSIS

- Achlorhydria (pernicious anemia atrophic gastritis)
- Pharmacologic inhibition of gastric acid secretion (proton pump inhibitors; H_2-receptor blockers)
- Vagotomy with retained antrum
- Antral G-cell hyperplasia
- Renal insufficiency

DIAGNOSIS

- Fasting serum gastrin level > 500 pg/mL (normal: < 100 pg/mL)

TREATMENT

- Proton pump inhibitor to alleviate symptoms
- Surgical resection (difficult because lesions are usually multiple)

Twenty-five percent of gastrinomas are associated with multiple endocrine neoplasia type 1 (MEN-1).

Typical scenario: A 40-year-old male complains of chronic epigastric pain shortly following meals and notices needing increasing doses of his anti-ulcer medication. *Think:* Gastrinoma.

VIPoma

DEFINITION

Overproduction of vasoactive intestinal peptide (VIP).

EPIDEMIOLOGY

- Also known as Verner–Morrison syndrome or WDHA syndrome: Watery diarrhea, hypokalemia, achlorhydria.
- Most are malignant; majority have metastasized to liver at time of diagnosis.

SIGNS AND SYMPTOMS

- Severe watery diarrhea
- Signs of hypokalemia

DIAGNOSIS

Fasting serum VIP level > 800 pg/mL (normal: < 200 pg/mL)

TREATMENT

- Surgical resection, chemotherapy
- Octreotide (somatostatin analogue)

Typical scenario: A 57-year-old male presents with a history of severe watery diarrhea characterized by hypokalemia and achlorhydria. His most recent bout required fluid resuscitation in the intensive care unit (ICU). *Think:* VIPoma.

Glucagonoma

DEFINITION

Rare tumor that results in overproduction of glucagon.

EPIDEMIOLOGY

Most are malignant, large primary tumors that have usually metastasized to lymph nodes and liver at the time of diagnosis.

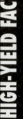

Necrolytic migratory erythema is the skin condition associated with glucagonoma.

SIGNS AND SYMPTOMS

- Hyperglycemia
- Anemia
- Mucositis
- Weight loss
- Severe dermatitis

DIFFERENTIAL DIAGNOSIS

- Hepatic insufficiency
- Severe stress
- Hypoglycemia
- Starvation
- Decompensated diabetes mellitus
- Renal insufficiency

DIAGNOSIS

- Fasting serum glucagon level > 1,000 pg/mL (normal: < 200 pg/mL)

TREATMENT

- Surgery and chemotherapy.

Somatostatinoma

DEFINITION

Overproduction of somatostatin.

EPIDEMIOLOGY

- Very rare tumor.
- Tumor is large and has metastasized at the time of diagnosis.

SIGNS AND SYMPTOMS

- Indigestion
- Diarrhea
- Abdominal cramps
- Weight loss
- Glucose intolerance/diabetes
- Gallstones
- Hypochlorhydria

- Fasting serum somatostatin level > 1,000 pg/mL (normal: < 100 pg/mL)

TREATMENT

Surgical resection, chemotherapy.

PANCREATIC TRAUMA

See trauma chapter.

PANCREAS TRANSPLANTATION

See transplant chapter.

The Spleen

DESCRIPTION

Immunologic organ without distinct lobes or segments that weighs about 100 to 175 g.

Twenty percent of patients have an accessory spleen.

ANATOMIC BOUNDARIES

Left upper quadrant (LUQ) of the abdomen, between the eighth and eleventh ribs (see Figure 18-1).

- Superior: Left diaphragm leaf
- Inferior: Colon, splenic flexure, and phrenocolic ligament

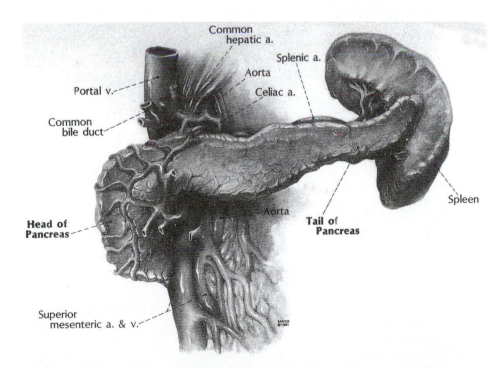

FIGURE 18-1. The spleen and its relationships. (Copyright 2003 Mayo Foundation.)

- Medial: Pancreas (tail) and stomach
- Lateral: Rib cage
- Anterior: Rib cage, stomach
- Posterior: Rib cage

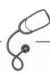

SPLENOMEGALY

DEFINITION

- Physical enlargement of the spleen.
- Normal spleen is palpable in only 2% of adults.

SIGNS AND SYMPTOMS

Palpation of spleen inferior to left costal margin with a notching on the anteromedial surface.

CAUSES

- Main cause of splenomegaly are disease states (can be transient) in which flow patterns become more circuitous, blood cells pool, and even normal cells can get trapped.
- These disease states can be primary or conditions associated with hypersplenism.

HYPERSPLENISM

DEFINITION

- A physiologic state characterized by splenomegaly and overactive splenic function, which results in excessive removal of any and all circulating blood elements
- Classified as primary (idiopathic) and secondary

CAUSES OF SECONDARY HYPERSPLENISM

Hemolytic Anemias

- Hereditary spherocytosis
- Hereditary elliptocytosis
- Glucose-6-phosphate dehydrogenase (G6PD)
- Thalassemia major
- Sickle cell anemia
- Idiopathic autoimmune hemolytic anemia
- ITP
- TTP

Neoplastic and Myeloproliferative States

- Lymphomas
- Leukemias (hairy cell, chronic lymphocytic leukemia [CLL], and chronic myelogenous leukemia [CML])
- Angiosarcoma
- Metastatic carcinoma
- Myelofibrosis with myeloid metaplasia
- Polycythemia vera

Chronic Inflammatory Diseases

- Felty syndrome (rheumatoid arthritis, splenomegaly, and neutropenia)
- Sarcoidosis (25% of patients develop splenomegaly and 5% hypersplenism)
- Porphyria erythropoietica
- Systemic lupus erythematosus (SLE)

Congestive Splenomegaly

- Portal hypertension
- Cirrhosis (60% of patients develop splenomegaly and 15% develop hypersplenism)
- Portal or splenic vein obstruction
- Splenic venous thrombosis
- Severe congestive heart failure (CHF)

Portal hypertension is the most common cause of hypersplenism.

Infection

- Mononucleosis
- Bacterial endocarditis
- Parasites
- Fungus
- Tuberculosis
- Brucellosis
- Malaria

Storage Diseases/Metabolic Abnormalities

- Gaucher's disease
- Letterer–Siwe disease
- Amyloidosis
- Niemann–Pick disease

SIGNS AND SYMPTOMS

Depend on the underlying condition.

DIAGNOSIS

- Decrease in number of circulating RBCs, neutrophils, or platelets
- Bone marrow hypertrophy (secondary to a decrease in circulating blood cells) and increased marrow production of the deficient cell type (unless there is disease)
- Hemolysis:
  - Increased lactic dehydrogenase (LDH), decreased haptoglobin, anemia, reticulocytosis, increased serum bilirubin
  - Schistocytes and helmet cells on peripheral smear

TREATMENT

- Splenectomy is absolutely indicated for primary hypersplenism.
- Splenectomy in secondary hypersplenism is relatively indicated, depending on the degree to which the hypersplenism is affecting the patient.

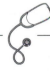

Patients who undergo splenectomy for any reason (hypersplenism or trauma) should receive vaccinations for *Pneumococcus*, *Hemophilus*, and *Meningococcus*.

HYPOSPLENISM

DEFINITION

Anatomic presence of spleen with peripheral blood smears characteristic of asplenism.

CAUSES

- Sickle cell anemia
- Inflammatory bowel disease
- Collagen vascular disease
- Autoimmune disease

SIGNS AND SYMPTOMS

Patients are at increased risk for infection, especially by encapsulated organisms.

DIAGNOSIS

Peripheral smear reveals fragments of old or diseased blood cells such as:
- Howell–Jolly bodies (remnants of nucleated RBCs)
- Pappenheimer bodies (iron granules)
- Acanthocytes (spur cells)
- Heinz bodies

TREATMENT

Prophylaxis against encapsulated organisms, such as pneumococcal and *Hemophilus influenzae* vaccines.

The spleen can be of any size in hyposplenism, which is a functional rather than anatomic state.

SPLENECTOMY

INDICATIONS

- Splenic rupture
- Hereditary spherocytosis (cures the disease)
- Primary tumors or cysts
- Parasitic cysts (e.g., echinococcal hydatid disease)
- Splenic abscess (can sometimes be drained laparoscopically)
- ITP
- Refractory TTP
- Symptomatic splenomegaly (pain, early satiety, severe anemia) associated with various hypersplenic states

COMPLICATIONS

- Atelectasis
- Pneumonia
- Pleural effusion (usually on the left)
- **Overwhelming postsplenectomy sepsis**
- Subphrenic abscess
- Injury to pancreas (because tail of pancreas "hugs" spleen)
- Postoperative hemorrhage
- Thrombocytosis

Conditions associated with rupture of the spleen:
- Mononucleosis
- Malaria
- Blunt LUQ trauma
- Splenic abscess

- Rare site for solid tumor metastatic disease.
- Rare primary nonlymphoid tumor originating in the spleen.
- A common site for metastases especially in lung and breast. However, it is rarely clinically significant and usually an autopsy finding.

Hodgkin's Lymphoma

DESCRIPTION

- Malignant lymphoid neoplasm, with giant multinucleated Reed–Sternberg cells in abnormal lymphoid tissue
- Localized origin, limited regional spread, systemic dissemination (late in disease), and spleen can be primary site

CLASSIFICATION

Major histologic types:
1. Nodular sclerosis
2. Lymphocyte predominant
3. Mixed cellularity
4. Lymphocyte depletion

SIGNS AND SYMPTOMS

Specific
- Pel–Ebstein cyclic fever
- Chest pain following alcohol ingestion

General
- Chest pain, cough, dyspnea, hoarseness, superior vena cava syndrome
- Weight loss, malaise, anorexia

DIAGNOSIS

Hallmark is presence of Reed–Sternberg cells.

STAGING

Can be done via clinical symptoms or laparotomy (more accurate) (see Table 18-1).

Reasons for staging:
- Lesion usually starts as a single focus and spreads along adjacent lymphatic channels.
- Prognosis related to clinical stage.
- Therapy dependent on stage.
- Clinical staging by laboratory values and radiographic studies are inaccurate.

HIGH-YIELD FACTS

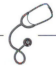

Adverse prognostic factors in Hodgkin's disease include:
- Bulky mediastinal disease
- Age > 40
- Male gender
- Significant weight loss, fevers

The Spleen

TABLE 18-1. Clinical and laparotomy staging of Hodgkin's lymphoma.

Stage	Clinical Staging	Laparotomy Staging
I	Limited to one anatomic region	Wedge liver biopsy
II	Two or more regions of disease on the same side of the diaphragm	Splenectomy
III	Disease on both sides of the diaphragm with disease limited to lymph nodes, spleen, Waldeyer's ring	Periaortic chain, mesentery, and hepatoduodenal lymph node sampling
IV	Metastatic disease	Iliac crest bone marrow biopsy

TREATMENT

- Stages IA and IIA with good prognostic factors: Can consider radiation alone.
- If adverse prognostic factors or advanced disease present: Add chemotherapy.

Non-Hodgkin's Lymphoma

DESCRIPTION

See Table 18-2.
- Systemic disease at the time of diagnosis.
- Primary disease limited to the spleen is rare.
- Two to four times more common in men.

SIGNS AND SYMPTOMS

- Superior vena cava syndrome
- Constitutional symptoms such as fever, weight loss, malaise

TREATMENT

- Chemotherapy.
- Splenectomy has a limited role in the management of lymphoma.

Hairy Cell Leukemia

DESCRIPTION

Lymphocytic leukemia.

RISK FACTORS

- More common in males 4:1
- Age > 50

TABLE 18-2. Classification of non-Hodgkin's lymphoma by aggressiveness and morphologic appearance of the tumor cells.

Classification	Description
Low-grade aggressiveness	Small lymphocytic Follicular small cleaved cell Follicular mixed cell
Intermediate-grade aggressiveness	Follicular large cell Diffuse small cell Diffuse mixed cell Diffuse large cell
High-grade aggressiveness	Lymphoblastic Small noncleaved cell Immunoblastic

- Abdominal fullness (due to splenomegaly)
- Easy bruising (due to thrombocytopenia)
- Recurrent infections (due to leukopenia)
- Weight loss, anorexia, weakness
- Splenomegaly
- Not much lymphadenopathy (unlike CLL)
- Variable hepatomegaly

DIAGNOSIS

- Ruffled leukocyte cell membranes and positive staining for tartrate-resistant acid phosphates, found predominantly in the red pulp (seen in 90% of patients)
- Peripheral smear: Predominance of mononuclear cells, hairy cells pancytopenia
- Definitive diagnosis made by bone marrow biopsy

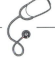

Hairy cell leukemia:
The cells are called "hairy" because of the filamentous cytoplasmic projections seen on electron microscopy.

TREATMENT

- Alpha-interferon is the preferred treatment, with a 80% response rate.
- Splenectomy for symptomatic hypersplenism can improve cell counts and decrease risk of hemorrhage.

Chronic Lymphoctytic Leukemia (CLL)

EPIDEMIOLOGY

- Occurs primarily in sixth decade
- More common in males 2:1

SIGNS AND SYMPTOMS

- Lymphadenopathy
- Splenomegaly due to autoimmune hemolytic anemia that frequently complicates CLL
- Hepatomegaly
- Late: Weakness, anorexia, weight loss, anemia, thrombocytopenia

DIAGNOSIS

- Peripheral smear: Leukocytosis with predominance of immature, abnormal lymphocytes
- Definitive diagnosis made by bone marrow biopsy

TREATMENT

- Chemotherapy
- Corticosteroids
- Radiation
- Splenectomy—improves symptoms but does not change disease course

HIGH-YIELD FACTS

The Spleen

Chronic Myelocytic Leukemia (CML)

DESCRIPTION

Myeloproliferative disorder resulting in overgrowth of granulocytes in bone marrow.

EPIDEMIOLOGY

More common in males 3:2.

SIGNS AND SYMPTOMS

Splenomegaly—most common physical exam finding.

DIAGNOSIS

- Ninety percent have Philadelphia chromosome t(9;22).
- Peripheral smear: Predominance of myeloblasts and basophils.
- Leukocyte alkaline phosphatase is low in CML cells.

TREATMENT

- Chemotherapy
- Splenectomy for selected patients for symptoms of hypersplenism; does not alter disease course or prolong survival

BENIGN TUMORS

Hemangioma

- Most common primary nonlymphoid tumor of the spleen.
- Main complications are risk of rupture and platelet sequestration with coagulopathy (with large ones).
- Splenectomy is both diagnostic and therapeutic.

Hamartoma

- Usually an incidental finding; can be cystic or solid
- Has no clinical consequence unless very large (mass effect)
- Splenectomy required for diagnosis

Lymphangioma

- Cystic mass associated with liver lymphangiomas and involve multiple body sites (lung, skin, and bone).
- Results in hypersplenism.
- Splenectomy is both diagnostic and therapeutic.

IDIOPATHIC THROMBOCYTOPENIC PURPURA (ITP)

DEFINITION

Immune-mediated thrombocytopenia of unknown etiology.

PATHOPHYSIOLOGY

Development of antibodies against a platelet surface antigen. The antibody–antigen complexes effectively decrease platelet count by being removed from circulation.

SIGNS AND SYMPTOMS

- Petechiae and purpura over trunk and limbs
- Guaiac-positive stool
- Mucosal bleeding

DIAGNOSIS

- Thrombocytopenia on complete blood count (CBC)
- Absence of other factors to explain thrombocytopenia (diagnosis of exclusion)

TREATMENT

- Corticosteroids acutely
- May also consider intravenous immunoglobulin for severe cases.
- Platelet transfusion if significant bleeding present.
- Splenectomy electively to decrease recurrence.
- Takes a few weeks to resolve; caution against strenuous activity during this time.

One unit of platelets increases platelet count by 10,000.

THROMBOTIC THROMBOCYTOPENIC PURPURA (TTP)

DEFINITION

A hemolytic anemia that results from deposition of abnormal von Willebrand factor (vWF) multimers into microvasculature.

PATHOPHYSIOLOGY

- Normally, when endothelial cell damage occurs, vWF and platelets migrate to the site and form clot.
- In TTP, abnormal vWF, in the form of multimers, is present. The presence of such multimers are thought to be due to a defective or missing protease.
- These abnormal vWF multimers migrate to site of endothelial damage and attract platelets as usual but, due to their size, cause clumping of the platelets at the site of repair.
- The clumping of large numbers of platelets effectively decreases their number in circulation.
- This mechanical obstruction within microvasculature causes a shearing of the RBCs as they pass through, resulting in a hemolytic anemia.

Typical scenario: A 27-year-old HIV-positive female presents with fever, waxing and waning mental status, and hematuria. CBC shows pancytopenia. *Think:* TTP.

E. coli 0157:H7 is an invasive gastroenteritis resulting in hemolytic uremic syndrome (HUS). HUS differs from TTP in severity and lack of neurologic symptoms.

Diagnostic pentad for TTP:
FAT RN
Fever
Anemia
Thrombocytopenia
Renal dysfunction
Neurologic dysfunction

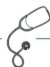

Transfusing platelets in TTP is thought to "fuel the fire" and exacerbate consumption of platelets and clotting factors, resulting in more thrombi in the microvasculature.

EPIDEMIOLOGY

- More common in women.
- Peak age is age 12 to 45 years.

RISK FACTORS

- Infection (especially HIV and *Escherichia coli* 0157:H7)
- Malignancy
- Drugs (antiplatelet agents, chemotherapy agents, contraceptives)
- Autoimmune disorders
- Pregnancy

SIGNS AND SYMPTOMS

Diagnostic Pentad
- Fever
- Altered mental status (waxing and waning, depending on location and movement of clot)
- Renal dysfunction (hematuria, oliguria)
- Thrombocytopenia—can be mild to severe
- Microangiopathic hemolytic anemia

Others
- Petechiae, purpura
- Pallor, jaundice

DIAGNOSIS

- Clinical features of pentad
- Laboratory:
  - Evidence of hemolysis on peripheral smear: Schistocytes, helmet cells.
  - Blood urea nitrogen (BUN) and creatinine may be elevated.
  - CBC: Elevated reticulocyte count, anemia, thrombocytopenia.
  - Decreased haptoglobin level.
  - Increased LDH.
  - May note casts or RBCs in urine.

TREATMENT

- **Do not transfuse platelets.**
- Plasmapheresis is mainstay of treatment (given daily, until platelet count rises to normal).
- May give fresh frozen plasma (FFP) if plasmapheresis not available.
- Transfuse packed red blood cells (PRBCs) if anemia is symptomatic (tachycardia, orthostatic hypotension, hypoxia).
- Consider corticosteroids, vincristine, antiplatelet agents, and splenectomy for refractory cases.
- Monitor for and treat acute bleeds (remember to look for intracranial bleed as well).
- Admit patients to the intensive care unit (ICU).

SPLENIC RUPTURE

See trauma chapter.

SPLENIC ABSCESS

CAUSES

- Sepsis seeding
- Infection from adjacent structures
- Trauma
- Hematoma
- Infection
- IV drug use

SIGNS AND SYMPTOMS

- Fever, chills.
- LUQ tenderness and guarding.
- Spleen may or may not be palpable.

DIAGNOSIS

- Ultrasound: Enlarged spleen with areas of lucency contained within.
- CT: Abscess will show lower attenuation than surrounding spleen parenchyma. Defines abscess better than ultrasound.

TREATMENT

- Splenectomy for most cases
- Percutaneous drainage for a large, solitary juxtacapsular abscess

COMPLICATIONS

- Spontaneous rupture
- Peritonitis
- Bacteremia
- Death

Hernia and Abdominal Wall Problems

OVERVIEW

- Hernias are a common health problem.
- It is estimated that 10% of the population develops some type of hernia during life and that they are present in 3–4% of the male population.
- Fifty percent are indirect inguinal hernias, 25% are direct inguinal, and 15% are femoral.
- The male-to-female ratio is 7:1.
- Abdominal wall hernias are the most common condition requiring major surgery.

The most common hernia in females is the indirect inguinal hernia.

DEFINITIONS

- Hernia: A protrusion of a viscus through an opening in the wall of a cavity in which it is contained
- Groin hernia: Protrusion of a peritoneal sac through the transversalis fascia that extends over the myopectineal orifice
- Hernia orifice: Defect in the innermost abdominal layer of the aponeurosis
- Hernia sac: Outpouch of peritoneum

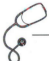

Groin hernias usually present with the complaints of a bulge in the inguinal region. The patient may describe minor pain or vague discomfort.

CLASSIFICATION OF HERNIAS

- **External hernia:** The sac protrudes completely through the abdominal wall. Examples: Inguinal (indirect and direct), femoral, umbilical, and epigastric.
- **Intraparietal hernia:** The sac is contained within the abdominal wall.
- **Internal hernia:** The sac is within the visceral cavity. Examples: Diaphragmatic hernias (congenital or acquired) and the duodenum herniating in the paraduodenal pouch.
- **Reducible hernia:** The protruding viscus can be returned to the abdomen.

Hernia Calendar

- 0 to 2 years—indirect inguinal hernia
- 2 to 20 years—hernia is uncommon
- 20 to 50 years—indirect inguinal hernia
- > 50 years—direct inguinal hernia

- **Irreducible (incarcerated) hernia:** The protruding viscus cannot be returned to the abdomen.
- **Strangulated hernia:** The vascularity of the viscus is compromised. Occurs frequently with small orifices and large sacs.

GENERAL GROIN ANATOMY

See Figure 19-1.

Layers of the Abdominal Wall

Skin, subcutaneous fat, Scarpa's fascia, external oblique muscle, internal oblique muscle, transversus abdominis muscle, transversalis fascia, peritoneal fat, and peritoneum.

Internal Structures

- Inguinal canal boundaries:
  - Anterior wall: External oblique aponeurosis
  - Posterior wall: Transverse abdominal muscle aponeurosis and transversalis fascia
  - Medial border: Transverse aponeurosis and transversalis fascia
  - Lateral border: Transverse abdominal muscle
  - Inferior crus: Transverse aponeuroticofascia
  - Superior crus: A portion of the transverse aponeurosis (transverse aponeurotic arch)

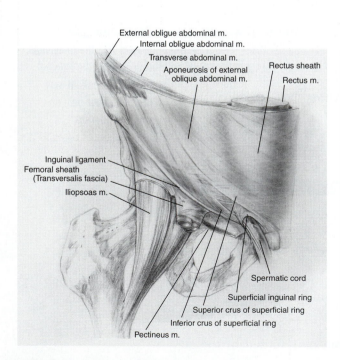
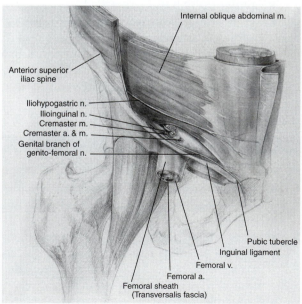

FIGURE 19-1. Groin anatomy. (From Schwartz.)

- Spermatic cord: Begins at the deep ring and contains the vas deferens and its artery (descend to the seminiferous tubules), one testicular artery and two to three veins, lymphatics (incline superiorly to the kidney region), autonomic nerves, and fat

Ligaments

- **Inguinal ligament:** Medial insertion—pecten pubis, which attaches to the adjacent iliopubic tract and transversalis fascia. All three strongly brace the myopectineal orifice, which separates inguinal from femoral herniation and constitutes the medial border of the orifice of the femoral canal.
- **Henle's ligament:** The portion of the tendon of the rectus abdominal muscle that curves laterally onto the pecten pubis.
- **Hesselbach's ligament:** Fascial condensation in the region of the inferior epigastric vessels.

Vasculature

Cremaster vessels: Arise from the inferior epigastric vessels and pass through the posterior wall of the inguinal canal via their own foramen. Supply: Cremaster muscle and the testis tunica.

Nerves

- Genital nerve:
  - Location: Travels along with the cremaster vessels to form a neurovascular bundle.
  - Originates: From L1 and L2.
  - Motor and sensory: Innervates the cremaster muscle, skin of the side of the scrotum and labia.
  - May substitute for the ilioinguinal nerve if it's deficient.
- Iliohypogastric, ilioinguinal nerves, and the genital branch of the genitofemoral nerve:
  - Iliohypogastric and ilioinguinal intertwine.
  - Originates: From T12 and L1.
  - Sensory: To skin of groin, base of penis, and medial upper thigh.
  - Genital branch of genitofemoral nerve: Located on top of the spermatic cord in 60% of people but can be found behind or within the cremaster muscle. Often cannot be found or is too small to be seen.

Femoral Canal Structures

From lateral to medial: **N**erve, **A**rtery, **V**ein, **E**mpty space, **L**ymph nodes

Anatomical Triangles

- **Hesselbach's triangle:** The triangular area in the lower abdominal wall. It is the site of direct inguinal hernia. The boundaries of Hesselbach's triangle are:
  - Inferior border: Inguinal ligament
  - Medial border: Rectus abdominis
  - Lateral border: Inferior epigastric vessels (lateral umbilical fold).

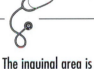

The inguinal area is examined with the patient standing and facing the physician. Presence of a discrete bulge in the inguinal area reveals the hernia. Valsalva's maneuver and cough may accentuate the bulge, making it clearly visible.

Memory aid for the femoral canal structures: **NAVEL.**

- **Triangle of Grynfeltt** (superior lumbar) bounded by the twelfth rib superiorly and the internal oblique muscle anteriorly, with the floor composed of fibers of the quadratus lumborum muscle.
- **Triangle of Petit** (inferior lumbar triangle) bounded by:
  - Posteriorly: Latissimus dorsi muscle
  - Anteriorly: External oblique muscle
  - Inferiorly: Iliac crest
  - The floor is composed of fibers from the internal oblique and transversus abdominis muscle.

INGUINAL HERNIA

- Hernias arising above the abdominocrural crease.
- Most common site for abdominal hernias.
- Male-to-female ratio: 25:1.
- Males: Indirect 2:1 direct.
- Female: Direct is rare.
- Incidence, strangulation, and hospitalization all increase with age.
- Cause 15–20% of intestinal obstructions.

RISK FACTORS

- Abdominal wall hernias occur in areas where aponeurosis and fascia are devoid of protecting support of striated muscle.
- They can be congenital or acquired by surgery or muscular atrophy.
- Female predisposition to femoral hernias: Increased diameter of the true pelvis as compared to men, proportionally widens the femoral canal.
- Muscle deficiency of the internal oblique muscles in the groin exposes the deep ring and floor of the inguinal canal, which are further weakened by intra-abdominal pressure.
- Connective tissue destruction (transverse aponeurosis and fascia): Caused by physical stress secondary to intra-abdominal pressure, smoking, aging, connective tissue disease, systemic illnesses, fracture of elastic fibers, alterations in structure, quantity, and metabolism of collagen.
- Other factors: Abdominal distention, ascites with chronic increase in intra-abdominal pressure, and peritoneal dialysis.

SYMPTOMS

- Nonsymptomatic: Some patients have no symptoms and don't know they have a hernia until they are told.
- Symptomatic: Wide variety of nonspecific discomforts related to the contents of the sac and the pressure by the sac on adjacent tissue.
- Pain: Worse at the end of the day and relieved at night when patient lies down (because the hernia reduces).
- Groin hernias do not usually cause testicular pain. Likewise, testicular pain doesn't usually indicate the onset of a hernia.

DIAGNOSIS

Physical exam: In the standing position, have patient strain or cough. The hernia sac with its contents will enlarge and transmit a palpable impulse.

Hydroceles can resemble an irreducible groin hernia. To distinguish, transilluminate (hernias will not light up).

DIFFERENTIAL DIAGNOSIS

- Abdominal wall mass
- Desmoids
- Neoplasm
- Adenopathy
- Rectus sheath hematoma

RADIOLOGY

- Plain radiography (see Figure 19-2)
- Ultrasound
- Computed tomography (CT)
- Magnetic resonance imaging (MRI)
- Herniography: Radiographic examination of a hernia following injection of a nonirritating contrast medium into the hernial sac.

MANAGEMENT

Principles of Treatment

- Restore the disrupted anatomy.
- Repair using fascia and aponeurosis, not muscle.
- Suture material used should hold until natural support is formed over it.
- Resuscitation in case of strangulated hernia with gangrene with shock or with intestinal obstruction.

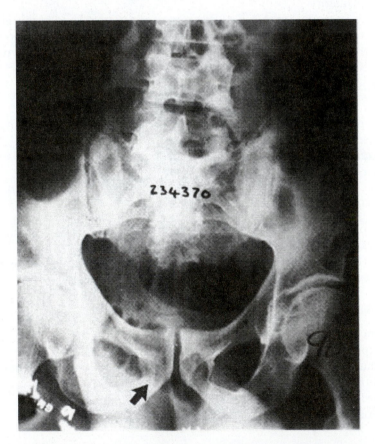

FIGURE 19-2. Abdominal x-ray demonstrating bowel gas pattern in pelvis, consistent with an inguinal hernia. (Reproduced, with permission, from Billitier AJ et al. Radiograhic imaging modalities for the patient in the emergency department with abdominal complaints. *Emerg Med Clinics of North America.* 1996; 14(4): 789–850.)

- Reduction of hernia under anesthesia.
- Repair of the defect.

Nonsurgical

- Can be considered in elderly or unstable patients.
- Support devices can be used but must be applied with hernia reduced.
- Must prevent reappearance of the hernia on straining.

Surgical

- Treatment modality of choice.
- Herniotomy is the operation of cutting through a band of tissue that constricts a strangulated hernia. This may be sufficient in young, muscular individuals and in children.
- Herniorrhaphy involves opening the coverings, returning the contents to their normal place, obliterating the hernial sac, and closing the opening with strong sutures. This can be considered in adults with good muscular tone. Examples:
  - Lytle's repair: Narrowing of the deep ring by suturing medial wall.
  - Bassini's repair: Suturing of conjoint tendon to the incurved part of inguinal ligament.
  - Shouldice repair: Double breasting of transversalis fascia.
  - Ogilvie's repair: Plication of transversalis fascia.
  - McVay's repair/Cooper's repair: Conjoint tendon sutured to Cooper's ligament.
  - Laparoscopic repair: Requires a very experienced and highly skilled surgeon, has decreased postop pain, requires general or regional anesthesia, and more expensive. Wound infection has been shown to decrease with laparoscopic repair.

INDICATIONS FOR SURGERY

- Generally, all hernias should be repaired unless the risks of surgery outweigh the benefits of the repair.
- Exception: A hernia with a wide neck and shallow sac that is expected to enlarge slowly.

COMPLICATIONS OF SURGERY

- Ischemic orchitis with testicular atrophy
- Residual neuralgia
- Both: More common with anterior groin hernioplasty because of the nerves and spermatic cord dissection and mobilization

PROGNOSIS

Recurrence:
- Expert surgeons 1–3% in 10-year follow-up
- Caused by excessive tension on repair, deficient tissue, inadequate hernioplasty, or overlooked hernias
- Decreased with relaxing incisions
- More common with direct hernias

- Direct
- Indirect

Direct Inguinal Hernia

A direct inguinal hernia enters the inguinal canal through its weakened posterior wall. The hernia does not pass through the internal ring.

- Lies posterior to the spermatic cord
- Practically never enters the scrotum
- Wide neck (almost never strangulates)
- Practically only in males
- Common in older age groups
- Common in smokers due to weakened connective tissue
- Predisposing factors: Hard labor, cough, straining, etc.
- Can lead to damage to the ilioinguinal nerve

SYMPTOMS

- Dull dragging pain in the inguinal region referred to testis.
- Pain increases with hard work and straining.

Indirect Inguinal Hernia

Herniation through the internal inguinal ring traveling to the external ring. If complete, can enter the scrotum while exiting the external ring.

- If congenital, is associated to a patent processus vaginalis.
- Bilateral in one third of cases.
- Most common hernia in both males and females.
- Occurs at all ages.
- More common in males than in females.
- In the first decade of life, the right-sided hernia is more common than left (because of late descent of right testis).

A form of indirect hernia arising out of the femoral canal beneath the inguinal ligament (medial to the femoral vessels).

- Female-to-male ratio of 2:1.
- Males affected are in a younger age group.
- Rare in children.
- Uncommon—around 2.5% of all groin hernias.
- Left side 1:2 right side: Secondary to the sigmoid colon tamponading the left femoral canal.
- Common in elderly patients.
- High incidence of incarceration due to narrow neck.
- Twenty-two percent strangulate after 3 months and 45% after 21 months.

- The femoral canal is 1.25 cm long and arises from the femoral ring to the saphenous opening.
- Femoral sac originates from the femoral canal through a defect on the medial side (common) or the anterior (uncommon) side of the femoral sheath.

SYMPTOMS

- Dull dragging pain in the groin, with swelling.
- If obstructed, can cause vomiting and constipation.
- If strangulated, can lead to severe pain and shock.
- Swelling arises from below the inguinal ligament.

DIFFERENTIAL DIAGNOSIS

- Inguinal hernia
- Saphenous varix
- Enlarged femoral lymph node
- Lipoma
- Femoral artery aneurysm
- Psoas abscess

ACQUIRED UMBILICAL HERNIA

- Abdominal contents herniate through a defect in the umbilicus.
- Common site of herniation, especially in females.

ASSOCIATED FACTORS

Ascites, obesity, and repeated pregnancies.

COMPLICATIONS

- Strangulation of the colon and omentum is common.
- Rupture occurs in chronic ascitic cirrhosis. Emergency portal decompression is needed.

TREATMENT

- Surgical repair:
  - Small partial defect: Closed by loosely placed polypropylene suture
  - Large partial defect: Managed with a prosthesis repair
- Mayo hernioplasty is the classical repair (not used often).

PEDIATRIC UMBILICAL HERNIA

- Secondary to a fascial defect in the linea alba with protruding abdominal contents, covered by umbilical skin and subcutaneous tissue.
- Caused by a failure of timely closure of the umbilical ring, and leaves a central defect in the linea alba.
- Common in infants.
- Incarceration is rare and reduction is contraindicated.

Usually close spontaneously within 3 years if the defect < 1.0 cm. Surgical repair indicated if:

- The defect > 2 cm.
- Child is > 3 to 5 years of age.
- Protrusion is disfiguring and disturbing to the child or parents.

ESOPHAGEAL HIATAL HERNIA

- A hernia in which an anatomical part (such as the stomach) protrudes through the esophageal hiatus of the diaphragm
- Two types:
  - Paraesophageal hernia
  - Sliding esophageal hernia

Sliding Esophageal Hernia (Type I)

- The gastroesophageal junction and the stomach herniate into the thoracic cavity.
- These account for more than 90% of all hiatal hernias.
- Can lead to reflux and esophagitis that can predispose to Barrett's esophagus.
- Management can be done medically with antacids and head elevation.
- Only 15% require surgery, consisting of wrapping of the stomach fundus around the lower esophageal sphincter (Nissen fundoplication).

Paraesophageal Hiatal Hernia (Type II)

- Herniation of the stomach into the thorax by way of the esophageal hiatus, without disruption of the gastroesophageal junction
- Rare (< 5%)
- High frequency of complications (i.e., obstruction, strangulation, and hemorrhage); warrants prompt surgical correction

OTHER HERNIAS

- **Richter's hernia:** Only part of the intestine wall circumference is in the hernia. May strangulate without obstruction. Seen commonly in femoral and obturator hernias.
- **Littre's hernia:** The hernial sac contains Meckel's diverticulum. It may become inflamed.
- **Garengoff's hernia:** The hernial sac has the appendix. Importance is that it may form an inflamed hernia.
- **Pantaloon hernia:** A combination of a direct and an indirect inguinal hernia.
- **Maydl's hernia:** W type of intestinal loop herniates; may strangulate with the gangrenous part being inside the abdomen, or may be reduced into the abdomen without noticing the gangrenous part.

HIGH-YIELD FACTS

Hernia and Abdominal
Wall Problems

The hernias associated with obesity are: Direct inguinal, paraumbilical, and hiatal hernias.

- **Spigelian hernia:** The sac passes through the spigelian or semilunaris fascia.
- **Cooper's hernia:** Hernia that involves the femoral canal and tracts to the labia majora in females and to the scrotum in males.
- **Lumbar hernias:** Divided into congenital, spontaneous, traumatic, and incisional. Can pass through the triangle of Grynfeltt, through the inferior lumbar triangle of Petit, or previous incision.
- **Perineal hernia:** Located through pelvic diaphragm, anterior (passes through labia majora—females only) or posterior (male: enters the ischiorectal fossa; female: close to the vagina) to the superficial transverse perineal muscle.
- **Incisional hernia:** Resulting as a surgical complication. These could enlarge beyond repair. Associated with obesity, diabetes, and infection.
- **Eventration:** Loss of integrity of the abdominal wall, reducing the intra-abdominal pressure and resulting in external herniation of bowel.

Surgical Subspecialties and Anesthesia

Pediatric Surgery

CARDIOVASCULAR SYSTEM

Shunts

- Ductus venosus
- Ductus arteriosus
- Foramen ovale

Shunts allow mixing of blood.

Fetal Circulation

- Blood from the placenta returns to the fetus by way of the umbilical vein through the ductus venosus directly into the inferior vena cava.
- Most of saturated blood is shunted directly through the foramen ovale to the left.
- Destuarted blood through the ductus arteriosus enters the placental circulation.

Highest O_2 saturation is in the umbilical vein.

Changes at Birth

- Systemic vascular resistance increases.
- Pulmonary vascular resistance decreases.
- Ductus arteriosus (DA) closes.

- Ductus arteriosus usually closes within the first 24 hours.
- Foramen ovale closes in first month.
- Prostaglandin keeps DA patent.
- Indomethacin facilitates DA closure.

CONGENITAL HEART DISEASE

Right-to-Left Shunts

GENERAL CONSIDERATIONS

Cyanotic type usually due to a combination of right-sided obstruction in addition to right-to-left shunt:
- Polycythemia (response to cyanosis)
- Hypoxic "spells"
- Squatting (helps to increase systemic vascular resistance, increase pulmonary blood flow)
- Clubbing

- Ventricular septal defect (VSD).
- Pulmonary stenosis.
- Overriding aorta.
- Right ventricular hypertrophy.
- Atrial septal defect (ASD) in 10–15% of cases (pentalogy of Fallot).
- Most common cyanotic malformation (accounts for 50%), fourth most common congenital heart defect.
- Small, "wooden shoe"–shaped heart (coeur en sabot); decreased pulmonary blood flow; cyanosis.
- Treatment guided by size of pulmonary arteries vs. ascending aorta; 1:3 ratio requires just one corrective procedure.
- Smaller pulmonary arteries (ratio < 1:3) requires two-step process:
  1. Palliative procedure: Enlargement of stenotic outflow tract or systemic to pulmonary shunt (via *Blalock–Taussig, Waterston,* or *Potts* techniques) (see Figure 20-1)

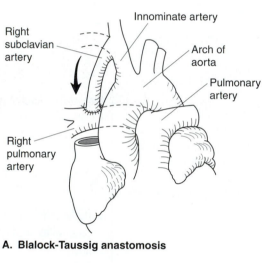

A. Blalock-Taussig anastomosis

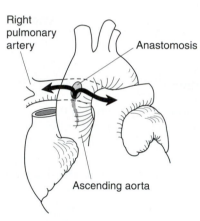

B. Waterston aortic-pulmonary anastomosis

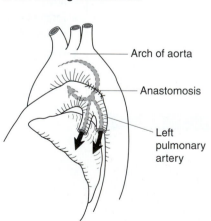

C. Potts anastomosis

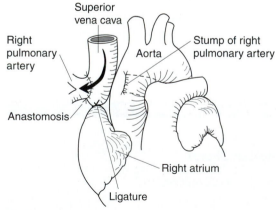

D. Glenn operation

FIGURE 20-1. Palliative operations to increase pulmonary arterial blood flow. **A.** Blalock–Taussig subclavian–pulmonary arterial anastomosis. **B.** Waterston aortic to right pulmonary arterial anastomosis. **C.** Potts anastomosis between the left pulmonary artery and the descending thoracic aorta. **D.** Glenn operation. The end of the right pulmonary artery is connected to the side of the superior vena cava, which is ligated caudad to the anastomosis. (Reproduced, with permission, from Way LW, Doherty GM, eds. *Current Surgical Diagnosis and Treatment,* 11th ed. New York: McGraw-Hill, 2003: 459.)

2. Corrective procedure: Patching to reduce outflow obstruction, resection and division of muscle to enlarge outflow tract, patching of VSD

Ninety to 95% success rate.

PULMONARY STENOSIS/PULMONARY ATRESIA WITH INTACT VENTRICULAR SEPTUM

- Stenosis alone fairly common (10% of all congenital heart defects).
- Pulmonary atresia with intact ventricular septum (PAIVS) is a more severe form of this process:
  - Total obstruction of outflow tract, valvular atresia, annular hypoplasia, maldevelopment of right ventricle
  - Accounts for 1–3% of congenital heart defects
- Patent foramen ovale or ASD required for compatibility with life.
- Stenotic lesions treated with *balloon dilation*.
- Surgical correction required for atresia: Valvulotomy or transannular patch (to relieve outflow obstruction) *plus* systemic–pulmonary shunt.
- More definitive correction may be made later in childhood if right ventricle develops adequately. Outflow tract is further enlarged and shunt may be closed.

TRICUSPID ATRESIA

- Atresia of tricuspid valve accompanied by:
  1. Atresia and hypoplasia of right ventricle
  2. ASD, patent foramen ovale, or VSD
  3. Transposition of great vessels in 30% of cases
  4. Pulmonary stenosis or atresia in 85% with normally located great vessels
  5. PDA in most cases
- Decreased pulmonary blood flow with normally located great vessels, unrestricted flow with transposed vessels
- Unrestricted flow leading to overperfusion of lungs: Single-ventricle complex
- Treatment: Emergency systemic–pulmonary shunt or enlargement of ASD/foramen needed in the newborn for palliation
- Later correction made via bidirectional Glenn shunt followed by modified Fontan (total cavopulmonary most often used)

EBSTEIN'S ANOMALY

- Malformed and downwardly displaced septal and posterior leaflets of tricuspid valve, leading to obstruction and incompetence.
- Patent foramen ovale (PFO) or ostium secundum defect.
- Tricuspid obstruction plus PFO/ASD lead to right-to-left shunting, cyanosis.
- "Atrialized" right ventricle: Area of right ventricle between the true annulus and displaced origin of tricuspid leaflets becomes morphologically and functionally a part of right atrium.
- May be associated with maternal lithium use during pregnancy.
- Arrhythmias are common.
- Treatment: Valve reconstruction or replacement, plication/oversewing of atrialized right ventricle if it bulges or contracts paradoxically, and closure of ASD.

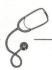

Arterial switch (Jatene procedure) involves transection of great vessels just superior to valves, then transfer of vessels to their correct locations. Right and left coronary artery ostia need to be cut out as separate "buttons" due to their close proximity to the valves.

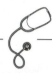

Rastelli procedure: Aorta is rerouted internally to left ventricle across VSD; pulmonary artery is attached to right ventricle externally.

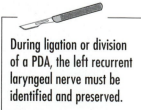

During ligation or division of a PDA, the left recurrent laryngeal nerve must be identified and preserved.

TRANSPOSITION OF THE GREAT ARTERIES (TGA)

- Abnormal division of bulbar trunk during embryogenesis leads to opposite origins of aorta and pulmonary artery. Caval inflow and pulmonary veins are normal.
- Systemic venous blood pumped back out to body via right ventricle through aorta; pulmonary circulation rages between lungs and left side of heart.
- Incompatible with life unless concurrent PDA, PFO, or VSD exists so that mixing can occur.
- Most common association: TGA with VSD (50% of TGAs).
- Four diagnostic groups:
  1. TGA with intact ventricular septum (worst). Treatment: Balloon septostomy of foramen ovale at birth, then arterial switch operation.
  2. TGA with VSD. Treatment: Arterial switch operation within first 2 weeks of life (before development of pulmonary congestion).
  3. TGA with VSD plus left ventricular outflow tract (LVOT) obstruction. Treatment: Palliative systemic–pulmonary shunt, then Rastelli procedure at age 4 or 5.
  4. Complex transposition (any of the above plus other severe cardiac defects). Treatment: Individualized.
- TGA four times as prevalent in males.
- "Egg-shaped" heart, narrow cardiac shadow, and marked pulmonary congestion on chest x-ray (CXR).

Left-to-Right Shunts

GENERAL CONSIDERATIONS

- Many left-to-right shunts progress to right-to-left shunts.
- Acyanotic (until shunt reversal).
- Increased pulmonary blood flow.
- Symptoms of pulmonary congestion often appear at first pregnancy.

PATENT DUCTUS ARTERIOSUS (PDA)

- Second most common congenital heart defect. Incidence varies inversely with birth weight and gestational age. It is two to three times more common in females.
- Derives embryologically from the sixth left aortic arch and arises just distal to left subclavian takeoff.
- Patients with PDA have increased susceptibility to bacterial endocarditis.
- Increased pulmonary blood flow leads to elevated pulmonary vascular resistance and pulmonary hypertension.
- Cyanosis can appear in PDA with pulmonary hypertension, but it may also be a sign of an associated cardiac defect.
- Treatment:
  - Indomethacin successfully treats 90% of cases.
  - Surgery indicated in premature infants with severe respiratory insufficiency who are refractory to indomethacin. Double ligation of ductus is performed.
  - Complete surgical division performed in older children.
  - Unless congestive heart failure (CHF) develops, surgery can be performed electively in full-term infants some time between 6 months and 2 years of age.

- Coil insertion performed in older children, unless large diameter or short length of ductus requires division.

VENTRICULAR SEPTAL DEFECTS (VSDs)

- Most common congenital heart defect (20–30%), results in left-to-right shunt that increases pulmonary blood flow and may lead to CHF, pulmonary hypertension, and Eisenmenger syndrome, as well as recurrent pneumonia and growth limitations.
- Classified according to *position:*
  1. Perimembranous (most common VSD requiring surgery).
  2. Posterior inlet or atrioventricular canal type (risk of heart block from repair due to close proximity to conduction bundle).
  3. Outlet or supracristal (often associated with aortic insufficiency).
  4. Muscular (most common, often closing on their own).
- Also classified by size of VSD in relation to aortic valve (i.e., how restrictive the defect is):
  1. Restrictive: Smaller defect, with normal-to-increased right ventricular systolic pressure
  2. Nonrestrictive: Larger defect, with right equaling left systolic pressure, on the road to Eisenmenger syndrome
- Treatment: Medical management for congestive symptoms.
- Fifty percent of small defects close on their own within the first 3 years of life, 90% by 8 years. Small defects still leave patient at higher risk of bacterial endocarditis.
- Surgical closure by patch if:
  - CHF is not controlled by medical management.
  - VSD does not close by 9 months and pulmonic pressure has reached two thirds of systemic pressure.
- If pulmonary, and systemic flow is > 2:1 after 4 years of age, closure is also indicated.

Surgical outcome for ventricular septal defects: One-third rule
- Regression of increased pulmonary vascular resistance in one third
- No change in one third
- Gradual decrease in one third

EISENMENGER SYNDROME

- Increased pulmonary blood flow leads to potentially irreversible hypertrophy of pulmonary arterioles.
- Hypertrophy increases pulmonary vascular resistance.
- Right-to-left shunting begins to develop commensurate with the progression of pulmonary resistance.
- Pulmonary hypertension in which pulmonary resistance exceeds systemic resistance leads to right-to-left dominance and cyanotic clinical picture.
- Heart–lung transplantation is the only hope.

ATRIAL SEPTAL DEFECTS (ASDs)

- Third most common congenital heart defect, more than twice as common in females.
- Left-to-right shunt results from greater distensibility of right ventricle than left ventricle and higher left-sided pressures. Increased pulmonary blood flow ensues as in VSD, but development of pulmonary hypertension is more gradual, except in *ostium primum* type (see below).
- Usually symptomatic in adult life, but growth retardation, fatigability, and recurrent pneumonia in those with large defects. Adults usually present with arrhythmia (due to enlarged right atrium) or CHF.

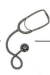
- *Secundum* type (middle or lower defect in area of ostium secundum—majority of ASDs).
- *Sinus venosus* type with partial anomalous pulmonary venous return ("high" defect near superior vena cava [SVC], usually associated with anomalous entry of pulmonary veins into right atrium, SVC, or inferior vena cava [IVC])
- *Ostium primum* type (also called "partial endocardial cushion defect" or "partial atrioventricular canal"), cleft in anterior mitral valve leaflet plus low, sickle-shaped septal defect; mitral insufficiency accompanies left-to-right shunt.
- Treatment: Patch, with leaflet reconstruction in ostium primum.
- Operative indications:
  - Pulmonic: Systemic flow > 1.5 to 2.1.
  - Asymptomatic ASD > 1 to 2 cm (operate at age 3 to 4 years).
  - Ostium primum type at 1 to 4 years, earlier if pulmonary hypertension and cardiac failure.
  - Complete atrioventricular canal (large VSD plus ostium primum that involves both mitral and tricuspid valves) requires surgery within first 6 to 9 months.
  - Little gain in patients with Eisenmenger syndrome.

Obstructive Left-Sided Lesions

COARCTATION OF THE AORTA

- Three times more common in males.
- Probably caused by same fibrotic mechanism that converts PDA to ligamentum arteriosum.
- Traditionally described in relation to ductus arteriosus (preductal, juxtaductal, postductal):
  - Usually located within 4 cm distal to takeoff of left subclavian
  - Complete occlusion in up to 25%
- Collateral circulation distal to coarctation usually causes marked dilation of intercostal arteries, creating "notching" of the ribs on CXR.
- Surgery performed immediately in neonates presenting with CHF. Otherwise, ideal age is 3 to 4 years, when the aorta has reached about 55% of expected size. This may obviate the need for reoperation.
- Subclavian flap arterioplasty or resection of coarctation with end-to-end anastomosis in infants and children.
- Older children tend to present as hypertensive but asymptomatic. Nonetheless, fibrosis, calcification, and thinning of the proximal aorta progress with age.
- In adults, due to long-standing fibrotic changes, an intervening prosthetic graft is needed to approximate the two ends at time of resection. Alternately, a bypass of the coarctation may be performed.

CONGENITAL AORTIC STENOSIS

- Up to four times more common in males.
- **Valvular:** Usually bicuspid valve with ensuing calcification by early adulthood; sometimes tricuspid with fused commissures, or even unicuspid (associated with other cardiac anomalies).
- **Subvalvular:** Rare, involving fibrosis that extends from the aortic valve cusps to varying degrees.

Lutembacher syndrome is an ostium secundum defect plus mitral stenosis.

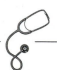

Ostium primum is uncommon except in Down syndrome.

Paraplegia is an uncommon but notorious complication of repair for coarctation of the aorta. This is attributed to ischemia of the spinal cord that results from cross-clamping the aorta during surgery. It is recommended that the occlusion not exceed 20 minutes and that the distal aortic pressure remain above 50 mm Hg.

- **Supravalvular:** Most rare, often with abnormalities of the aortic valve cusps and coronary arteries.
    - Hourglass type
    - Diffuse hypoplastic type
    - Membranous type
- Concentric left ventricular hypertrophy, cardiomegaly, and CHF are the eventual results of aortic stenosis.
- Fatigue, angina, and syncope are common presentations. In the supravalvular type, children may have "elfin facies" and mental retardation. All may present with sudden death.
- Treatment: See section on valvular heart disease, aortic stenosis.
    - In neonates presenting with CHF, emergent valvulotomy is performed, which seeks to provide an aortic valve orifice that is appropriate for the child's body size.
    - Surgery for subvalvular lesions involves excision of the fibrotic area.
    - Among the supravalvular lesions, the hourglass type is most amenable to surgical treatment. The stenosis is divided, and an intervening patch extends the diameter of the vessel.
- **Idiopathic hypertrophic subaortic stenosis:**
    - Genetic disease in which asymmetric septal hypertrophy creates obstruction to aortic outflow tract.
    - Same presentation as with other forms of aortic stenosis, though atrial fibrillation and systemic emboli are also common.
    - Treatment: Medical, unless symptoms are refractory and ventricular–aortic gradient exceeds 50 mm Hg. Then septal myomectomy is performed.

HYPOPLASTIC LEFT HEART SYNDROME

- **L/S ratio < 2:** Risk of respiratory distress syndrome (RDS).
- **Lungs reach full maturity at 8 years.**

- Left side of heart is underdeveloped, with ineffective contractile function and a valveless aortic remnant.
- Blood enters systemic circulation after leaving the lungs via PDA. Once ductus closes, this is incompatible with life; thus, most die within the first 10 days.
- Palliative surgery with 80% survival.
- Norwood plan:
    1. Anastomosis of pulmonary artery to aortic arch in order to establish flow from right ventricle to systemic circulation. Resection of atrial septum is performed to mix blood. Subclavian–pulmonary artery shunt is created to control pulmonary blood flow.
    2. After 6 to 18 months of age, the pulmonary vascular resistance has dropped enough to take down the shunt and establish a direct atrial–pulmonary artery connection. (Can be done in 1 or 2 stages known as a Glenn (hemi-Fontan) or Fontan procedure.)

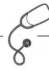

- Glucocorticoids are given to mothers if birth is imminent before 34 weeks.

PULMONARY SYSTEM

Lecithin/Sphingomyelin (L/S) Ratio

- Marker for fetal lung maturity
- Delayed lung maturation:
    - Diabetes mellitus
    - Rh isoimmunization

Neonates are primarily nasal breathers.

Gastric and tracheal tubes should be oral.

Normal Arterial Blood Gas (ABG) for Neonates

$PaO_2 = 75$ mm Hg
$PaCO_2 = 35$ mm Hg
pH = 7.30 to 7.35

Neonatal Total Body Water (TBW)

Eighty percent of weight.

Urine Concentration

- 600 mOsm/kg (neonates)
- 1,200 mOsm/kg (adults)

Glomerular Filtration Rate (GFR)

- 50 mL/min/m² (neonates)
- 100 mL/min/m² (adults)

- Urine production starts at 9 to 12 weeks gestation.
- Nephrogenesis is complete by 35 weeks.

Urine Output

1 to 2 mL/kg/hr.

Fluid Bolus

20 mL/kg lactated Ringer's (LR) or normal saline.

Fluid bolus should not contain dextrose.

Maintenance Fluid

- 100 to 120 mL/kg/day (full term)
- 140 mL/kg/day (preterm infant)

CONGENITAL NECK LESIONS

TYPES

- Congenital
- Inflammatory
- Traumatic
- Neoplastic

Inflammatory masses are the most common congenital neck lesions. Common causes:
- Lymphadenopathy
- Cervical adenitis
- Hematoma
- Benign tumors (lipoma)

LOCATION

Location provides the most information regarding the diagnosis.

Midline
- Thyroglossal duct remnants
- Dermoid cyst

HIGH-YIELD FACTS

Pediatric Surgery

- Submental lymph node
- Goiter

Lateral
- Cystic hygroma
- Branchial cyst
- Lymph adenitis
- Lymphoma

Thyroglossal Duct Cyst and Sinus

DEFINITION

Midline neck mass that arises from base of tongue at foramen cecum.

SIGNS AND SYMPTOMS

- Most commonly present as infection
- Usually painless, smooth, mobile, and cystic

TREATMENT

- Complete excision of cyst
- Resection of central portion of hyoid bone
- High ligation of duct at foramen cecum
- Complete excision necessary to prevent recurrence
- Radionuclide scans prior to surgery to rule out ectopic thyroid gland
- Follow-up screening for hypothyroidism

Branchial Cleft Cysts and Sinuses

DEFINITION

Remnants of the four paired branchial arches, clefts, and pouches.

SIGNS AND SYMPTOMS

- Lateral neck mass at anterior border of sternocleidomastoid muscle
- Usually painless
- Fluctuant, mobile, and nontender
- May present with drainage

DIAGNOSIS

Ultrasound.

TREATMENT

- Complete excision of cyst and entire tract
- Antibiotics if infected

Cystic Hygroma

DEFINITION

Congenital lymphangioma.

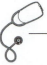

Life-threatening causes of congenital neck lesions:
- Hematoma secondary to trauma
- Subcutaneous emphysema plus airway or pulmonary injury
- Non-Hodgkin's lymphoma with mediastinal mass and airway compromise

Thyroglossal duct cyst moves with swallowing and tongue protrusion; however, absence of this finding does not exclude the diagnosis.

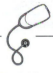

Second branchial cleft cyst is the most common branchial cyst.

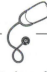

Probing of branchial cyst may lead to infection.

Cystic hygroma is the most common lymphatic malformation in children.

SIGNS AND SYMPTOMS

- Most are identified at birth.
- May be recognized after injury or upper respiratory infection.
- Painless, soft, and mobile.
- Transilluminate brightly.
- May compress trachea or spread into the floor of mouth, causing upper airway obstruction.
- Do not regress spontaneously.

DIAGNOSIS

Computed tomography (CT) scan (extent and involvement of surrounding structures).

TREATMENT

Surgical excision.

Congenital diaphragmatic hernia is more common on the left.

Typical scenario: A newborn presents with respiratory distress and a scaphoid abdomen. *Think:* Diaphragmatic hernia.

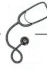

- Positive pressure ventilation must be delivered by endotracheal (ET) tube, *never by mask.*
- Bag and mask ventilation may cause respiratory compromise.

CONGENITAL DIAPHRAGMATIC HERNIA

DEFINITION

Patent pleuroperitoneal canal through the foramen of Bochdalek.

SIGNS AND SYMPTOMS

- Significant respiratory distress within first few hours of life
- Scaphoid abdomen

DIAGNOSIS

- Ultrasound (prenatally)
- CXR:
  - Bowel gas pattern in hemithorax
  - Mediastinal shift

TREATMENT

- Respiratory and metabolic support
- Gastric decompression
- Surgical correction
- Extracorporeal membrane oxygenation (ECMO)

PROGNOSIS

- Survival rates are 50% at best.
- Predictors of mortality:
  - Pulmonary hypoplasia
  - Pulmonary hypertension

CONGENITAL LOBAR EMPHYSEMA

DEFINITION

Hyperexpansion of one or more lobes of the lung.

SIGNS AND SYMPTOMS

- Respiratory distress at birth or soon after
- Tachypnea
- Cyanosis

DIAGNOSIS

CXR:
- Hyperaerated lobe
- Hyperlucency (air trapping)
- Mediastinal shift

TREATMENT

- Observation for small cysts
- Selective ventilation of uninvolved lung
- Resection of affected lung lobe

PULMONARY SEQUESTRATION

DEFINITION

- A nonfunctioning embryonic and cystic pulmonary tissue that receives its entire blood supply from the systemic circulation.
- Most do not communicate with functional airways.

TYPES

- Intralobar:
  - No pleural covering.
  - Present with infection.
  - CXR may reveal mass lesion and air–fluid level.
  - Venous drainage via pulmonary veins.
- Extralobar:
  - Pleural covering present.
  - Associated with diaphragmatic hernia.
  - Incidental finding on CXR.
  - Venous drainage via pulmonary veins.
  - Venous drainage via azygous veins.

DIAGNOSIS

Magnetic resonance imaging (MRI) or aortography to demonstrate sequestration of lung tissue within systemic venous drainage.

TREATMENT

Surgical removal.

Congenital cystic adenomatoid malformation is the second most common congenital lung lesion (lobar emphysema is the most common).

Presentation of congenital cystic adenomatoid malformation similar to diaphragmatic hernia.

Where is the NG tip?
- Tip in thorax: CDH
- Tip in abdomen: CCAM

This makes the difference between a thoracic and an abdominal surgery!

Most common malformation is esophageal atresia with a TE fistula (85%).

Fifty percent of infants with esophageal atresia have associated anomalies:
- Polyhydramnios
- Preterm birth
- Small for gestational age

CONGENITAL CYSTIC ADENOMATOID MALFORMATION

DEFINITION

Congenital pulmonary malformation involving varying degrees of adenomatosis and cyst formation.

SIGNS AND SYMPTOMS

- Neonatal respiratory distress
- Recurrent respiratory infection

DIAGNOSIS

- CXR:
  - Characteristic "Swiss cheese" appearance of affected lung
  - May be difficult to distinguish from air-filled loops of bowel associated with congenital diaphragmatic hernia (CDH)
- Location of nasogastric (NG) tube is key.

TREATMENT

Surgical resection.

TRACHEOESOPHAGEAL (TE) MALFORMATIONS

DEFINITION

Failure of complete separation of trachea from esophagus.

EMBRYOLOGY

- Esophagus and trachea originate from a single diverticulum and divide at fifth week of gestation.
- The esophagus ends blindly 10 to 12 cm from the nares.

SIGNS AND SYMPTOMS

- Respiratory distress or choking following first feeding
- Infant drools and is unable to swallow saliva

TYPES

1. Esophageal atresia and tracheoesophageal fistula
2. Pure esophageal atresia
3. H-type tracheoesophageal fistula

DIAGNOSIS

- Attempts to pass feeding tube unsuccessful
- CXR: Tube to end or coil in the region of thoracic inlet
- Abdominal x-ray (AXR)
- Contrast x-ray studies

TREATMENT

- Decompress blind esophageal pouch and control oral secretions with sump tube on constant suction.

- Parenteral antibiotics.
- Evaluate for other anomalies (primarily cardiac and renal)—cardiac echo to define aortic arch.
- If cardiac and respiratory stable, may repair surgically.
- Surgical repair:
  - Ligation of fistula and insertion of gastrostomy tube
  - Anastomosis of two ends of esophagus

ABDOMINAL WALL DEFECTS

Gastroschisis

DEFINITION

Centrally located, full-thickness abdominal wall defect.

DIAGNOSIS

- Often detected during prenatal ultrasound.
- No covering over bowel.
- Umbilical cord is an intact structure.
- Defect is usually to the right of umbilicus.
- Not usually associated with other anomalies.

TREATMENT

- Temperature regulation
- Sterile covering of warm saline-soaked sponges and plastic wrap to minimize evaporative loss
- Nasogastric decompression
- Broad-spectrum antibiotics
- Total parenteral nutrition (TPN)
- Surgical correction

Omphalocele

DEFINITION

- Herniation of abdominal contents into the base of the umblical cord.
- Protective membrane present.
- Elements of the umbilical cord course individually over the sac and come together at its apex to form a normal-appearing umbilical cord.

ASSOCIATED ANOMALIES

- Beckwith–Wiedemann syndrome (gigantism, macroglossia, umbilical defect, hypoglycemia)
- Trisomy 13 and 18
- Pentalogy of Cantrell (omphalocele, diaphragmatic hernia, cleft sternum, absent pericardium, intracardiac defects)
- Exstrophy of the bladder or cloaca

TYPES

- Small: Contain only intestine
- Large: Contain liver, spleen, and GI tract

Typical scenario: An infant has excessive oral secretions, and chokes and has apneic episodes during feedings. *Think:* TE malformation.

H-type fistula most likely to be seen in emergency department (others usually picked up earlier, while infant is still in hospital).

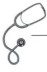

- Tubes < 10 F may coil, giving a false sense of passage.
- The absence of gas in gastrointestinal (GI) tract implies esophageal atresia without tracheoesophageal fistula (TEF).

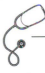

- Esophageal atresia is a surgical emergency.
- Determine the status of the anastomosis before feeding by esophagography.

Seven percent have coexistent intestinal atresia—important to search for this at surgery.

TREATMENT

- Ruptured sac:
    - Cared as for gastroschisis.
    - Emergent surgical correction.
- Intact sac:
    - Less urgent.
    - Timing of surgery depends on size of defect, size of infant, and presence of other anomalies.

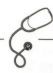

No difference in outcomes for gastrochisis whether infant is delivered vaginally or via c-section.

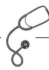

A common error is presuming that bowel is nonviable based on its dark color due to meconium.

Pyloric Stenosis

DEFINITION

- Narrowing of the pyloric canal due to hypertrophy of the musculature
- Occurs 1 in 250 births
- Male-to-female ratio: 4:1

CAUSES

Unknown.

SIGNS AND SYMPTOMS

- Starts third to fifth week of life
- Nonbilious vomiting:
    - Progressive
    - Projectile (±)
    - Hungry after vomiting
- Dehydration
- Midepigastric mass ("olive")
- Visible peristaltic wave (left to right) hypochloremic metabolic alkalosis

Ruptured omphalocele may be confused with gastroschisis, but remember, the latter does not have an intact umbilical cord at the level of abdominal wall.

DIAGNOSIS

- Ultrasound (90% sensitivity):
    - Elongated pyloric channel (> 14 mm)
    - Thickened pyloric wall (> 4 mm)
- Radiographic contrast series:
    - **String sign**—from elongated pyloric channel
    - **Shoulder sign**—bulge of pyloric muscle into the antrum
    - **Double tract sign**—parallel streaks of barium in the narrow channel

TREATMENT

- Correction of fluid and electrolyte and acid–base balance
- IV fluid 5% dextrose in normal saline plus potassium chloride 3 to 5 mEq/kg
- Surgical correction: Ramstedt pyloromyotomy

Pyloric stenosis:
- Children of affected parents have a 7% chance of disease.
- Twenty percent of male and 10% of female children have an affected mother.
- Most common in first-born male.

Biliary Atresia

DEFINITION

- Progressive obliterative cholangiopathy
- Obliteration of the entire extrahepatic biliary tree at or above the porta hepatis

SIGNS AND SYMPTOMS

- Neonatal jaundice (beyond first week)
- Conjugated hyperbilirubinemia

DIAGNOSIS

- Radioisotope scanning
- Ultrasound
- Direct bilirubin
- > 2 mg/dL
- > 10% of total bilirubin

TREATMENT

Laparotomy, liver biopsy, and operative cholangiography should be done in any suspicious case.

Correctable Type
- Blind-ending cystic dilation of the common hepatic duct
- Repaired by direct anastomosis with Roux-en-Y loop of jejunum

Noncorrectable Type
- Kasai procedure—hepatoportoenterostomy

Postoperative Rx
- Prophylactic antibiotics
- Phenobarbital
- Liver transplantation

Malrotation and Midgut Volvulus

DEFINITION

- Incomplete rotation of the intestine during fetal development
- May cause complete or partial duodenal obstruction

EMBRYOLOGY

- Midgut = duodenum to mid-transverse colon.
- Develops extraperitoneally and migrates intraperitoneally at 12 weeks.
- During this migration, the midgut rotates 270° counterclockwise around the superior mesenteric artery (SMA).
- Problem results from abnormal fixation of the mesentery of the bowel.

SIGNS AND SYMPTOMS

- Acute onset of bilious vomiting
- Abdominal distention
- Lethargy
- Skin mottling
- Hypovolemia
- Bloody stool (late sign)

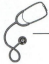
Vomitus in hypertrophic pyloric stenosis is never bile stained.

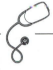
There is a total body potassium deficit but normal serum potassium level in hypertrophic pyloric stenosis.

Biliary atresia accounts for 90% of extrahepatic obstruction in neonates.

Optimal time of surgery for biliary atresia is at < 8 weeks of age.

Malrotation without volvulus may present with intermittent vomiting and abdominal distention.

DIAGNOSIS

- AXR:
  - Presence of bowel loops overriding liver
  - Air in stomach and in duodenum (double bubble sign)
  - No gas in GI tract distal to volvulus
- Upper GI series:
  - Duodenal C-loop does not extend to the left.

TREATMENT

- Surgical emergency
- Reduced with counterclockwise rotation
- Ladd procedure
- Appendectomy—because cecum will remain in the right upper quadrant (RUQ) and future appendicitis may have misleading presentation

PROGNOSIS

Ten percent chance of recurrent volvulus.

Intestinal Atresia

DEFINITION

Failure of the duodenum to recanalize during early fetal life.

ASSOCIATED ANOMALIES

- Down syndrome
- Esophageal atresia
- Imperforate anus

SIGNS AND SYMPTOMS

- Small for gestational age
- Polyhydramnios
- Bilious vomiting
- Abdominal distention

DIAGNOSIS

Plain abdominal film:
- Dilated bowel proximal to obstruction
- Double bubble sign (air in stomach and duodenum)

TREATMENT

- Fluid resuscitation
- Gastric decompression
- Broad-spectrum antibiotics
- Duodenal atresia: Side-to-side anastomosis (avoids injury to bile and pancreatic duct)
- Jejunoileal atresia: End-to-end anastomosis

- Duodenal atresia is the most common type of intestinal atresia.
- Most common site of atresia is at the papilla of Vater.

Passage of meconium does not rule out intestinal atresia.

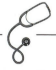

Since malrotation/volvulus has the same radiographic double bubble sign, get upper GI for confirmation.

Intussusception

DEFINITION

Invagination of one portion of the bowel into itself—proximal portion usually drawn into distal portion by peristalsis.

EPIDEMIOLOGY

- Incidence 1 to 4 in 1,000 live births
- Male-to-female ratio: 2:1 to 4:1
- Peak incidence 5 to 12 months
- Age range: 2 months to 5 years

CAUSES

- Idiopathic.
- Viral (enterovirus in summer, rotavirus in winter).
- A "lead point" (or focus) is thought to be present in older children 2–10% of the time. These lead points can be caused by:
  - Meckel's diverticulum
  - Polyp
  - Lymphoma
  - Henoch–Schönlein purpura
  - Cystic fibrosis

SIGNS AND SYMPTOMS

- Classic triad:
  - Intermittent colicky abdominal pain
  - Bilious vomiting
  - Currant jelly stool
- Neurologic signs:
  - Lethargy
  - Shock-like state
  - Seizure-like activity
  - Apnea
- RUQ mass:
  - Sausage shaped
  - Ill defined
  - Dance's sign—absence of bowel in right lower quadrant (RLQ)

DIAGNOSIS

- AXR:
  - Paucity of bowel gas
  - Loss of visualization of the tip of liver
  - "Target sign"—two concentric circles of fat density
- Ultrasound:
  - "Target" or "donut" sign—single hypoechoic ring with hyperechoic center
  - "Pseudokidney" sign — superimposed hypoechoic (edematous walls of bowel) and hyperechoic (areas of compressed mucosa) layers
- Barium enema

TREATMENT

- Correct dehydration
- NG tube for decompression

- Most common cause of acute intestinal obstruction under 2 years of age.
- Most common site is ileocolic (90%).

Intussusception and link with rotavirus vaccine led to withdrawal of vaccine from the market.

Intussusception:
- Classic triad is present in only 20% of cases.
- Absence of currant jelly stool does not exclude the diagnosis.
- Neurologic signs may delay the diagnosis.

HIGH-YIELD FACTS

Pediatric Surgery

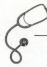

Barium enema for intussusception is both diagnostic and therapeutic. Rule of threes:
- Barium column should not exceed a height of 3 feet
- No more than three attempts
- Only 3 minutes/attempt

Meckel's diverticulum is the most frequent congenital GI abnormality.

Meckel's diverticulum:
- 2% of population
- 2 inches long
- 2 feet from the ileocecal valve
- Patient is usually under 2 years of age
- 2% are symptomatic

Meckel's diverticulum may mimic acute appendicitis and also act as lead point for intussusception.

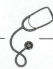

If a Meckel's diverticulum is found within a hernia sac, it is called a Littre's hernia.

- Hydrostatic reduction
- Barium enema:
  - Cervix-like mass
  - Coiled spring appearance on the evacuation film
  - Contraindications:
    - Peritonitis
    - Perforation
    - Profound shock
- Air enema:
  - Decreased radiation
  - Fewer complications

RECURRENCE

- With radiologic reduction: 7–10%
- With surgical reduction: 2–5%

Meckel's Diverticulum

DEFINITION

Persistence of the omphalomesenteric (vitelline) duct (should disappear by seventh week of gestation):
- Arises from the antimesenteric border of ileum
- Contains heterotopic epithelium (gastric, colonic, or pancreatic)
- A true diverticulum in that it contains all layers of bowel wall

SIGNS AND SYMPTOMS

Usually in first 2 years:
- Intermittent painless rectal bleeding
- Intestinal obstruction
- Diverticulitis

DIAGNOSIS

Meckel's scan (scintigraphy) has 85% sensitivity and 95% specificity. Uptake can be enhanced with cimetidine, glucagon, or gastrin.

TREATMENT

Surgical: Diverticular resection with transverse closure of the enterotomy.

Inguinal Hernia

DEFINITION

- Protrusion of a viscus or part of a viscus through an abnormal opening in the walls of its containing cavity.
- Indirect inguinal hernia is most common.

EPIDEMIOLOGY

- Male-to-female ratio: 4:1
- Higher incidence in premature infants (30%)

CAUSES

Patent processus vaginalis.

SIGNS AND SYMPTOMS

Bulge in the groin, scrotum, or labia, especially with increased intra-abdominal pressure (coughing, crying, straining, and blowing up a balloon).

TREATMENT

Operative repair:
- Should be repaired shortly after diagnosis except in premature infants.
- Increased risk of incarceration in first few months of life.
- Major risks include incarceration of a loop of bowel, an ovary, or a fallopian tube.

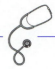

Correction of inguinal hernia is the most frequent surgical intervention in children.

Imperforate Anus

DEFINITION

Lack of an anal opening of proper location or size.

CAUSES

Results from a failure of the urinary and hindgut systems to separate.

ASSOCIATED ANOMALIES

Anomalies of sacrum and spinal and genitourinary tracts.

TYPES

High and low: Classification depends on whether the rectum ends above (high) or below (low) the puborectalis sling.

TREATMENT

- Colostomy for high lesions
- Perineal anoplasty or dilatation of fistula for low lesions

PROGNOSIS

The higher the lesion, the poorer the prognosis.

Hirschsprung's Disease (Congenital Aganglionosis Coli)

DEFINITION

- Congenital absence of ganglion cells in the plexuses of Auerbach (myenteric) and Meissner (submucosal)
- Results in functional intestinal obstruction

Hirschsprung's disease is the most common cause of lower intestinal obstruction in the neonate.

EPIDEMIOLOGY

- One in 5,000 to 8,000 live births
- Male-to-female ratio: 4:1

TYPES

- Rectosigmoid (75%)
- Entire colon (10%)

SIGNS AND SYMPTOMS

- In neonatal period:
  - Delayed passage of meconium
  - Rectal examination
  - An empty vault that is not dilated
  - Explosive release of feces
  - Most ominous presentation is enterocolitis
- Presentation later in childhood:
  - Bilous vomiting
  - Chronic constipation
  - Abdominal distention
  - Failure to thrive

DIAGNOSIS

- AXR to look for evidence of obstruction
- Barium enema to look for transition zone (may not be present until 1 to 2 weeks of age)
- Rectal biopsy to demonstrate absence of ganglion cells

TREATMENT

Surgical repair:
- Temporary colostomy proximal to transition zone at diagnosis
- Definitive repair when the infant is 6 to 12 months old
- Closure of colostomy 1 to 3 months postop

Necrotizing Enterocolitis (NEC)

DEFINITION

- An end expression of serious intestinal injury following a combination of vascular, mucosal, and toxic insults to a relatively immature gut.
- Predominantly a disorder of preterm infants.
- Incidence increases with decreasing gestational age.
- Increased incidence in conditions of low cardiac output and diastolic run-off lesions (e.g., CHD that is PBA dependent).

SIGNS AND SYMPTOMS

- Lethargy
- Feeding intolerance
- Hematochezia
- Fever
- Hypothermia
- Apneic spells
- Bloody diarrhea
- Abdominal pain and distention
- Presentation is identical to sepsis

Typical scenario: A premature infant born at 33 weeks' gestation now at 1 week of age has developed feeding intolerance, is febrile, and has hematochezia and a distended belly. *Think:* Necrotizing enterocolitis.

DIAGNOSIS

- AXR: Pneumatosis intestinalis (gas within the bowel wall)
- Lateral decubitus or cross-table lateral:
  - Probable NEC:
    - Thickened bowel loop
    - Fixed position loops on serial films
    - Ascites
  - Definite NEC:
    - Intramural gas
    - Portal gas
  - Free air

TREATMENT

- Nothing by mouth.
- Bowel decompression.
- Antibiotics/sepsis evaluation.
- TPN.
- Monitor vital signs and abdominal girth.
- Monitor fluid intake and output.
- Surgical resection for:
  - Perforation
  - Full-thickness necrosis of bowel

PROGNOSIS

Variable (depends on extent of injury). Overall > 95% survival rate.

NEOPLASTIC DISEASE

Wilms' tumor

DEFINITION

- Nephroblastoma—originates intrarenally
- Most common intra-abdominal malignancy in childhood

ASSOCIATION

- Hemihypertrophy
- Aniridia
- Genitourinary abnormalities, mental retardation

SIGNS AND SYMPTOMS

- Triad:
  - Flank mass
  - Hematuria
  - Hypertension
- Most occur by the age of 6 years

DIAGNOSIS

- Intravenous urography (intrarenal solid mass)
- Ultrasound of abdomen (extension into renal vein and IVC)

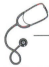

Presence of abdominal mass in infant or child is always abnormal and requires evaluation.

Lung is the most common site of metastasis.

- CT scan (metastasis—nodal enlargement and liver nodule)
- CXR or CT scan (lung metastasis)

TREATMENT

- Surgical resection of tumor, exploration of abdomen, evaluation of contralateral kidney
- Chemo/radiotherapy postop
- 90% survival rate

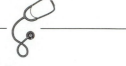
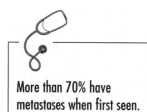
Neuroblastoma

DEFINITION

- Arises from neural crest cells.
- May arise in adrenal glands, sympathetic ganglia, and organ of Zuckerkandl.
- Most common tumor in infants under 1 year of age.
- Second most common solid tumor of childhood.
- Abdominal tumors are most common presentation: 65% in adrenal gland.
- Thoracic tumors are next most common presentation: < 8 years old (50% < 2 years old)

SIGNS AND SYMPTOMS

- Abdominal pain and mass
- Fever, failure to thrive, and proptosis
- Neurological symptoms (ataxia, opsomyoclonus)
- Hypertension (25%)

DIAGNOSIS

- Urine: Raised catacholamines (vanillylmandelic acid [VMA], homovanillic acid [HVA])
- Intravenous pyelography (inferior displacement of opacified calyces—"drooping lily sign")
- CT abdomen with contrast
- CXR or bone scan to evaluate metastases

TREATMENT

- Patient often presents with unresectable metastases.
- Aggressive chemo/radiotherapy
- Better prognosis if child < 1 year old

Anesthesia

ALGORITHM FOR RAPID-SEQUENCE INTUBATION

1. **Prepare** the necessary equipment:
   - IV access, cardiac monitor, pulse oximetry.
   - Bag–valve mask (Ambu bag).
   - Suction equipment (make sure it works!).
   - Laryngoscope with blade (check light bulb!).
   - Endotracheal (ET) tube (7.0 adult female/8.0 adult male).
   - Insert ET tube stylet (if desired).
   - Medications.
   - Prepare adjunct airway if unsuccessful.
   - Laryngeal mask airway (LMA), cricothyroidotomy tray, etc.
2. **Pretreat:**
   - Lidocaine for head injury patients (decreases intracranial pressure [ICP] given 90 sec prior to intubation for maximal effect)
   - Atropine for children (prevents bradycardia)
3. **Position** the patient:
   - Raise bed to height appropriate for intubation.
   - Place head in "sniffing position" with neck extended (except when C-spine injury suspected).
4. **Preoxygenate** the patient:
   - Bag–valve mask with 100% oxygen.
   - Pulse oximetry should read 100%.
   - Hyperventilate patient to accomplish nitrogen washout.
5. **Pressure** on cricothyroid cartilage:
   - Sellick maneuver compresses esophagus to limit risk of aspiration.
6. **Sedation/induction:** Many agents available including:
   - Thiopental (can cause hypotension; good for hemodynamically stable patients or those with elevated ICP)
   - Etomidate (minimal hepatic and renal effects; good for patients with decreased cardiac output)
   - Midazolam (can cause hypotension)
   - Ketamine (can cause tachycardia and increased ICP; good for patients with bronchospasm)

   Paralyze the patient:
   - Succinylcholine (1.5 mg/kg IV push [IVP]) onset 45 to 60 sec, duration 5 to 10 min. Do not use in burn injuries, crush injuries, or history of neuromuscular diseases.
   - Vecuronium (0.2 mg/kg IVP) onset 1 to 2 min, duration 40 to 60 min.
7. **Place** the tube:
   - Open the mouth and displace the jaw inferiorly.

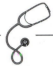

The **8Ps** of rapid-sequence intubation:
Prepare = equipment
Pretreat = drugs
Position = sniffing position
Preoxygenate = pulse oximetry of 100%
Pressure = Sellick
Paralyze = drugs
Placement of the tube
Position of the tube = confirm by two methods

- Holding the laryngoscope in the left hand, insert the blade along the right side of the tongue, and the tongue is swept toward the left.
- If using a curved (Macintosh) blade, the tip should be inserted to the vallecula (the space between the base of the tongue and the epiglottis).
- If using a straight (Miller) blade, the tip is inserted beneath the epiglottis.
- The laryngoscope is used to lift the tongue, soft tissues, and epiglottis to reveal the vocal chords. (Remember: It is a lifting motion, not a rocking motion.)
- Upon direct visualization of the chords, the tube is directed through the chords, the stylet (if used) is removed, the tube is connected to an oxygen source, and it is secured.

8. **Position** of tube: Confirm by two methods:
  - Direct visualization
  - Bilateral breath sounds (check both apical lung fields!)
  - Absence of breath sounds in abdomen
  - End tidal carbon dioxide detection
  - Portable chest x-ray (CXR)
  - Condensation in ETT

PULSE OXIMETRY

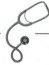

- Noninvasive probe placed on a digit or ear lobe.
- Measures arterial oxygen saturation by spectrophotometry. Two light sources of different wavelength emitted and at each frequency oxyhemoglobin and deoxyhemoglobin absorb light differently. Oximeter analyzes this difference to obtain a measure of arterial saturation.
- **Falsely lowers reading:**
  - **Methylene blue**
  - **Indigo carmine dye**
  - **Certain fingernail polish**
- **Falsely raises reading:**
  - Carboxyhemoglobin
- **Falsely reads 85%:**
  - Methemoglobin

SPINAL AND EPIDURAL ANESTHESIA

ANATOMY

- Spinal canal extends from foramen magnum to sacral hiatus.
- Spinal cord ends at L1–L2.
- Subarachnoid space lies between arachnoid and pia mater, which contains cerebrospinal fluid (CSF).
- Iliac crests are at level of L4.

SPINAL ANESTHESIA

- For surgeries of lower extremities, lower abdomen, genitourinary and anal region.
- Insert needle at L3–L4 or L4–L5 (at this level cauda equina is present and spinal cord has already ended).

- Order of structures traversed with needle:
  - Skin
  - Subcutaneous layer
  - Supraspinous ligament
  - Interspinous ligament
  - Ligamentum flavum
  - Epidural space
  - Dura mater
  - Subarachnoid space (CSF)

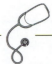

EPIDURAL ANESTHESIA

- Indicated for same surgeries as with spinal anesthesia
- Differs from spinal anesthesia in that needle is placed in epidural space (outside of CSF); commonly an indwelling catheter is left in place
- With catheter, can have continuous anesthesia (can periodically bolus the catheter for prolonged surgeries)
- Takes longer to obtain effect and requires higher dosages than spinal anesthesia
- Technically more difficult and requires more time to place than spinal anesthesia

COMPLICATIONS

See Table 21-1.

TABLE 21-1. Complications of spinal and epidural anesthesia.

Complication	Spinal	Epidural
Hypotension (from sympathetic nervous system blockade)	More common	Less common
Nausea (from unopposed parasympathetic activity)	More common	Less common
Postspinal headache (due to CSF leak)	Less common	Occurs only with inadvertent dural puncture during epidural placement
Urinary retention	Common	Common
Backache	Common	Common
Permanent neurologic injury	Very rare	Very rare
Epidural abscess or hematoma	n/a	Rare

GENERAL ANESTHESIA

ASA DEFINITION

- Drug-induced loss of consciousness during which patients are not arousable, even by painful stimulation.
- Ability to independently maintain ventilatory function is often impaired, therefore airway assistance by way of intubation, laryngeal mask airway, or other adjunct is usually necessary.
- Cardiovascular function may be impaired.

INDUCTION

See Table 21-2.

TABLE 21-2. Induction agents.

Induction Agent	Onset of Action	Duration of Action	IV Push Dose	Contraindications/ Caveats
Thiopental	< 1 min	5–10 min	3.0–5.0 mg/kg	Hypotension, asthma
Methohexital	< 1 min	5–10 min	1.0–2.0 mg/kg	Seizures, hypotension, asthma
Etomidate	< 1 min	5 min	0.3 mg/kg	Age < 10, pregnant/ lactating
Fentanyl	2–4 min	45 min	2–5 µg/kg	Hypotension
Midazolam	30 sec	6–15 min	0.05–0.1 mg/kg (6 mos–5 yrs) 0.025–0.05 mg/kg (6–12 yrs) 5–10 mg (adults)	■ Narrow-angle glaucoma ■ Decrease dosage in elderly and patients receiving concurrent erythromycin or drugs that inhibit P_{450} system
Ketamine	1 min	10–20 min	1.0–1.5 mg/kg	Head trauma, elevated intracranial pressure
Propofol	40 sec	3–6 min	2–2.5 mg/kg	■ Propofol comes as a lipid emulsion ■ Use with caution in patients with disorders of lipid metabolism ■ Use of aseptic technique especially important to prevent sepsis (emulsion is a great growth medium!)

- Intravenous agents are the most common way of inducing patients.
- Inhalation agents (with a mask) are used more commonly in pediatric patients.

NEUROMUSCULAR BLOCKADE

- Used to paralyze patients during surgical procedures.
- Postsynaptic receptors: Located in the neuromuscular junction, they are the site of action of neuromuscular blockers, blocking acetylcholine transmission.
- Can be classified as depolarizing (noncompetitive) or nondepolarizing (competitive) agents (see Table 21-3).
- Anticholinesterases prevent breakdown of acetylcholine, thus allowing acetylcholine to compete more effectively with the paralyzing agents. Can be used to "reverse" neuromuscular blockade of nondepolarizing agents (at end of surgery).

MAINTENANCE

Involves use of inhalational agents (e.g., nitrous oxide, isoflurane, sevoflurane, desflurane) and IV agents (e.g., opiates, ketamine, propofol).

EMERGENCE

- Return of patient to an awake state.
- Patient should have full muscle strength and protective airway reflexes before extubation.
- Recovery from effects of sedation occurs in postanesthesia care unit (PACU).

Nitrous oxide can diffuse into closed spaces/lumens, causing expansion of bowel or worsening of pneumothorax.

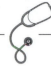

During emergence, patient is at risk for **aspiration** and for **laryngospasm** (involuntary spasm of laryngeal musculature, resulting in the inability to ventilate the patient).

TABLE 21-3. Classes of drugs used in anesthesia.

Drug Class	Examples	Properties	Remember . . .	Antidote
Benzodiazepines	Midazolam Diazepam Lorazepam	Amnesia Anxiolysis Skeletal muscle relaxant	NO ANALGESIA	Flumazenil
Opiates	Morphine Meperidine Fentanyl	Analgesia Sedation	NO PARALYSIS	Naloxone
Neuromuscular blockers	NONCOMPETITIVE: Succinylcholine COMPETITIVE: Atracurium Pancuronium Rocuronium Vecuronium	Paralysis (skeletal muscle relaxant)	NO ANALGESIA NO SEDATION	Anticholinesterases (e.g., neostigmine, pyridostigmine, edrophonium)

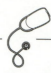

Halothane hepatitis is an immune-mediated hepatotoxicity associated with use of halothane (an inhalational anesthetic). Incidence is 1/22,000 to 1/35,000.

Platelet dysfunction is a qualitative defect that affects bleeding time only. Does not affect prothrombin time (PT) or partial thromboplastin time (PTT).

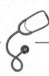

It is important to limit intraoperative fluid replacement in ESRD to prevent risk of pulmonary congestion.

Infants and children are *not* just small adults; their physiology is dramatically different, affecting their anesthetic management during surgery.

Hepatic Insufficiency

- Hypoalbuminemia: Results in less drug binding, causing an increase in unbound active drug
- Coagulopathy: Decreased production of coagulation factors results in prolonged aPTT. Splenomegaly can cause sequestration of platelets.
- Drug metabolism: P_{450} microsomal enzyme activity is decreased, resulting in prolonged elimination of many drugs.
- Hepatic blood flow: Both cirrhosis and inhaled anesthetics decrease hepatic blood flow, resulting in slower clearance of drugs.
- Chronic alcoholism: Increases anesthetic requirements.
- Acute alcohol intoxication: Decreases anesthetic requirements.
- Hypoglycemia: Seen in severe hepatic dysfunction.

Renal Insufficiency

- Anemia: Common in those with end-stage renal disease (ESRD).
- Coagulopathy: Decreased platelet adhesiveness from uremia.
- Hyperkalemia: Increased risk for cardiac arrhythmias.
- Metabolic acidosis: Due to impaired renal excretion of hydrogen ions, which can also worsen hyperkalemia.
- Hypertension: Often resulting from fluid overload.
- Lactated Ringer's (LR) solution: Avoid LR and other potassium-containing solutions in ESRD.
- Succinylcholine: Potential for elevating serum potassium.
- Renally excreted drugs: Must be carefully titrated because effects may be prolonged.

Pediatric Patients

- Increased oxygen consumption: High metabolic rate in neonates.
- Left shift of oxyhemoglobin dissociation curve: This left shift in neonates results in decreased release of oxygen from fetal hemoglobin to tissues.
- Alveolar ventilation: In neonates, it is doubled, resulting in an increased respiratory rate.
- Functional residual capacity is lower.
- Cardiac output: In infants is mainly dependent on heart rate not increased stroke volume.
- Extracellular fluid volume: Much higher in neonates (40% vs. 20% in adults).
- Temperature regulation: Impaired in neonates in the operating room (immature thermogenesis).
- Renal: Urine concentrating ability decreased until 6 to 12 months of age; low glomerular filtration rate (GFR).
- Volatile anesthetics: Neonates require less than infants and adults.
- Nondepolarizing muscle relaxants (e.g., vecuronium, atracurium, pancuronium): Neonates and infants are more sensitive to these drugs.
- Succinylcholine: Associated with risk of bradycardia and very rarely malignant hyperthermia in this population.

TABLE 21-4. Ways pediatric airway differs from adult.
■ Larger occiput
■ Large tongue
■ Larynx is higher up (C3 vs. C4–5) and funnel shaped so narrowest portion of airway is beyond what you see!
■ Vocal cords are at a slant and more anterior

- Airway: Due to anatomy of pediatric airway, intubation can be more challenging (see Table 21-4).

Obstetric Patients

- Cardiac output/stroke volume: Both are increased by 50% in pregnancy.
- Blood volume: Increased.
- Minute ventilation: Increased.
- Functional residual capacity (FRC): Decreased, making patients more susceptible to hypoxemia.
- Minimum alveolar concentration (MAC): The MAC of inhalational agents is decreased (therefore decreased anesthetic requirements).
- Demerol (meperidine): Better than morphine for analgesia as respiratory center of newborn is less sensitive to it.
- Spinal or epidural anesthesia: Preferred for labor because of decreased chance of fetal depression and maternal aspiration.
- Hypotension: Can treat with ephedrine because it preserves uterine blood flow (avoid pure vasoconstrictors such as phenylephrine).

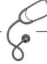

Remember, the narrowest part of a child's airway is at the glottic opening, beyond what is visualized with a laryngoscope.

Obstetric patients are at increased risk for aspiration when general anesthesia is undertaken.

LOCAL ANESTHESIA

- Used for local infiltration of operative site, during spinal or epidural anesthesia, and peripheral nerve blocks.
- Classification: Ester or amide anesthetic.
- Mechanism of action: Through blockade of sodium channels.
- Myelinated fibers: More susceptible to blockade.
- Sensory fibers: More readily blocked than motor nerves.
- Nonionized form: Needed to cross nerve sheath while the ionized form is the active form.
- Acidosis: Local tissue acidosis as from infection increases ionized drug form and limits anesthetic activity of the drug. Therefore, local infiltration into an area of infection may not produce adequate analgesia.
- Epinephrine: Adding this to the local anesthetic prolongs duration of action by vasoconstriction. Avoid epinephrine in areas with lack of collateral blood flow.
- Toxicity: Initially central nervous system (CNS) effects (tinnitus, restlessness, vertigo, seizures), then cardiovascular effects (hypotension, PR prolongation, QRS widening, dysrhythmias)

Amide anesthetics have **"i"** before **"caine"** (e.g., prilocaine, lidocaine, bupivacaine).

Do not use epinephrine in these areas: **SPF-10**
Scrotum
Penis
Fingers
Toes
Ears
Nose

MONITORED ANESTHESIA CARE VERSUS MAC

- **Monitored anesthesia care:** Intravenous sedation is provided usually with local anesthetic infiltration of surgical site. Commonly used in inguinal hernia repair, breast biopsy, lipoma excision.
- **Minimum alveolar concentration (MAC):** The minimum concentration necessary to prevent movement in 50% of patients in response to a surgical stimulus (refers to inhalational agents, such as nitrous oxide, isoflurane).

MALIGNANT HYPERTHERMIA

DEFINITION

Autosomal dominant inherited hypermetabolic syndrome occurring after exposure to an anesthetic agent (very rare, but life threatening).

ETIOLOGY

Impaired reuptake of calcium by sarcoplasmic reticulum in muscles.

SIGNS AND SYMPTOMS

- Tachycardia
- Hyperthermia
- Hypercarbia
- Hypoxemia
- Acidosis
- Muscle rigidity
- Ventricular dysrhythmias

TREATMENT

- Discontinue anesthetics.
- Benzodiazepines (work fastest to control hypermetabolic state).
- Dantrolene (considered more definitive treatment, but onset of action takes about 30 minutes).

POSTOPERATIVE NAUSEA AND VOMITING

- Common after general anesthesia
- Also seen in hypotension with spinal/epidural anesthesia
- More common with high doses of opiates, in young women, after laparoscopy, and strabismus surgery
- Antiemetic agents:
  - Metoclopramide (Reglan)
  - Prochlorperazine (Compazine)
  - Droperidol
  - Ondansetron (Zofran)
  - Dolasetron

See Table 21-5.

TABLE 21-5. Postoperative analgesia.

Route	Drug	Side Effects
IV	Morphine	Respiratory depression Nausea
IM/IV	Meperidine (Demerol): Best avoided in renal failure patients because of potential for accumulation of toxic metabolites (seizures)	Pruritis Pupillary constriction
PO	Percocet: Acetaminophen with oxycodone	
PO	Tylenol #2 (Tylenol #3, Tylenol #4): Acetaminophen with varying doses of codeine	
PO	Darvocet: Acetaminophen with propoxyphene	
PO	Vicodin: Acetaminophen with hydrocodone	
PO/IM/IV	Ketorolac (Toradol): A nonsteroidal anti-inflammatory drug (NSAID) that can be administered parenterally	Dyspepsia Gastritis Reversible inhibition of platelets
IV	Patient-controlled analgesia (PCA)	Renal insufficiency

HIGH-YIELD FACTS

Anesthesia

Ear, Nose, and Throat

Anatomy

See Figure 22-1.

EXTERNAL EAR

- Auricle: Funnels sound waves into external auditory meatus.
- External auditory meatus: About 2.5 cm long. Internal two thirds made of bone; external one third made of cartilage. The skin in the bony portion lacks a subcutaneous layer and is attached directly to the periosteum.
- Tympanic membrane: Conducts sound waves from external ear to middle ear. Has three layers: Cutaneous outer layer, fibrous intermediate layer, and a mucousal inner layer.

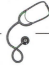

Cartilaginous portion of the external auditory meatus has ceruminous glands that secrete cerumen (ear wax).

Cone of light found in anterior–inferior quadrant of tympanic membrane.

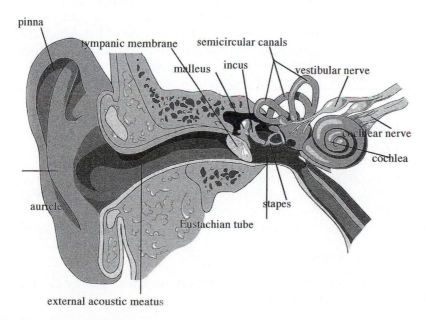

FIGURE 22-1. Anatomy of the ear.

MIDDLE EAR

- Transmits sound waves from tympanic membrane to inner ear via the ossicles. Impedance match air and inner ear perilymph to transmit the force of the sound waves. The eustachian tube connects the nasopharynx to the anterior wall of the middle ear cavity. Mastoid air cells communicate with the middle ear cavity via the aditus ad antrumon, which lies on the posterior wall of the cavity.
- Ossicles: Tympanic membrane → malleus → incus → stapes → oval window → perilymph of scala vestibuli of the inner ear. The ossicles are joined by synovial joints.
- Malleus: Manubrium is fused to tympanic membrane; head articulates with incus in the epitympanic recess. Tensor tympani muscle is attached to the manubrium and is innervated by cranial nerve (CN) V3.
- Incus: Articulates with the other two ossicles. No muscular attachments.
- Stapes: Neck serves as attachment for stapedius muscle, which is innervated by the stapedial branch of CN VII. Footplate attached to oval window.
- Eustachian tube: Connects nasopharynx to middle ear. Balances pressure in middle ear by allowing passage of air. Opened by contraction of two muscles: Tensor vali palatini (CN V3) and salpingopharyngeus (CN X). Adenoids are in close proximity to nasopharyngeal opening of tube.

INNER EAR

- Acoustic apparatus: Includes the cochlea, which consists of the scala vestibuli and scala tympani, both of which are filled with perilymph. The oval window transmits vibrations to the scala vestibuli at the base of the cochlea, which, via the helicotrema at the apex of the cochlea, transmits the pressure waves to the scala tympani. The scala tympani transmits the waves to the round window, where they are dissipated. The scala media, which contains the spiral organ of Corti, is the sensory portion of the inner ear and is filled with endolymph. The spiral organ of Corti contains the nerve terminals of the cochlear nerve.
- Vestibular apparatus: Includes the vestibule (utricle and saccule) and semicircular canals all contributing to the sense of balance. Utricle and saccule contain maculae, and the anterior, lateral, and posterior semicircular ducts have dilatations called ampullae. The utricle and saccule as well as the semicircular ducts are filled with endolymph.

Evaluation of Hearing Loss

PHYSIOLOGY

Sound waves can reach the cochlea in two ways: Through air conduction using the ear canal, tympanic membrane, and middle ear structures; or through bone conduction, vibrating the temporal bone and therefore the cochlea which lies within it, bypassing the external and middle ear structures.

AIR-CONDUCTED HEARING

Depends on the condition of the external ear, middle ear, inner ear, CN VIII, and central auditory pathways.

BONE-CONDUCTED HEARING

- Depends on the condition of the inner ear, CN VIII, and central auditory pathways, skipping the external and middle ear structures.
- If hearing by air conduction is decreased while hearing by bone conduction is normal, the lesion can be isolated to the external or middle ear structures.
- If hearing by both air and bone conduction is decreased, the lesion can be isolated to the inner ear, CN VIII, or central auditory pathways.
- Remember that there could be coexisting lesions that independently affect either air or bone conduction. If both are on the same side, air conduction will decrease to a greater extent than bone conduction.

WEBER TEST

Use a 256-Hz or a 512-Hz fork and place on midline of head while vibrating. Ask patient if tone is heard better by one ear. If sound lateralizes, either a conductive hearing loss in same ear, or sensorineural hearing loss in opposite ear.

RINNE TEST

- Compares the ability to hear by air conduction to that of bone conduction.
- Ask patient to indicate if ringing is heard louder when a vibrating fork is placed on mastoid process or when placed near opening of external auditory meatus. Normally, sound is heard louder by air conduction than by bone, but with conductive hearing loss bone conduction is louder (positive test). With sensorineural hearing loss this test is normal, although technically both bone and air sound perceptions are reduced.

Conductive Hearing Loss

DIAGNOSIS

- Due to a lesion in the structures that conduct the waves into the inner ear. These structures include the external auditory meatus, tympanic membrane, and middle ear structures all the way up to the oval window.
- Weber test lateralizes to affected ear; Rinne test positive.

CAUSES

- Obstruction of external auditory meatus by cerumen, foreign body, or debris.
- Swelling of lining of canal, neoplasms, or stenosis of canal.
- Perforation of tympanic membrane (as in chronic otitis media).
- Disruption of middle ear structures such as ossicles (e.g., otosclerosis).
- Fluid scaring or neoplasms of middle ear.

Sensorineural Hearing Loss

DIAGNOSIS

- Due to a lesion in the inner ear, CN VIII, or central auditory structures.
- Weber test lateralizes to unaffected ear; Rinne test normal.

Ménière's disease:
Intermittent vertigo, tinnitus, hearing loss, and aural fullness due to excess endolymph.

CAUSES

- Intense noise, damaging the hair cells of the organ of Corti
- Viral infections (e.g., human herpes virus)
- Ototoxic drugs (e.g., aminoglycosides)
- Temporal bone fractures
- Meningitis
- Cochlear otosclerosis
- Ménière's disease
- Acoustic neuromas (schwannomas)

Myringotomy

PROCEDURE

- Opening the tympanic membrane to remove fluid from the middle ear. Frequently a tube is left to maintain drainage. Usually, tympanic membrane heals fully after removal of tube if infection is prevented.
- Hearing should improve noticeably almost immediately.

INDICATIONS

- Severe/recurrent acute otitis media
- Hearing loss > 30 dB in patients with otitis media with infusion
- Otitis media with poor response to antibiotics
- Impending mastoiditis or intracranial complication due to otitis media
- Otitis media with effusion > 3 months
- Recurrent episodes of acute otitis media

Tinnitus might be the presenting sign in an acoustic neuroma.

Tinnitus

DEFINITION

- Perception of sound when there is no sound in the environment. Does not interfere with hearing, although it may affect attention span.
- Usually associated with hearing loss whether it be conductive or sensorineural, but can be associated with almost any hearing problem. Stress or tension makes tinnitus worse.
- Can be described as ringing, buzzing, or roaring, and can even be pulsatile, raising suspicion of a vascular cause.
- Vascular causes of tinnitus include glomus jugulare tumors, aneurysms, and stenotic lesions.

TREATMENT

- Treatment of tinnitus can be difficult. Masking of tinnitus with music can help. Tinnitus maskers present a more pleasant sound that the patient focuses on instead of the tinnitus. Usually followed by a period of tinnitus inhibition.
- Treatment for anxiety, depression, or insomnia with medications can also help. Behavioral habituation therapy is also available, wherein the patient learns to ignore the tinnitus.

Anatomy

- Nasal cavity opens on the face through the nares (nostrils).
- Choanae are the posterior openings of the nasal cavity that communicate with the nasopharynx.
- The vestibule is lined with skin.
- Boundaries of nasal cavity:
  - Medial wall: The nasal septum. Seven bones plus septal cartilage contribute to the septum: Perpendicular plate of the ethmoid, vomer, palatine, maxillary, frontal, sphenoid, and nasal bones.
  - Lateral wall: Formed mostly by the superior and middle concha of the ethmoid bone and the inferior concha. A corresponding meatus is found below each respective concha, and the sphenoethmoidal recess is located superior to the superior concha. The sphenopalatine foramen is found on the posterior edge of the middle concha and contains the corresponding artery, which is a terminal branch of the maxillary artery.

> Incisive foramen in floor of nasal cavity transmits the nasopalatine nerve and branches of the sphenopalatine artery.

Structure	Opening
Sphenoethmoidal recess	Sphenoid sinus
Superior meatus	Posterior ethmoidal air cells
Middle meatus	Frontal sinus, maxillary sinus, middle ethmoidal air cells, anterior ethmoidal air cells
Inferior meatus	Nasolacrimal duct

- Floor: Formed by the palatine process of the maxilla and the horizontal plate of the palatine bone.
- Roof: Curved and narrower than the floor. Formed by the cribriform plate of the ethmoid, body of the sphenoid, nasal, and frontal bones. Cribriform plate transmits terminal branches of the olfactory nerve.

Epistaxis

CAUSES

Local Causes
- Trauma: Nose picking of a dried mucosa is most common. Barometric pressure changes can also traumatize mucosa.
- Septal perforations as with cocaine use.
- Polyps and tumors.
- Infections: Rhinitis, vestibulitis, and sinusitis.
- Angiofibroma of the nasopharynx.

Systemic Causes
- Inflammation and infectious diseases such as scarlet fever, malaria, and typhoid fever
- Vascular lesions such as arteriosclerosis, hereditary hemorrhagic telangiectasis (Osler–Weber–Rendu disease—autosomal dominant), and coarctation of aorta
- Bleeding disorders such as hemophilia and platelet disorders
- Overdose with anticoagulants or antiplatelet agents

MANAGEMENT AND TREATMENT

- Patient will usually present with an anxious and bloody appearance, making diagnosis impossible until bleeding is controlled.
- Have patient pinch nostrils against nasal septum with head flexed anteriorly for at least 5 minutes. This will stop bleeding originating from Kiesselbach's plexus or any origin anterior to the pinch. If bleeding is behind the pinch, blood will collect in the nasal cavity and start spilling over into the nasopharynx. This blood will be coughed up.
- Next, try to make a geographic diagnosis of the bleed. If bleeding origin is identified, it is usually in Kiesselbach's plexus and will stop with the 5-minute pinch, cauterization, or an anterior nasal pack. If the origin is not identified, must treat as a diffuse bleed by packing.
- Bleeding posterior to Kiesselbach's plexus will need a speculum and good light to locate, and possibly an endoscope.
- Bleeding can be controlled temporarily by applying pressure with a cotton pledget impregnated with a vasoconstrictor, such as phenylephrine, and a topical anesthetic, such as lidocaine, until the site is anesthetized.
- Cautery of the hemorrhagic point: When visible, the bleeding site may be cauterized with silver nitrate or electrocautery. Do not use cautery for bleeding due to a bleeding disorder.
- For epistaxis due to a bleeding disorder, use petrolatum gauze to apply pressure as atraumatically as possible.
- If bleeding is in the anterior nasal cavity, an anterior nasal pack should be used.
- If bleeding is in the posterior nasal cavity, an anterior–posterior pack should be used.
- Ligation of arteries such as the sphenopalatine should be reserved for the most severe cases in which packing does not stop the bleeding.
- Arterial embolization can be considered instead of ligation.

THROAT

Anatomy

MUSCULATURE

- The pharynx extends from the base of the skull to the cricoid cartilage of the larynx. Consists of a set of circular constrictor muscles and a set of longitudinal "pharyngeus" muscles.
- Circular muscles: Superior, middle, and inferior constrictors. All are innervated by the vagus via the pharyngeal plexus.
- Longitudinal muscles: Stylopharyngeus, palatopharyngeus, salpingopharyngeus. All but the stylopharyngeus are innervated by the vagus via the pharyngeal plexus. The stylopharyngeus is innervated by the glossopharyngeal nerve.

NASOPHARYNX

- Borders are from base of skull to soft palate. Communicates with nasal cavity via choanae; with middle ear via eustachian tube. Contains the pharyngeal tonsils (adenoids) in posterior wall, and are nearly continuous with the tubal tonsils, which surround the eustachian tube openings.

OROPHARYNX

Borders from soft palate to epiglottis. Communicates with oral cavity via oropharyngeal isthmus. Contains tonsillar fossa in which the palatine tonsils lie.

LARYNGOPHARYNX

- Borders are from epiglottis to cricoid cartilage. Contains the larynx. A piriform recess is found on each side of the larynx, in which swallowed foreign bodies may be lodged.
- Waldeyer's ring is a tonsillar ring formed by the lingual, palatine, tubal, and pharyngeal tonsils. Offers an immune barrier at the oropharyngeal isthmus.

TONSILLECTOMY

- Commonly refers only to the palatine tonsils, but the adenoids can be removed in cases of airway or eustachian tube obstruction.
- Usually a last resort to all other nonsurgical interventions.
- Major complication is bleeding at the tonsillar bed after removal. One to 2% of cases will have severe bleeding, half of which will need to go back into OR to stop bleeding.
- Damage to underlying glossopharyngeal nerve is possible, as well as to the internal carotid artery which lies lateral to the tonsil.

INDICATIONS

- Chronic tonsillitis: Guidelines are six to seven infections in 1 year, or two to three infections per year for a few years.
- If tonsils block breathing.
- Cases of obstructive sleep apnea due to enlargement.
- Carriers of diphtheria.
- If only one tonsil is enlarged, in order to biopsy the tissue.
- In regards to the adenoids: In cases of chronic middle ear infections due to spread to tubal tonsils and eustachian tube blockage.

Salivary Gland Tumors

- No specific risk factors or environmental carcinogens have been identified.
- Can arise from the major (parotid, submandibular, sublingual) or minor salivary glands. Parotid tumors are the most common.
- Most parotid tumors are benign, but half of submandibular and sublingual gland tumors, and most minor salivary gland tumors, are malignant.
- Have a tendency to recur after resection.
- All parotid gland tumors can affect the facial nerve and cause a unilateral facial palsy.

TUMOR TYPES

- **Pleomorphic adenoma:**
  - Most frequent tumor
  - Most commonly affects the parotid, but can be found in the submandibular or minor glands
  - Benign but recurs; rarely undergoes malignant transformation

Tonsillar fossa is bordered by the palatoglossal fold anteriorly and the palatopharyngeal fold posteriorly.

Bleeding can be due to tonsillar branches of ascending palatine artery or facial artery, but most commonly due to the large external palatine vein.

Sialadenitis: Inflammation of the salivary glands.

- **Warthin's tumor:**
  - Papillary cystadenoma lymphomatosum
  - Benign and affects the parotid gland
- **Oncocytoma:**
  - Benign
  - Affects the parotid
  - Elderly
- **Mucoepidermoid carcinoma:**
  - Can vary from benign to highly malignant
  - Affects the parotid
- **Adenoid cystic carcinoma:**
  - Malignant but slow growing; late metastasis
  - Commonly affects the minor salivary glands
  - Has a tendency to recur along the nerve tracks and cause severe pain

TREATMENT

- Benign tumors treated with surgical incision.
- Invasive tumors with surgery and radiation.
- Neutron radiation is particularly effective.
- Watch for frequent recurrences.
- Determine status of facial nerve before and after surgery.
- Chemotherapy with doxorubicin or cisplatin for metastatic disease.

Oropharyngeal Carcinoma

- Most head and neck cancers are of the squamous cell variety and may be preceded by various precancerous lesions.
- Etiology: Clearly related to tobacco consumption, heavy ingestion of alcohol, and the use of chewing tobacco. Poor oral hygiene, mechanical irritation, and the Plummer–Vinson syndrome can also contribute. Mouthwash with a high alcohol content increases chance of malignancy.
- Location of lesion determines prognosis: Lips have the best prognosis, while the hypopharynx has the worst.

DIAGNOSIS

- Nasopharyngeal endoscopy, together with esophagoscopy and laryngoscopy. This is done because there is a high rate of synchronous primary tumors presenting at the same time as the symptomatic tumor.
- Biopsy and histopathologic confirmation.
- MRI to evaluate extent of primary tumor and metastasis to lymph nodes.

TREATMENT

- Combination of surgery and radiation, or either one, depending on extent of functional impairment the surgery will cause.
- Most often, radiation therapy is used postoperatively. Advanced inoperable patients may be palliated with radiation therapy.
- Chemotherapeutic clinical trials in advanced cases.

Lower airway involvement is better evaluated with a scan (x-ray, CT, MRI) than bronchoscopy.

Esophagus is most common site of a subclinical second primary tumor.

Neurosurgery

Cranial Foramina

Optic canal: Optic nerve and ophthalmic artery
Superior orbital fissure: Cranial nerves (CN) III, IV, VI, and V_1
Foramen rotundum: CN V_2
Foramen ovale: CN V_3
Carotid canal: Internal carotid artery
Internal acoustic meatus: CN VII and VIII
Stylomastoid foramen: CN VII and stylomastoid artery
Jugular foramen: Internal jugular vein and CN IX–XI
Hypoglossal canal: CN XII
Foramen spinosum: Middle meningeal artery and vein
Foramen magnum: Spinal cord, CN XI (spinal accessory) and vertebral, posterior, and anterior spinal arteries

Internal carotid artery (ICA) does not produce branches until it enters the petrous bone where it gives off angiographically occult feeders to the middle and inner ear.

Major ICA Branches Visible with Angiography (in order)
- Meningohypophyseal
- Inferolateral trunk
- Ophthalmic
- Posterior communicating
- Anterior choroidal
- Middle cerebral
- Anterior cerebral

Anterior Cerebral Artery (ACA) Branches (in order)
- Medial lenticulostriates
- Anterior communication

- Recurrent artery of Heubner
- Orbitofrontal
- Frontopolar
- Pericallosal
- Callosomarginal

Middle Cerebral
- Lateral lenticulostriates
- Anterior temporal
- Posterior cerebral
- Ascending frontal
- Lateral orbitofrontal
- Precentral
- Central
- Anterior parietal
- Posterior parietal
- Angular

Vertebral Artery
- Posterior meningeal
- Anterior spinal
- Posterior inferior cerebellar
- Vertebrals fuse to form the basilar artery

Basilar Artery
- Anterior inferior cerebellar
- Pontine perforators
- Superior cerebellar
- Posterior cerebral

Posterior Cerebral
- Posterior thalamoperforators
- Medial posterior choroidal
- Lateral posterior choroidal
- Thalamogeniculates
- Inferior temporals
- Parieto-occipital
- Calcarine
- Posterior pericallosal

Arterial

Circle of Willis is complete in only approximately one fifth of persons (see Figure 23-1).

Hydrocephalus

Enlargement of the ventricles with excess CSF.

GENERAL

- ~1% prevalence; 1/1,000 congenital incidence
- Three general categories:
  - **Communicating:** All ventricles affected. Defect in absorption at the arachnoid granulations.

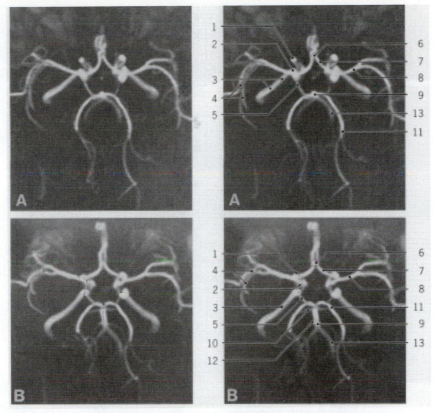

Cerebral arteries, MR angiography, circle of Willis

1: Internal carotid artery, "siphon"
2: Internal carotid artery in cavernous sinus
3: Internal carotid artery in carotid canal
4: Insular branches of middle cerebral artery
5: Posterior communicating artery

6: Anterior communicating artery
7: Anterior cerebral artery
8: Middle cerebral artery
9: Basilar artery
10: Superior cerebellar artery

11: Posterior cerebral artery
12: Anterior inferior cerebral artery (AICA)
13: Vertebral artery

FIGURE 23-1. MR angiography demonstrating circle of Willis. (Reproduced, with permission, from Fleckenstein P, Tranum-Jensen J. *Anatomy and Diagnostic Imaging,* 2nd ed. Philadelphia, PA: WB Saunders, 2001: 244.)

- **Noncommunicating (obstructive):** Block in CSF flow proximal to arachnoid granulations. May not affect all ventricles depending on the location of the block (e.g., aqueductal stenosis spares the fourth ventricle).
- **Ex vacuo:** Atrophic parenchymal tissue loss results in dilated ventricles. Not pathologic hydrocephalus.

IMAGING CRITERIA

See Figure 23-2.
- Width of frontal horns at anterior tips should not exceed one-half of the parenchymal width at that point.
- **Evan's ratio:** Width of frontal horns at anterior tips should not exceed 30% of maximum bipariental diameter.
- On MRI, increased T2 signal in periventricular white matter is suggestive of transependymal flow secondary to hydrocephalus (indicates increased pressure).

In a young person ≤ 35 to 40 years of age, appearance of the temporal tips of the lateral ventricles is one of the earliest manifestations of hydrocephalus ("boomerang" sign).

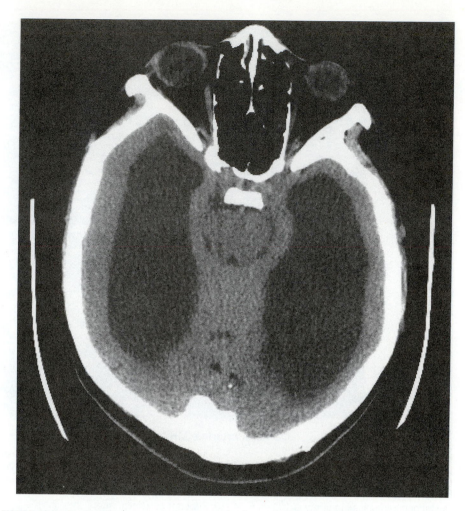

FIGURE 23-2. Brain CT demonstrating gross hydrocephalus. Note massive dilatation of lateral and third ventricles. The fourth ventricle is decompressed. There is a VP shunt tip in the body of the right lateral ventricle. Note deformity of calvarium, which is consistent with long-standing hydrocephalus.

Macewen's sign: Tapping on the head of a hydrocephalic infant produces a cracked pot sound. (*Tip:* Don't perform this exam tip in front of the parents.)

ETIOLOGIES

- Congenital
- Acquired:
  - Hemorrhage
  - Infectious/inflammatory
  - Obstructing masses
  - Postoperative (particularly in pediatric posterior fossa procedures)

CLINICAL PRESENTATION

- That of increased ICP: Headache, nausea/vomiting, ataxia, abducens palsy, Parinaud syndrome
- In children, check for bulging anterior fontanelle, increase in head circumference, irritability, poor feeding, and engorged scalp veins.

TREATMENT

- Acetazolamide to reduce CSF production and furosemide to promote diuresis (both only temporizing).

- Shunt placement:
  - Most commonly a ventriculoperitoneal shunt is placed. Alternatives include ventriculoatrial and ventriculopleural shunts.
  - Shunts are placed similar to an extraventricular drain except that the catheter is subcutaneously tunneled behind the ear where a valve is attached and placed in the subgaleal space. The catheter is then tunneled over the clavicle and to the destination outsource.

COMPLICATIONS

- Obstruction (usually proximal).
- Infection.
- Patient growth—possible need for replacement of the distal catheter as the infant/child grows (shunt tip will pull out of peritoneal cavity).
- Undershunting: Occurs in ~15–20% of cases due to obstruction, kinking or disconnection. Suspect this should shunting not resolve signs/symptoms of hydrocephalus or should they return.
- Overshunting: Creates symptoms similar to elevated ICP except ameliorated with recumbency (similar to post–lumbar puncture [LP] headache).
- Subdural hematoma: Collapse of ventricles may tear bridging veins. Treat these subdural hematomas only if symptomatic.
- **Slit ventricle syndrome:** Chronic overshunting may result in a theoretical decrease in ventricular compliance. Higher pressures are required to effect small changes in ventricular volume. Symptoms are of increased ICP without accompanying radiographic evidence of hydrocephalus. This syndrome occurs in the minority of patients with slit ventricles following shunting. May require revision of the shunt.

POSTOPERATIVE RADIOGRAPHIC EVALUATION

- **Shunt series:** Plain films to assess location of ventricular catheter, shunt tubing continuity, and distal catheter tip location. Valves typically have a series of radiopaque arrows to confirm direction of flow.
- **Shunt-o-gram** (see Figure 23-3): Injection of radioisotope into shunt to confirm both proximal catheter patency and distal flow (contrast "washes out" of ventricles and into peritoneum over time).

Carotid Artery Stenosis

GENERAL

- Differentiate based on asymptomatic or symptomatic.
  - Asymptomatic: No history of TIA-like symptoms
  - Symptomatic history of:
    - Amaurosis fugax
    - MCA syndrome
    - ACA syndrome
- Syncope is not considered "symptomatic" because unilateral carotid occlusion rarely results in impairment of consciousness.

EVALUATION

Duplex Doppler Ultrasound
- Detects increased flow in stenotic lesions.
- Not reliable in very high-grade stenoses.
- Near-complete stenosis results in "trickle" flow.

A carotid bruit detected in isolation is not a reliable indicator of carotid stenosis. In the presence of symptoms suggestive of stroke, a carotid bruit is highly correlated with significant stenosis.

Typical scenario: An 83-year-old female with a history of diabetes, hypertension, and atherosclerosis presents with painless, monocular vision loss that lasted a few minutes and has now completely resolved. She has no other neurologic deficits. *Think:* Amaurosis fugax.

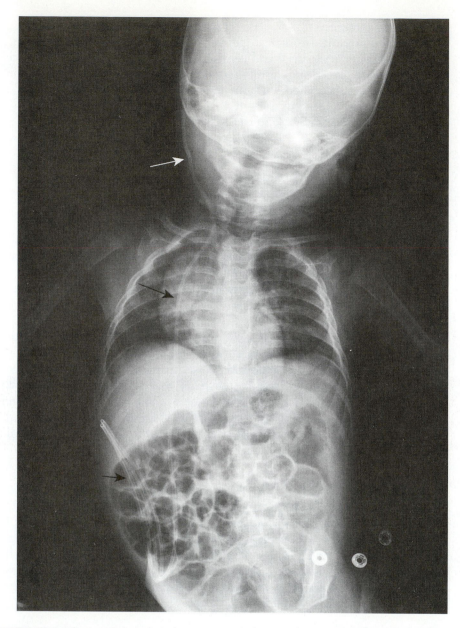

FIGURE 23-3. Plain radiograph ("shunt-o-gram") demonstrating VP shunt catheter coiled in the upper abdomen without evidence of kinks in this 8-month-old girl.

- May be mistaken for complete occlusion.
- Cannot assess carotids above the mandible.

MR Angiogram
- Detects functional flow
- Can estimate plaque thickness
- Can evaluate intracranial vasculature
- May not resolve trickle flow

Carotid Angiogram
- Gold standard
- Reveals trickle flow
- Cannot discern thickness of plaque

Ocular Pneumoplethysmography (OPG)

- Measures of orbital pressure are surrogate of ophthalmic artery pressure.
- Correlate with brachial artery pressure.
- If OPG pressure is lower than expected, correlated with significant stenosis of ICA.

TREATMENT

- Medical therapy:
  - Aspirin
  - Aspirin plus dipyridamole
  - Clopidogrel
  - Control of:
    - Hypertension
    - Diabetes mellitus
    - Hyperlipidemia
  - Smoking cessation
- Surgical therapy—carotid endarterectomy (CEA):
  - Beneficial over medical therapy alone in stroke risk reduction in asymptomatic men if ≥ 60% stenosis and performed by a surgeon with a complication rate ≤ 3%.
  - Beneficial over medical therapy alone in symptomatic patients with ≥ 70% stenosis. Possibly more beneficial if stenosis 50–69% and surgeon complication rate low.
  - Procedure:
    - Patient is maintained on aspirin preoperatively.
    - Timing is generally 4 to 6 weeks after CVA.
    - Intraoperative electroencephalogram (EEG) and sensory evoked potentials routinely monitored in case ischemia develops.
    - After intraoperative ICA occlusion, measurement of retrograde flow from opposite circulation ("stump pressure") should yield mean arterial pressure (MAP) ≥ 50 mm Hg. ICA shunt may be indicated if the stump pressure is < 50 mm Hg.
  - Risks/complications:
    - Hoarseness (recurrent laryngeal nerve injury)
    - Horner syndrome
    - Partial tongue paresis (hypoglossal nerve injury)
    - Hematoma causing airway compromise
- Cerebral hyperperfusion syndrome:
  - Unilateral headache due to poor autoregulation
  - May cause seizures
  - Often self-limited as autoregulation is restored
- Carotid occlusion (100% stenosis) of chronic nature usually has little benefit from surgical intervention. Typically, slowly progressive carotid stenosis affords development of alternative collateralization to the anterior cerebral circulation (e.g., through external carotid artery [ECA] anastomoses).
- Emergency CEA may be indicated in symptomatic cases of recent onset with angiographically proven occlusion or loss of a known previous bruit.

> Only superficial layers should be closed primarily after carotid endarterectomy. Closure of deep fascia creates an enclosed space capable of retaining hematoma under high pressures. Should an arterial leak develop, the airway may be rapidly compromised.

Carotid Dissection

DEFINITION

Tear in media layer of vessel

EPIDEMIOLOGY

Male > female incidence.

ETIOLOGIES

- Trauma
- Connective tissue disease
- Iatrogenic (angiogram)
- Vasculitis

PRESENTATION

- Headache
- Ipsilateral Horner syndrome
- Symptoms of SAH or stroke

EVALUATION

- MRA—not high sensitivity
- Angiogram—gold standard
- Vessel "beaking"
- String and pearl sign
- Double-lumen sign

TREATMENT

- If dissection is extradural, medical therapy is employed (anticoagulation).
- If dissection involves intradural portion of carotid, endovascular stenting or surgical bypass of ECA to ICA (e.g., superficial temporal artery to middle cerebral artery—STA-MCA bypass) is indicated.

HERNIATION SYNDROMES

Central (Transtentorial)

Diencephalon is forced through tentorial incisure.
- Early decrease in level of consciousness
- Occlusion of PCAs (cortical blindness)
- Parinaud syndrome
- Cheyne–Stokes respirations as progresses
- Finally, decorticate rigidity → decerebrate rigidity × flaccid paralysis and apnea

Uncal

Uncus forced medially over edge of tentorial incisure usually by mass effect from a lesion in the middle fossa or temporal lobe.
- CN III palsy (blown pupil, "down and out eye").
- Level of consciousness may not be impaired early.

- May be rapid direct midbrain compression.
- Contralateral weakness—pressure on cerebral peduncle.

Cingulate (Subfalcine)

Cingulate gyrus forced beneath falx cerebri.
- Often clinically occult
- May lead to ACA occlusion—produces abulia

Cerebellar (Upward)

Usually due to posterior fossa mass.
- May occlude superior cerebellar arteries (SCAs) against tentorium—ataxia.
- Can ultimately compress brain stem.

Tonsillar

Herniation of hindbrain through foramen magnum.
- Due to supra- or infratentorial lesions.
- May be early-onset apnea.
- Level of consciousness may be preserved.
- Can be rapidly progressive and fatal.

Uncal herniation may produce contralateral or ipsilateral weakness:
- Direct pressure of uncus on ipsilateral peduncle causes contralateral arm/leg weakness (most common).
- Midbrain shift forcing contralateral peduncle against tentorial incisure causes ipsilateral arm/leg weakness (Kernohan's phenomenon).

CENTRAL NERVOUS SYSTEM TUMORS

GENERAL

- Most brain tumors present with progressive neurologic deficit, motor weakness headache or seizure.
- Tumor headache is usually due to elevated ICP.
- Any new-onset seizure in adulthood should prompt an aggressive search for a brain tumor.
- Presentation:
  - Posterior fossa mass:
    - Headache
    - Nausea/vomiting
    - Ataxia
    - Diplopia
    - Parinaud syndrome
    - Cranial nerve paresis
    - Rotatory/vertical nystagmus
  - Supratentorial mass:
    - Headache
    - Nausea/vomiting
    - Diplopia
    - Parinaud syndrome
    - Motor weakness
    - Aphasia
    - Tumor TIA (hemorrhage/vascular compression)
- Dexamethasone may halt/reverse neurologic deterioration caused by to vasogenic edema.

Low-Grade Astrocytoma

EPIDEMIOLOGY

- Approximately 12% of primary brain tumors.
- Children are more likely to have low-grade forms.

LOCATION

- Cerebral hemispheres
- Cerebellum

PATHOLOGY

- Fibrillary
- Juvenile pilocytic
- Pleomorphic xanthroastrocytoma
- Dysembryoplastic neuroepithelial (DNET)

NATURAL HISTORY

- No uniform presentation among varieties
- Often diagnosed following a seizure

IMAGING

- Hypointense on T1; hyperintense on T2.
- Most low-grade forms lack enhancement.

TREATMENT

- Follow asymptomatic lesions.
- Cerebellar juvenile pilocytic astrocytomas can be resected for cure.
- Surgery not curative for most low-grade gliomas, but utilized if lesion is symptomatic.
- Diagnostic biopsy at minimum in all cases.
- Radiotherapy for most postoperatively.
- Radiation can be held until recurrence.
- Chemotherapy if above fail to stabilize.

Malignant Glioma

TYPES

- Anaplastic astrocytoma
- Glioblastoma multiforme (GBM)

EPIDEMIOLOGY

- Approximately 40% of primary brain tumors
- More common in elderly
- Often de novo generation
- Less frequently due to malignant degeneration of low-grade forms

LOCATION

Anywhere in CNS.

PATHOLOGY

- Highly pleomorphic cells
- Invasive
- Necrosis in GBM

NATURAL HISTORY

Rapidly progressive

IMAGING

- Inhomogenous low T1 signal/high T2 signal.
- Enhancing rim.
- Highly vascular.
- Usually significant surrounding edema.
- GBMs often have a necrotic core.
- Rarely calcific.
- May be difficult to differentiate from abscess.

TREATMENT

- Treatment is palliative, not for cure.
- Surgical excision.
- Postop radiotherapy.
- Postop chemotherapy.
- Brain stem gliomas are presumed malignant—surgery is not typically an option.

OUTCOME

- Surgery and radiotherapy prolong survival by a few months.
- Chemotherapy is of no proven benefit.
- These lesions are almost invariably fatal with nearly 0% 5-year survival for GBMs.

Meningioma

EPIDEMIOLOGY

- 12% of all primary brain tumors
- 1.8:1 female-to-male ratio
- Arise from arachnoid cells

LOCATION

- Superior convexities
- Sphenoid wing
- Orbital rim
- Cerebellar tentorium
- Intraventricular

PATHOLOGY

- Meningotheliomatous (most common)
- Fibrous
- Angioblastic
- Atypical
- Anaplastic
- Psammoma bodies

NATURAL HISTORY

- Slowly progressive growth
- Rarely invasive or metastatic
- Symptoms secondary to pressure on surrounding structures
- Many discovered incidentally

IMAGING

- Isointense on T1/hyperintense on T2.
- Homogenous enhancement with CT/MRI.
- Dural tail may be apparent.
- CT may demonstrate calcifications.
- May cause hyperostosis of adjacent bone.

TREATMENT

- Observe if asymptomatic
- Surgical excision if symptomatic
- External beam radiotherapy/gamma knife if subtotal resection or unresectable

OUTCOME

- Five-year survival > 90%.

Pituitary Adenoma

EPIDEMIOLOGY

- 10% of primary brain tumors
- Male = female incidence
- Associated with multiple endocrine neoplasia (MEN) syndrome

LOCATION

- Sella turcica
- Parasellar extension
- May envelop carotid arteries

PATHOLOGY

- Chromophobe (null-cell or prolactin)
- Acidophil (prolactin or growth hormone [GH])
- Basophil (adrenocorticotropic hormone [ACTH])

NATURAL HISTORY

- Pituitary apoplexy may be an emergent presentation.
- Generally slow, progressive enlargement.

- Bitemporal hemianopsia (superior to inferior loss).
- May compromise cranial nerves in cavernous sinuses.
- Stigmata of endocrine abnormalities:
  - Galactorrhea
  - Cushing's disease
  - Acromegaly
  - Addisonian hypoadrenalism

IMAGING

- Low T1/high T2 signal on MRI
- Nonenhancing mass (remainder of pituitary enhances).
- Microadenoma may not be visualized.

TREATMENT

- Perform preoperative visual field testing.
- Preop endocrinological evaluation.

PROLACTINOMAS

- Medical treatment (dopamine agonists)
- Surgical excision if no response to therapy

ACROMEGALY

- Surgical resection—50% cure
- Avoid surgery in asymptomatic eldery patients as no survival benefit
- Medical therapy with octreotide (somatostatin analogue)

CUSHING'S DISEASE

Surgery is the treatment of choice—85% cure.

THYROID-STIMULATING HORMONE (TSH) ADENOMAS

Medical therapy with octreotide.

NONFUNCTIONAL ADENOMAS

- Observe if asymptomatic
- Surgical resection otherwise

Neuroma

EPIDEMIOLOGY

- 8–10% of primary brain tumors
- 1 in 100,000 incidence

LOCATION

- CN VIII affected most frequently.
- Any cranial nerve can be involved.
- Usually unilateral.
- Bilateral CN VIII neuromas pathognomonic for neurofibromatosis 2 (NF2).

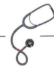

Patients with bitemporal hemianopsia (tunnel vision) may admit to increased clumsiness if asked.

PATHOLOGY

Antoni A and B fibers.

NATURAL HISTORY

- Unilateral progressive hearing loss (sensorineural)
- Tinnitus
- Dysequilibrium
- Possible vertigo
- Growth rate unpredictable, but generally slow

IMAGING

- MRI reveals homogenously enhancing lesion.
- Often protrudes into porous acousticus (CN VIII neuroma).

TREATMENT

- Perform pretreatment audiometric and vestibular testing.
- Surgical excision or stereotactic radiosurgery.
- Conventional radiotherapy.

Ependymoma

EPIDEMIOLOGY

- Six percent of primary brain tumors.
- Most occur in children.

LOCATION

- Fourth ventricle (most common)
- Spinal cord
- Lateral ventricles

PATHOLOGY

- Papillary
- Myxopapillary (only at filum terminale)
- Subependymoma
- Ependymoblastoma

NATURAL HISTORY

- Usually presents as a posterior fossa mass
- Infrequently presents with seizure
- Tends to disseminate through CSF ("seeding")

Preop imaging of the spinal neuraxis should be performed to detect CSF seeding.

IMAGING

- Inhomogenous T1 signal/high T2 signal.
- Moderate inhomogenous enhancement.
- Arises from floor of fourth ventricle.
- Cystic components are common.

HIGH-YIELD FACTS

Neurosurgery

TREATMENT

- Surgical resection
- Radiation if in fourth ventricle or spinal cord
- Chemotherapy of little benefit

OUTCOME

- 80% 5-year survival (adult) with surgery and radiation
- 30% 5-year average survival in children

Oligodendroglioma

EPIDEMIOLOGY

- 4% of primary brain tumors
- Male > female (3:2)
- Mostly occur in middle-aged adults

LOCATION

- Predilection for frontal lobes.
- Nearly all occur in cerebral hemispheres.

PATHOLOGY

- Uniform cells with round nuclei
- May have mixed astrocytic component
- Classically, "fried egg" or "chicken wire" pattern—a fixation artifact not routinely seen

NATURAL HISTORY

- Slowly progressive
- Most frequently presents with a seizure

IMAGING

- Hypointense on T1; hyperintense on T2.
- Low-grade forms tend to lack enhancement.
- CT may reveal extensive calcification in 90%.

TREATMENT

- Observe if asymptomatic
- Surgery for:
  - Symptomatic lesions
  - Lesions > 5 cm
- Postop radiotherapy employed in most—not necessary to use immediately
- Chemotherapy perhaps of some value

OUTCOME

- 75% 5-year survival
- 30% 10-year survival

Craniopharyngioma

EPIDEMIOLOGY

- Three percent of primary brain tumors.
- Most occur in childhood.
- No gender predilection.

LOCATION

- Anterior superior pituitary margin
- Third ventricle
- May extend into contiguous regions

PATHOLOGY

- Benign
- Epithelial–squamous
- Calcified cystic tumor
- Arises from remnants of the craniopharyngeal duct or Rathke's cleft

NATURAL HISTORY

- Headache and visual disturbance
- Benign, but difficult to cure

IMAGING

- Hypointense T1; hyperintense T2
- May be cystic regions
- Strong heterogenous enhancement

TREATMENT

- Preop endocrinological evaluation
- May be observed
- Surgical resection if symptomatic

OUTCOME

- 5% mortality (hypothalamic injury)
- 5-year survival perhaps 70%

Hemangioblastoma

EPIDEMIOLOGY

- 2% of primary brain tumors
- Tend to appear clinically in middle adulthood
- Associated with Von Hippel–Lindau disease

LOCATION

- Most common adult posterior fossa tumor
- Spinal cord

PATHOLOGY

- Benign
- May disseminate in CSF after surgery

NATURAL HISTORY

- Present with typical posterior fossa symptoms
- Hemorrhage extremely rare

IMAGING

- MRI may show serpiginous flow voids.
- Surrounding hemosiderin deposition.
- Intensely enhancing.
- Angiogram reveals marked vascularity.

TREATMENT

- Surgery curative in sporadic cases
- Radiation treatment to slow growth if surgically unresectable

Pineal Tumors

EPIDEMIOLOGY

- One to 2% of primary brain tumors.
- More frequent in children than adults.
- Germinomas and teratomas have a male preponderance.

LOCATION

- Pineal region
- Third ventricle

PATHOLOGY

- Multiple cell lineages
- Pineal cysts
- Pineocytoma
- Pineoblastoma
- Germinoma (most common)
- Embryonal carcinoma
- Choriocarcinoma
- Teratoma

NATURAL HISTORY

- Pineal cysts are seen in up to 40% of persons.
- Pineal tumors present with hydrocephalus.
- Parinaud syndrome.

IMAGING

Varied.

Von Hippel–Lindau disease:

- Autosomal dominant (chromosome 3).
- Multiorgan angiomatosis.
- CNS tumors are benign hemangioblastomas.
- Other organs: Spinal cord, eye, adrenal glands, kidneys, pancreas.

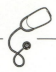
TREATMENT

- Observe pineal cysts unless HCP develops.
- Measure serum AFP and beta-human chorionic gonadotropin (HCG).
- Germinomas are highly radiosensitive.
- May give a test dose of radiation to determine responsiveness.
- Surgery if:
  - Well-encapsulated and symptomatic
  - No evidence of metastases
  - Unresponsive to radiotherapy

CNS Lymphoma

EPIDEMIOLOGY

- 1% of primary brain tumors
- May be primary or result of secondary spread
- Incidence increasing
- Male > female (1.5:1)
- Associated with:
  - AIDS
  - Connective tissue diseases
  - Chronic immunosuppression
  - Epstein–Barr virus infection

LOCATION

- Frontal lobes
- Basal ganglia/thalami
- Typically contact a CSF space

PATHOLOGY

- Appear similar to systemic lymphomas.
- Most are B-cell lineage.

NATURAL HISTORY

- May present with multiple cranial nerve palsies (lymphomatous meningitis)
- Seizure
- Spinal cord compression
- Tends to be rapidly progressive

IMAGING

- No pathognomonic features
- Can have varied appearance ("the great imitator" of brain tumors)
- Typically strongly, homogenously enhancing
- May have a wispy appearance
- Will vanish on imaging after a dose of steroids—"ghost tumor"

TREATMENT

- These tumors tend to melt away with an initial round of steroid treatment.
- Radiation therapy is the mainstay of treatment.

- Methotrexate and CHOP (cyclophosphamide, hydroxydaunorubicin, oncovin, and prednisone) chemotherapy.
- The main role of surgery is a diagnostic biopsy.
- Surgery does not improve survival.

Ganglioglioma

EPIDEMIOLOGY

- 1% of primary brain tumors
- Primarily occur in children and young adults

LOCATION

Nearly anywhere.

PATHOLOGY

- Ganglioneuroma (neural predominance, more benign)
- Ganglioglioma (glial predominance)

NATURAL HISTORY

Major presentation is seizure.

IMAGING

High T1 and low T2 signal on MRI.

TREATMENT

- Follow if asymptomatic
- Surgical resection if symptomatic
- Radiation therapy if recurrence

Epidermoid and Dermoid Tumors

Non-neoplastic.

EPIDEMIOLOGY

- 1% of primary brain masses
- May be congenital or result from trauma

LOCATION

- Calvarium
- Suprasellar region
- Spinal canal
- Cerebellopontine (CP) angle (epidermoid)
- Near midline (dermoid)

PATHOLOGY

- Epidermoid—squamous epithelium with keratin center
- Dermoid—same as an epidermoid with skin appendages (sebaceous glands, hair follicles)

NATURAL HISTORY

- Proliferates at a rate like normal epithelium.
- Presents as typical intracranial mass.
- Rupture of a cyst may produce a chemical meningitis.

IMAGING

- T1 and T2 signal similar to CSF
- Lucent on CT with occasional calcification

TREATMENT

- Surgical excision if symptomatic
- Caution to avoid spilling contents
- May pretreat with steroids to limit aseptic meningitis in case of cyst rupture

Primitive Neuroectodermal Tumors (PNET)

EPIDEMIOLOGY

- < 1% of all primary brain tumors
- Most common malignant pediatric brain tumor
- Extremely rare in adults
- Male > female (2:1)

LOCATION

- Cerebellar vermis
- Arises from roof of fourth ventricle

PATHOLOGY

- Densely cellular
- Small blue cells

NATURAL HISTORY

- Presents as a typical posterior fossa mass
- May cause early obstructive hydrocephalus
- May disseminate through CSF like ependymoma
- Tends to metastasize early

IMAGING

- Low inhomogenous T1 signal; variable T2 signal.
- Variable contrast enhancement.
- Cystic components are common.
- Arises from roof of fourth ventricle.

TREATMENT

- Surgical resection
- Postop radiotherapy
- Chemotherapy of questionable value

Outcome

Seventy-five percent 5-year survival if complete surgical excision followed by radiotherapy.

Choroid Plexus Papilloma

Epidemiology

- < 1% of primary brain tumors.
- Preponderance of cases are in infants.

Location

- Usually fourth ventricle
- Lateral ventricles

Pathology

- Benign
- Frond-like papillae
- Rosettes

Natural History

- Sometimes grow rapidly
- May result in overproduction of CSF
- Present mostly due to hydrocephalus

Imaging

- Isointense on T1/T2
- Intensely enhancing
- Intraventricular; deform ventricles

Treatment

Surgical resection.

Outcome

Five-year survival 85%.

Glomus Tumors

Tumors arising from paraganglion cells:
- Carotid body tumors
- Glomus jugulare tumors
- Pheochromocytomas

Epidemiology

- Rare, < 1% of all head and neck tumors
- Female preponderance (6:1)

Location

- Carotid bulb
- Jugular glomus body

> Preop imaging of the spinal neuraxis should be performed to detect CSF seeding.

PATHOLOGY

- Benign
- Locally invasive
- Highly vascular
- May secrete catecholamines
- Tend to grow along vasculature
- May be multiple

NATURAL HISTORY

- Slow growing
- May present with:
  - Pulsatile tinnitus
  - CN VIII–XII palsies

IMAGING

- Similar to neuromas on MRI
- Intense vascularity

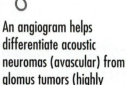

An angiogram helps differentiate acoustic neuromas (avascular) from glomus tumors (highly vascular).

TREATMENT

- Audiometric and vestibular testing preop
- 24-hour urine collection for catecholamines
- Surgical excision for smaller tumors
- Alpha and beta blockade preop
- Radiation therapy for large tumors

OUTCOME

- Recurs in > 25% of cases
- Risk of significant intraoperative hemorrhage

Chordoma

EPIDEMIOLOGY

- Neoplasm of notochord
- Rare: 1 in 1,000,000

LOCATION

- Clivus
- Vertebral column (usually sacral)

PATHOLOGY

- Low-grade malignancy
- Physaliphorous cells

NATURAL HISTORY

- Slow growing
- Osseodestructive
- Locally invasive

IMAGING

- Osseolytic on CT
- Frequently calcified
- "Ivory vertebra"

TREATMENT

- Wide en bloc excision.
- Avoid tumor—surgery can disseminate cells.
- Postoperative radiation/proton beam therapy.

METASTATIC TUMORS

- More than 50% of brain tumors are metastatic in origin.
- Most disseminate hematogenously.
- Incidence of cerebral metastases is increasing.
- Common sources:
    - Bronchogenic lung cancer
    - Melanoma (predilection for CNS metastasis)
    - Breast cancer
    - Renal cell carcinoma
    - Colon adenocarcinoma
- Most present with progressive focal neurologic deficit or signs/symptoms of increased ICP.
- Certain metastases are more likely to hemorrhage:
    - Melanoma
    - Renal cell carcinoma
    - Choriocarcinoma
- Most metastases occur in the cerebral hemispheres at the gray–white junction or in the cerebellum.

IMAGING

- Typically, metastases are well-circumscribed.
- Usually significant surrounding edema greater than that seen with primary brain tumors.
- Metastases usually enhance (completely or ring enhancement).

EVALUATION

Search for a primary source:
- Chest x-ray (CXR)
- CT chest/abdomen/pelvis
- Bone scan
- Mammogram in women
- Guaiac for occult blood

MANAGEMENT

- Biopsy for diagnosis if no other source identified.
- Resect most solitary symptomatic lesions and treat with radiotherapy postoperatively.
- If multiple metastases, proceed directly to radiotherapy.

RADIOSENSITIVE METASTASES

- Small cell lung carcinoma
- Lymphoma
- Multiple myeloma
- Germ-cell tumors

MEDICAL THERAPY

- Dexamethasone to relieve vasogenic edema.
- Anticonvulsants may be used for cerebral hemispheric lesions if seizures occur.
- Chemotherapy may be advantageous in certain cases.

OUTCOME

- Varies depending on type of metastasis.
- Survival averages 1 to 3 months if symptomatic at presentation.

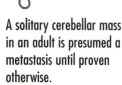

A solitary cerebellar mass in an adult is presumed a metastasis until proven otherwise.

PHAKOMATOSES

Neurofibromatosis

- Two major types: NF1 (von Recklinghausen's) and NF2
- Both autosomal dominant
- Incidence 1 in 3,000

COMMON FINDINGS

- Café-au-lait spots
- Neurofibromas
- Lisch nodules
- Family history

ASSOCIATED COMORBIDITIES

- Acoustic neuromas (bilateral in NF2 is pathognomonic)
- Multiple astrocytomas throughout CNS
- Syringomyelia
- Neuroblastoma
- Leukemia
- Wilms' tumor

MANAGEMENT

- Observe.
- Resect symptomatic lesions.
- May attempt early intervention in acoustic neuromas of NF2 to preserve hearing.

Tuberous Sclerosis

- Autosomal dominant
- Rare; 1 in 200,000 incidence

FINDINGS

- Pachygyria/microgyria.
- Subependymal "tuber" (hamartoma)—calcific.
- "Ash leaf" spots on skin.
- Adenoma sebaceum appears in later childhood.
- Giant cell astrocytoma.

MANAGEMENT

- Observation.
- Resect symptomatic lesions.
- Medical or surgical control of seizures.

Von Hippel–Lindau

- Incidence 1 in 40,000
- Autosomal dominant; 90% penetrance

Findings

- Multiple CNS hemangioblastomas
- Retinal angiomas
- Pheochromocytomas
- Renal cell carcinomas

MANAGEMENT

- Observation
- Surgical excision of symptomatic lesions

Sturge–Weber

Autosomal recessive or sporadic.

FINDINGS

- Port-wine facial nevus (V_1 distribution)
- Cortical atrophy
- Seizures

MANAGEMENT

- Anticonvulsants
- Surgical lobectomy/hemispherectomy if seizures are intractable

Tuberous sclerosis clinical triad:
- Mental retardation
- Adenoma sebaceum (actually perivascular fibromata)
- Seizures

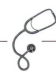

Calcification of cortex may appear as "tram tracks" on plain films.

CYSTIC LESIONS

Rathke's Cleft Cyst

- Non-neoplastic lesion in the parasellar region
- Often an incidental finding
- No treatment necessary unless symptomatic → surgical decompression

Colloid Cyst

- Benign tumor usually in anterior portion of the third ventricle.
- May obstruct foramen of Monro and lead to sudden death from hydrocephalus.
- Treatment is temporary lateral ventricular shunting followed by surgical excision.

RADIOSURGERY

External Beam Radiotherapy

- Conventional treatment
- Entire region within the treatment ports receives an equivalent dosage of radiation.
- Typically fractionated over several days to minimize injury to healthy tissue.
- Treatment instituted 2 to 3 weeks after surgery to allow time for wound healing.
- Avoid use in young children where possible—decreases IQ ~25 points.
- In younger patients, early-onset dementia may develop many years after treatment. Avoid multiple cycles of radiation treatment.
- May induce secondary tumors:
  - Gliomas
  - Meningiomas
  - Neuromas
  - Malignant transformation of treated tumor
- **Postradiation somnolence syndrome:** Lethargy for a period of 2 to 6 months after treatment is common.
- **Radiation necrosis:**
  - Four months to several years later.
  - White matter changes that may appear as recurrent tumor.
  - MRI, single photon emission computed tomography (SPECT) or positron emission tomography (PET) may help differentiate from tumor.
  - May require biopsy to be certain.
  - If necrotic area exerts mass effect, excise tissue.

Stereotactic Radiosurgery

- Radiation delivered from multiple points with intent of focusing beams on central focus to maximize radiation dosage to treatment area while minimizing surrounding tissue exposure.
- Gamma knife: 201 point sources of radiation focused on a central point. Requires stereotactic MRI imaging of the head.
  - Advantages:
    - Outpatient procedure.
    - Entire dose of radiation given in one session.
    - Radiation beams intersecting sensitive neural structures can be left out.
    - Unit accurate to 0.3 mm.
    - Allows treatment of lesions in surgically inaccessible sites.

- Disadvantages:
    - Requires precise positioning within unit.
    - Resolution of MRI is a limiting factor, ~3 mm.
- Patient may need to be repositioned multiple times to adjust beam focus to capture maximum volume of lesion.
- Avoid use when lesion < 3 mm from a sensitive structure (e.g., optic nerve, artery, venous sinus, or cranial nerves).
- Useful for lesions up to 3 cm (max < 4 cm).
- Linac: Slightly less precise than Gamma knife. Delivers radiation in a series of arcs through a fixed target focus.

Brachytherapy

- Implantation of radioactive beads into treatment bed
- Seldom used except as a last resort.

Definitions

- Spondylosis: Degenerative changes in spine; arthritis
- Spondylolisthesis: Subluxation of one vertebral body on another
- Spondylolysis:
    - Fracture or defect in pars interarticularis.
    - Mostly congenital at L5 level (spina bifida occulta).
    - Spondylolysis due to congenital/degenerative etiology generally does not require surgical intervention.
    - Traumatic spondylolysis requires spinal fusion.

Spondylolisthesis grading: Measured by percentage of vertebral body width that has subluxed anteriorly.

Grade 1	0–25%
Grade 2	25–50%
Grade 3	50–75%
Grade 4	75%–100%

Low Back Pain

GENERAL

- One of the most common chief complaints in medicine.
- Only 10–20% will ever have a specific cause found.
- Most are medically managed with pain control and physical therapy (PT).
- Protracted bed rest is actually detrimental; encourage early ambulation and return to work and activities.
- Over 90% improve in 1 month with no intervention.

TYPES

- Mechanical (myofascial or musculoskeletal):
    - Muscle/ligament strain
    - Facet joint injury
    - Disc pain
    - Generally, no anatomically identifiable source
- Radiculopathy:
    - Nerve root impairment
    - May be a combination of pain, paresthesia, weakness, and decreased muscle tendon reflexes in nerve territory

Lumbar spine
Straight leg raise: Radicular symptoms produced with leg elevation in supine position.
Crossed straight leg raise: Radicular symptoms produced in affected leg with elevation of opposite leg.
Cervical spine
Spurling's sign: Radicular pain produced with downward pressure on head when neck extended and tilted toward affected side.

Herniated disc terminology:
Bulge: Symmetric extension
Protrusion: Asymmetric extension
Extrusion: Free disc fragment
Degenerated: Narrowed disc space with decreased T2 (water) signal (i.e., desiccation).

ASSESSMENT

- Red flags:
  - Recent fever
  - Recent weight loss
  - Pain awakening patient from sleep
  - History of cancer
  - IV drug use
  - Symptoms extending below the knee
  - Bowel/bladder dysfunction
  - Sensory loss to perineum
- Physical exam:
  - Vertebral body tenderness
  - Fever
  - Specific weakness patterns in root distribution
  - Straight leg raise test causing radicular pain
- Further testing is indicated for those with red flags or significant neurologic deficits.
- Imaging:
  - Generally perform only if there may be a surgical consideration. Otherwise, imaging does little to influence choices in medical management.
  - Many asymptomatic patients have very abnormal-appearing spine imaging (spondylosis, disc herniations, etc.).
  - Imaging is useful only for supporting clinical suspicion.
  - Plain films:
    - Perform if trauma/tumor/infection suspected
    - Shows only bony alignment and some bony pathology
  - MRI:
    - Test of choice except in bony pathology
    - Ideal for demonstrating herniated discs or soft tissue abnormalities
    - Allows imaging in sagittal plane
  - CT:
    - Poor for soft-tissue imaging
    - Test of choice for bony pathology
  - CT/myelogram:
    - May help in instances in which MRI is equivocal.
    - Invasive—dye is injected into spinal canal.
    - Dye will reveal any functional block in the canal.
  - Bone scan:
    - Useful when suspecting tumor, infection, or occult fracture
    - Not useful for most acute presentations
  - Electromyogram (EMG):
    - May help diagnose radiculopathy.
    - Not necessary if physical exam reliable.
    - Nerve conduction may be normal for first 3 weeks.

CONSERVATIVE TREATMENT

- Bed rest for no more than 2 to 4 days (immobility will aggravate muscle stiffness and pain).
- Low-impact exercise: Walking, swimming.
- Avoid heavy lifting/pushing/pulling (e.g., > 10 to 20 lbs.).
- Pain control: Nonsteroidal anti-inflammatory drugs (NSAIDs); opioids/muscle relaxants if supplemental control necessary.
- Spinal manipulation: May help in acute setting as long as no radicular symptoms or neurological deficit present.

Herniated Disc (see Table 23-1)

- Typically, the nerve root with same name as lower vertebral body of interspace involved is impinged.
- Radicular symptoms may increase with flexion of the lumbar spine or extension of the cervical spine.
- Valsalva maneuvers may increase symptoms.
- Lying supine ameliorates most lumbar radiculopathy pain.
- Resting arm in flexed position behind head often lessens pain in cervical radiculopathy.
- Most common lumbar level: L5–S1, then L4–5
- Most common cervical level: C6–7, then C5–6
- An extreme lateral disc herniation will impact the nerve root exiting at that interspace (special case violation of rule above).
- Eighty-five percent of symptomatic herniated discs improve without surgery.

Surgical Indications

- Emergent:
  - Cauda equina syndrome (lumbar disc)
  - Conus medullaris syndrome (lumbar disc)
  - Myelopathy (cervical/thoracic disc)
  - Progressive neurologic deficit
- Elective:
  - Pain refractory to medical therapy and PT
  - Motor weakness

TABLE 23-1. Herniated disc syndromes.

Disc Level	Root Compressed	Pain Distribution	Sensory Pattern	Motor Weakness	Reflex Affected
C4–5	C5	Shoulder	Shoulder	Shoulder abduction	Deltoid
C5–6	C6	Upper arm, lateral forearm, and first two digits	Upper arm, lateral forearm, and first two digits	Forearm flexion	Biceps and brachioradialis
C6–7	C7	Second to fourth digits	Second to fourth digits and all fingertips	Forearm, wrist, and finger extension	Triceps
C7–T1	C8	Upper arm, medial forearm, and last two digits	Upper arm, medial forearm, and last two digits	Wrist and finger flexion	Finger jerk
L3–4	L4	Anterior thigh	Anterior thigh to medial malleolus	Quadriceps	Patellar
L4–5	L5	Posterolateral leg to hallux	Lateral thigh to dorsum of foot and great toe	Tibialis anterior and extensor hallucis longus	Medial hamstring
L5–S1	S1	Posterior leg and lateral and plantar aspects of the foot	Posterior thigh and leg to lateral malleolus	Gastrocnemius/ soleus	Achilles

Surgical Approaches

- Lumbar: Typically posterior trans-canal approach with patient in lordotic prone position.
- Operations mostly involve a combination of:
  - Laminectomy (hemi or bilateral)
  - Discectomy
  - Foraminotomy (if neural foramen stenotic)
  - Microdiscectomy (operating microscope utilized)
- Dural tear is a common complication. Requires a water-tight closure with suture and possibly fibrin glue.
- Cervical:
  - Anterior discectomy and cervical fusion (ADCF) for pathology involving C3–7:
    - Only means to remove central disc herniation
    - Fusion not necessary, but advisable if myelopathy present
    - Same operative risks as carotid endarterectomy (CEA) with additional risk of esophageal injury
  - Posterior laminectomy (only for lateral disc herniations):
    - If more than two levels involved
    - If patient is a professional singer/speaker
- Thoracic:
  - Transpedicular
  - Costotransversectomy
  - Transthoracic

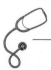

Examples:
In cervical spine, C5–6 disc herniation typically impacts C6 nerve root, which exits at the same interspace as level of herniation. In lumbar spine, L4–5 disc herniation typically impacts L5 nerve root, which exits at the interspace below the disc herniation (L5–S1 level).

Failed Back Syndrome

- Unsatisfactory postoperative improvement.
- Factors:
  - Incorrect initial diagnosis/operation
  - Continued nerve compression (incomplete resection)
  - Recurrent herniation/scar formation
  - Permanent nerve injury (preoperatively)
  - Nonorganic factors (psychosocial)
- As many as 10–15% of operated herniated lumbar discs may reherniate.
- Evaluation: MRI with and without contrast to reevaluate for recurrent disc herniation or root compression secondary to scar formation (typically enhances).

Spinal Stenosis

Narrowing of spinal canal.

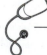

Emergent conditions should be operated in less than 48 hours. Most neurosurgeons will do no later than the next morning.

LUMBAR

- Etiology: Congenital and/or acquired
- Presentation: Neurogenic claudication
  - Lower extremity discomfort with walking/standing.
  - Tends to be circumferential (polyradicular).
  - May start distally and progress proximally.
  - Relieved by changing position.
  - Sitting or flexion of lumbar spine often alleviates pain.
  - Pain remits in 5 to 15 minutes.

- Evaluation: MRI test of choice. Decreased width of CSF signal about spinal cord and dural sac in stenotic areas.
- Spinal canal may have a cloverleaf shape secondary to:
  - Hypertrophied facet joints
  - Hypertrophied ligamentum flavum
  - Disc herniations
  - Spondylolisthesis
- Course: Hypertrophic changes creating neurogenic claudication do not improve and tend to progressively worsen.
- Treatment: Conservative management including analgesics and PT may be useful in some cases and should be tried initially in most patients.
- Surgical decompression indicated if:
  - Progressive neurologic deficit
  - Intractable pain or activity limitation despite medical therapy
- Procedure: Posterior bilateral laminectomy of involved levels with partial facetectomies and discectomies as needed. No need for spinal fusion if facet joints are not compromised.
- Outcome:
  - > 95% will experience pain relief and increased activity tolerance.
  - Of those with failure to respond, most are due to poor correlation of clinical and radiographic findings.

CERVICAL

- Etiology: Mostly congenital with superimposed acquired degenerative changes.
- Presentation:
  - Myelopathy
  - Radiculopathy
  - Diffuse head, neck, and shoulder pain
  - Typically, slowly progressive over time
- Evaluation: MRI test of choice
  - Decreased width/absence of CSF signal around spinal cord.
  - Spinal cord may be effaced by disc anteriorly, causing deformation— "banana cord."
  - Increased T2 signal may be evident within spinal cord.
- Treatment: Conservative management initially as with lumbar stenosis
- Surgical indications: Same as for lumbar stenosis.
- Urgent surgical decompression without attempt at medical management when:
  - Signs of myelopathy
  - Increased T2 signal in spinal cord

Surgical procedure is decompressive posterior bilateral laminectomies and facetectomies as needed.

- Laminectomies of several levels (≥ 4) may predispose to swan-neck deformity of cervical spine over time. Pedicle screw and rod fixation may be necessary to prevent/ameliorate this condition.

Atlantoaxial Dislocation

- Rheumatoid arthritis underlies 25% (see Figure 23-4).
- Presents with local pain and possibly hyperreflexia.
- May be signs of a C2 radiculopathy (suboccipital neuralgia).
- Acquire a lateral C-spine plain film to assess atlantodental interval— should be ≤ 4 mm.

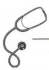

Surgery improves radicular symptoms of pain, but does not generally help back pain. Advisable to **not** operate on patients with chief complaint solely or mostly of back pain unless a significant radicular component extending below the knee is present.

"Shopping cart" sign: Patient may be able to walk further if there is something to lean on.

Differentiate from spinal stenosis from vascular claudication by:

1. Stopping and standing do not relieve pain in neurogenic claudication.
2. Sitting and resting does not result in near-immediate relief.
3. Vascular claudication will affect patients with any activity involving the lower extremities, including bicycling. Neurogenic claudication typically does not cause symptoms while cycling (lumbar spine flexed).

HIGH-YIELD FACTS

Neurosurgery

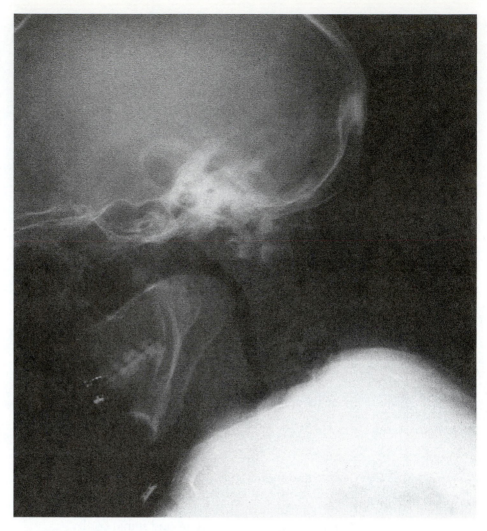

FIGURE 23-4. Atlantoaxial subluxation in a patient with rheumatoid arthritis.

When assessing reflexes, hyperreflexia with an increased jaw jerk indicates a diffuse condition (generally, a benign normal variant). Pathological diffuse hyperreflexia is suggested if the jaw jerk reflex is of normal responsiveness (no bulbar involvement—indicative of distal lesion).

- An interval ≥ 4 mm suggests compromise of the transverse ligament.
- If symptomatic or atlantodental interval ≥ 6 to 8 mm in asymptomatic patient, C1–2 surgical fusion indicated.

Ossification of the Posterior Longitudinal Ligament (PLL)

- Sclerosis of the PLL may cause impingement on the spinal cord. Slowly progressive. Myelopathy may develop.
- If symptomatic, treatment is ADCF and corpectomy of involved levels.

Diffuse Idiopathic Skeletal Hyperostosis

- Forestier syndrome.
- Includes osteophytic growth along spinal column.
- Plain films may reveal "bamboo spine"—osteophytic growth over intervertebral discs connecting adjacent vertebrae.
- May cause dysphagia.
- If symptomatic, can drill off bone over disc space to "disconnect" vertebral bodies.

Syringomyelia

- Cystic cavitation with the spinal cord
- "Syringobulbia" if cavity ascends into brain stem.
- Highly variable clinical presentation with varying patterns of sensory/motor dysfunction.
- Most are asymptomatic.
- Has high T2 signal on MRI; nonenhancing.
- Surgical decompression techniques if symptomatic:
  - Needle aspiration
  - Shunt
  - Excision

Peripheral Neuropathy

- May be single or multiple depending on etiology.
- Mononeuritis multiplex—neuropathy of two separate nerves.

ETIOLOGY

Drugs/DM
Alcohol/AIDS
Nutrition (vitamins E and B_{12})
Guillain–Barre
Traumatic
Hereditary
Entrapment
Radiation/Renal
Amyloid
Paraneoplastic/Porphyria/Psychological
Infectious
Sarcoidosis
Toxic (heavy metals)

BRACHIAL PLEXOPATHY

- Usually shoulder girdle weakness and varying patterns of arm weakness.
- Most common etiologies:
  - Idiopathic
  - Pancoast tumor (inferior trunk)
  - Infectious (viral)
  - Vasculitic
- EMG can help localize the portion of the plexus involved if no improvement is seen after 2 to 3 weeks.
- Perform MRI if no improvement in 2 to 3 weeks (rule out mass lesion).
- Traumatic brachial plexopathy.

LUMBAR PLEXOPATHY

- Same etiologies as above.
- May be very difficult to differentiate radiculopathy from plexopathy. With lumbar plexopathy, paraspinal musculature is not involved, but is affected with radiculopathies.

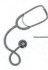

An atlantodental interval > 6 mm increases the chance of myelopathic deterioration, which may be irreversible.

Erb–Duchenne palsy— C5/6 injury: Arm medially rotated with wrist and fingers flexed. "Bellhop/waiter's tip palsy." Think of how Flintstones arms hang.

Klumpke's palsy—C8/T1 injury: "Claw hand." In an adult with insidious progressive development, think Pancoast tumor. There may be an associated Horner's syndrome.

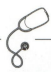

Nerve entrapment pain may start distally at source of stenosis and radiate retrograde as opposed to most radicular pains.

Median neuropathy due to carpal tunnel syndrome often involves the fingers but spares the palm unlike compression at the pronator teres (palmar cutaneous branch of median nerve is outside the carpal tunnel).

PERIPHERAL NERVE ENTRAPMENTS

- Pain and paresthesia are the main early symptoms. Weakness may develop.
- Demyelination occurs early, but may progress to axonal injury and wallerian degeneration later.
- Greater occipital: Caused by C1–3 fractures, atlantoaxial subluxation or local trauma. Presents with occipital neuralgia.
- Median: Compression at either the carpal tunnel (transverse carpal ligament) or more proximally in the forearm as it emerges between the heads of the pronator teres.
  - C5–T1 components.
  - Affects females > males.
  - Most common in middle age.
  - History of repeated hand movements.
  - Check Phalen's/Tinel's tests.
  - EMG may be helpful to differentiate from C6 radiculopathy.
  - Treat with rest.
  - Surgical decompression if motor weakness present or clinically intractable despite rest.
- Ulnar: Compression usually at the elbow or Guyon's canal at the wrist (not covered by transverse carpal ligament).
  - C7–T1 components.
  - Dysesthesias of last two digits.
  - Abducted fifth digit is an early sign.
  - Flexion of the distal phalanx of thumb may be weak.
  - Treat with rest.
  - Surgical transposition at elbow if weakness or clinically intractable.
- Radial: Compression either in axilla (crutches/thoracolumbosacral orthosis [TLSO]—triceps weakness and wrist drop) or spiral groove of humerus (Saturday night palsy—wrist drop). Remove compressive devices. If deltoid weakness present as well, indicative of brachial plexus lesion.
- Axillary: Generally due to shoulder dislocation. Deltoid weakness. Relocate humerus in glenoid to treat.
- Suprascapular: Entrapment in suprascapular notch (transverse scapular ligament overlies notch. Causes supra- and infraspinatus weakness. Surgical lysis of ligament to treat.
- Lateral femoral cutaneous: Meralgia paresthetica—entrapment as nerve emerges through inguinal ligament causing lateral thigh paresthesia. Due to:
  - Diabetes mellitus
  - Obesity
  - Previous surgery
  - Tight clothing

  Most remit without treatment. Because a purely sensory nerve, most treatment is medical (analgesics, local anesthetics, diabetes mellitus control, weight reduction, looser clothing). If above fail, surgical decompression of the inguinal ligament (difficult) or transection of the nerve is possible.
- Peroneal: Most common acute compression neuropathy. Occurs with pressure applied to lateral aspect of knee where peroneal nerve is very superficially positioned. May mimic an L5 radiculopathy except foot inversion is strength spared (L5 via tibial nerve).

Thoracic Outlet Syndrome (TOS)

- Subclavian artery/vein and brachial plexus pass through a space defined by the clavicle and first rib (thoracic outlet).
- Vascular compromise is more common than neurologic compromise.
- Etiologies:
  - Fibrous band compressing C8/T1 roots (inferior trunk)
  - Elongated C7 transverse process—"cervical rib"
- Treatment is to surgically lyse fibrous band or remove C7 transverse process by either transaxillary or supraclavicular approach to thoracic outlet.

Rotating head away from affected side with elevation of arm producing paresthesia/pain is suggestive of neurologic TOS. Concomitant reduction of radial pulse suggests vascular TOS.

BASIC NEUROSURGICAL OPERATIVE APPROACHES

Pterional and Frontotemporal

- Most common neurosurgical approaches employed.
- Allows access to anterior and middle fossae, lateral frontal lobe, anterior temporal lobe, parasellar region, and cavernous sinus. Pterional approach superiorly stops at the level of the pterion, but frontotemporal extends upward to the midpupillary line.
- Skin is incised 1 cm anterior to tragus (to avoid superficial temporal artery) in a "question mark" fashion over the pinna and forward superiorly above the orbit.
- Keyhole entry points at the pterion and in the frontal and temporal bones used for craniotomy.
- Orbitozygomatic and orbito-optic are further variations allowing additional anterior and lateral exposure about the orbit.

Subtemporal

A subtemporal craniotomy is utilized to access the posterior middle fossa, temporal lobe, petrous bone, cavernous sinus, and tentorium. A curvilinear incision superiorly located anterior and posterior to the pinna is fashioned.

Petrosal

An adjunct to pterional, frontotemporal, and subtemporal approaches where increased access to posterior fossa is required. Involves partial resection of the petrous portion of the temporal bone with care to avoid the facial and vestibulocochlear nerves as well as the inner ear structures within this region.

Suboccipital

Provides access to cerebellum, pineal region, dorsal brain stem, cerebellopontine angle, fourth ventricle, and foramen magnum. Incision is carried along the middle cervical raphe toward the inion. The incision is carried ~2 cm beyond the inion for bilateral suboccipital access. The incision may be carried in a curvilinear fashion toward the superior aspect of the pinna for a unilateral exposure.

Retromastoid

Allows access to the lateral brain stem. A "hockey stick" incision is placed posterior to the mastoid process. The mastoid is drilled off to provide exposure. Useful in providing access to posterior circulation aneurysms.

Frontal

Exposes the anterior fossa (planum sphenoidale), sella, lesions involving the posterior orbit or orbital canals. An incision is carried superiorly from 1 cm anterior to the pinna roughly along the trajectory of the coronal suture. This may be extended bilaterally (bicoronal incision).

Interhemispheric

Useful for exposure of midline lesions in the anterior fossa, sella, and third ventricle. Precallosal or transcallosal approaches may be utilized depending on location of the lesion. A horizontal incision is made in the superior forehead crease. Planning for the craniotomy should avoid the frontal sinus were possible.

Transsphenoidal

Accesses sella turcica. Approach through the sphenoid is narrowly placed between cavernous sinuses laterally. Bony osteotomy must be carefully performed. Preferred approach for most pituitary adenomas and some craniopharyngiomas.

Transoral

Provides exposure to the clivus and anterior portions of C1 and C2. May be useful for screw fixation of type II odontoid fracture.

Cardiothoracic Surgery

ISCHEMIC HEART DISEASE

DEFINITION

Myocardial injury caused by chronic or acute episodes of ischemia.

CAUSES

Disorders that affect coronary blood flow:
- Atherosclerotic coronary artery disease (most common)
- Valvular heart disease
- Vasculitis
- Congenital coronary anomalies
- Aortic dissection with involvement of ostia

ANATOMY

Right coronary dominance (90% of patients): Right coronary artery gives rise to posterior descending artery.

Left coronary dominance (10%): Left circumflex artery gives rise to posterior descending artery.
- *Consider how a lesion from either side will affect the posterior and inferior walls.*

PATHOPHYSIOLOGY

- Ischemic areas arise from lack of blood flow relative to the metabolic demands of the myocardium.
- The oxygen extraction already being high under normal metabolic conditions (75%), the heart must rely on increased blood flow to meet heightened demand.
- Determinants of demand: Wall tension (vis à vis preload, afterload, wall thickness), heart rate, level of contractility.
- An atherosclerotic plaque impedes flow significantly when coronary cross-sectional area is reduced by 75% (a 50% reduction in diameter).
- Coronary atherosclerotic lesions are usually multifocal, multivessel.
- Plaque rupture is the main cause of escalation of symptoms. Intermittent closure of dynamic plaques underlies symptoms of unstable angina.

Coronary atherosclerosis most common cause of cardiovascular morbidity and mortality in the Western world. Before age 70, men are more commonly affected than women by a ratio of 4:1. After age 70, it is 1:1.

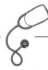

Severity of heart failure graded by **NYHA Classification:**

- Class I—no symptoms (fatigue, dyspnea, palpitations, anginal pain)
- Class II—symptoms with severe exertion
- Class III—symptoms with mild exertion
- Class IV—symptoms at rest

RISK FACTORS

- Hypertension
- Smoking
- Hypercholesterolemia
- Obesity
- Diabetes
- Family history

SIGNS AND SYMPTOMS

- Fatigue
- Angina pectoris
- Dyspnea
- Edema
- Palpitations
- Syncope
- Abnormal heart sounds
- Seventy-five percent present with classic angina, 25% present atypically, many have "silent" myocardial infarctions (MIs) (particularly diabetics and elderly).

DIAGNOSIS

- Electrocardiogram (ECG) may reveal ST segment elevations or depressions, inverted T waves, or Q waves.
- Stress test (to look at myocardial response when myocardial demand is increased).
- Echocardiography (localize dyskinetic wall segments, valvular dysfunction, estimate ejection fraction).
- Cardiac catheterization with angiography and left ventriculography (specifies coronary anatomy and sites of lesions to qualify the severity of the disease and vulnerable areas of myocardium, as well as to provide a roadmap for surgical or percutaneous intervention).

TREATMENT

- Medical—aspirin, beta blockers, calcium channel blockers, angiotensin-converting enzyme (ACE) inhibitors, diuretics, nitrates
- Percutaneous transluminal coronary angioplasty (PTCA)
- Surgical—coronary bypass grafting

CORONARY ARTERY BYPASS GRAFTING (CABG)

DESCRIPTION

- Bypass of discrete areas of obstruction in coronary vessels using the internal mammary artery, radial artery, a reversed segment of saphenous vein, inferior epigastric artery, or gastroepiploic artery.
- Internal mammary artery used in 95% of CABGs, usually to LAD.
- Three or four grafts are used on average.
- Minimally invasive CABG (MIDCAB): Fewer incisions, no cardiopulmonary bypass or cardioplegia are used (performed on a beating heart, limited to single-vessel disease). Minimizes pain, recovery time, and chances of wound infection.

- Port access technique: Endovascular aortic occlusion and cardiopulmonary bypass with cardioplegia allows for broader use of MIDCAB (multivessel disease, combined valve–coronary artery surgery).
- Vessel acronyms:
  - LAD—left anterior descending
  - RCA—right coronary artery
  - LCA—left main coronary artery
  - LCX—left circumflex artery
  - PDA—posterior descending artery
  - OMn—oblique marginal artery number 1, 2, 3, etc.
  - (L)(R)IM—(left)(right) internal mammary artery

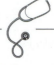

Diffuse patterns of coronary vessel obstruction, as can occur in diabetes, may not be amenable to CABG.

INDICATIONS

- Stable angina refractory to medical therapy
- Unstable angina
- Post-infarct angina
- Double- or triple-vessel disease with decreased left ventricular function
- Left main coronary disease
- During elective valve replacement with critical vessel occlusions
- During surgery for complications of MI (e.g., post-infarct ventral septal defect [VSD])
- Complications of PTCA stent replacement (rupture, dissection, thrombosis)

CONTRAINDICATIONS

- Chronic congestive heart failure (CHF)
- Ischemic cardiomyopathy with no signs of angina or *reversible* ischemia

PTCA VERSUS CABG

PTCA is preferred over CABG when:
- Low-risk obstruction (single vessel, mild double vessel) present causing severe symptoms.
- Patients at higher risk for complications from CABG.

PREOPERATIVE CONSIDERATIONS

- Evaluation for concurrent carotid disease (pre-CABG carotid endarterectomy may be required to reduce chances of perioperative stroke).
- Patencies of potential conduits are verified.
- Invasive monitoring (Swan–Ganz, central venous pressure [CVP], arterial line.)
- Broad-spectrum antibiotics as needed
- Aspirin discontinued 1 to 2 weeks preop
- Warfarin discontinued 1 week preop
- Antianginal meds continued until day of surgery
- Intra-aortic balloon pump for those who need it (augments cardiac output)

The **intra-aortic balloon pump (IABP)** sits in the descending aorta (just distal to where the left subclavian takes off). It works by inflating during diastole and deflating during systole. Inflation increases coronary blood flow. Deflation creates a negative pressure gradient in the aorta, thereby reducing afterload.

POSTOPERATIVE CONSIDERATIONS

Short-Term
- Continued monitoring of cardiac parameters
- Chest tubes
- Atrial fibrillation prophylaxis

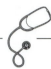

- Broad-spectrum antibiotics

Long-Term
- Rehabilitation
- Sternum heals in 3 to 6 months
- Anticipate incisional pain
- Risk factor modification (hyperlipidemia, smoking, sedentary lifestyle)
- Antiplatelet therapy

COMPLICATIONS

- MI
- Arrhythmias
- Infection (particularly mediastinitis and sternal infection)
- Hemorrhage
- Graft thrombosis
- Sternal dehiscence
- Tamponade
- Postpericardiotomy syndrome
- Stroke

PROGNOSIS

- 92% 4-year survival rate overall.
- 95% in those under 65 years, ejection fraction more than 40%, and/or undergoing elective procedure.
- Over 10 years, 84% in those with normal ventricle, 54% with severe cardiac impairment.
- Risk factors for mortality: Severe left ventricular dysfunction, advanced age, emergent CABG for acute MI or unstable angina.
- Multivessel disease and left main disease demonstrate greater survival with surgical intervention over medical therapy.
- Inferior mesenteric artery (IMA) has 95% 10-year patency.
- Saphenous vein has 60–70% 10-year patency.

VALVULAR HEART DISEASE

Mitral Stenosis

ETIOLOGY

- Rheumatic heart disease (most common)
- Congenital (rare)

EPIDEMIOLOGY

More common in women.

PATHOPHYSIOLOGY

- Mitral leaflets become thickened and calcified due to inflammation, resulting in commissural fusion in severe cases.
- Leads to pulmonary congestion and pulmonary hypertension, left atrial dilation, atrial fibrillation, reduced cardiac output.

SIGNS AND SYMPTOMS

- Dyspnea, DOE (dyspnea on exertion)
- Rales
- Cough
- Hemoptysis
- Systemic embolism (secondary to stagnation of blood in enlarged left atrium)
- Loud S1, opening snap
- Accentuated right ventricle precordial thrust
- Signs of right ventricular failure
- Hoarse voice (secondary to enlarged left atrium impinging on recurrent laryngeal nerve)

DIAGNOSIS

- Murmur is mid-diastolic with opening snap, low-pitched rumble.
- Best heard over left sternal border between second and fourth interspace.
- Chest x-ray (CXR) may show straight left heart border secondary to enlarged left atrium and Kerley B lines from pulmonary effusion.
- ECG may show left atrial enlargement, right ventricular hypertrophy, atrial fibrillation.
- Echocardiography demonstrates diseased valve, fish-mouth opening, decreased cross-sectional area (< 2 to 2.5 cm^2) on echo, and elevated transmitral pressure gradient (> 10 mm Hg)

TREATMENT

Medical
- Endocarditis prophylaxis.
- Treat for heart failure (diuretics, digitalis) and dysrhythmias as needed.
- Anticoagulation for atrial thrombus/fibrillation if present.
- Percutaneous mitral valve balloon valvuloplasty.

Surgical
- Indications for surgery:
  - NYHA Class III or IV symptoms
  - Atrial fibrillation
  - Worsening pulmonary hypertension
  - Systemic embolization
  - Infective endocarditis
  - Class II patients over age of 40
  - *Open commissurotomy:*
    - Will suffice in 30–50% of cases.
    - Fused leaflets are incised, calcifications are debrided, problematic chordae are resected, papillary muscle heads may be split, and mitral ring added to prevent regurgitation (annuloplasty).
- *Valve replacement* employed when excessive debridement would be required.
- *Percutaneous balloon valvuloplasty* not as effective in the long term, possibly because fused chordae cannot be corrected.
- Minimally invasive mitral valve surgery (port access technique) has recently been introduced.

Remember: Dilation of the left atrium is a major cause of atrial fibrillation.

Auscultatory triad of mitral stenosis:
- Increased first heart sound
- Opening snap
- Apical diastolic rumble

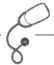

Balloon valvuloplasty in mitral stenosis is an effective intervention, as it has a low incidence of restenosis, in contrast to aortic stenosis.

HIGH-YIELD FACTS

Cardiothoracic Surgery

PROGNOSIS

- Ten years after commissurotomy, 7% require valve replacement.
- Yearly reoperation rates are 12% (balloon), 4% (commissurotomy), and 1.2% (valve replacement).
- Five-year survival after mitral valve replacement (MVR) 60–90%, 40–75% after 10 years (varies widely due to effect of risk factors, such as age, NYHA functional status, associated mitral insufficiency, additional need for CABG).

Mitral Insufficiency

ETIOLOGY

- Papillary muscle dysfunction from either ischemia or infarction (post-MI papillary muscle rupture causes massive regurgitation).
- Rupture of chordae tendineae (can happen spontaneously in otherwise healthy individuals).
- Valve destruction—scarring from rheumatic heart disease or destruction from endocarditis.
- Prolapse frequently progresses to valvular incompetence.

SIGNS AND SYMPTOMS

- Dyspnea
- Fatigue
- Weakness
- Cough
- Atrial fibrillation
- Systemic emboli
- Leads to pulmonary congestion, right-sided failure, left atrial dilation, atrial fibrillation, and volume overload of left ventricle. Cardiac output increases, then decreases.

Carpentier's functional classification of mitral insufficiency:
Type I — annular dilation or leaflet perforation with normal leaflet motion
Type II — increased leaflet motion and prolapse
Type III — restricted leaflet motion

DIAGNOSIS

- Murmur is loud, holosystolic, high-pitched, apical radiating to the axilla.
- Wide, splitting of S2 with inspiration (widening occurs in severe cases due to premature emptying of left ventricle [LV]).
- S3 due to rapid filling of LV by blood regurgitated during systole.
- ECG shows enlarged left atrium.
- Echocardiography demonstrates diseased/prolapsed valve and can be used to quantify MR.

TREATMENT

Medical

- Not definitive but used until surgery or in poor surgical candidates
- Diuretics to reduce volume load
- Vasodilators to reduce afterload favoring aortic forward flow
- Anticoagulation for atrial fibrillation

Surgical

- Valve replacement or repair
- Indications for surgery: At the first sign of symptoms, no symptoms with decline in systolic function, atrial fibrillation, left atrium > 4.5 to 5 cm.

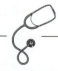

Mitral insufficiency has a good prognosis if LV function is preserved.

- *Mitral valve reconstruction:*
    - Involves resection of redundant areas of leaflets, chordal shortening, and ring annuloplasty (this corrects annular dilatation and stabilizes the repair).
    - Preferable to MVR in degenerative disease; MVR better in advanced deformity not amenable to reconstruction (e.g., due to rheumatic disease).

PROGNOSIS

- Better late survival in nonrheumatic patients undergoing reconstruction vs. replacement
- Opposite in rheumatic patients

Aortic Stenosis

ETIOLOGY

- Degenerative calcific disease (idiopathic, older population)
- Congenital stenosis
- Bicuspid aortic valve
- Rheumatic heart disease

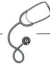

Congenital malformations account for about 50% of aortic valve operations.

PATHOPHYSIOLOGY

Obstruction of flow leads to left ventricular hypertrophy (LVH) (concentric type) and decreased LV compliance, then to LV dilation and congestion.

SIGNS AND SYMPTOMS

Usually asymptomatic early in course, then:
- Dyspnea
- Angina and syncope—particularly during exercise. Peripheral resistance falls; LV pressure remains the same due to stenotic valve; CO cannot maintain BP, causing syncope; low BP to coronary arteries causes angina.
- Heart failure
- Hypertension (consider associated aortic coarctation)

Mean survival for patients with aortic stenosis and:
Angina—5 years
Syncope—2 to 3 years
Heart failure—1 to 2 years

DIAGNOSIS

- Forceful apex beat with normally located point of maximal impulse (PMI).
- Loud systolic ejection murmur, crescendo–decrescendo, medium pitched, loudest at second R interspace, radiates to carotids.
- S4 (presystolic gallop) frequently present secondary to reduced LV compliance.
- Paradoxical splitting of S2.
- Narrow pulse pressure.
- ECG may show left ventricular strain pattern.
- Echocardiography demonstrates diseased valve and quantifies severity
- Calcification of aortic valve may be seen on CXR.

Left ventricular strain pattern is ST segment depression and T wave inversion in I, AVL, and left precordial leads.

TREATMENT

Medical
- Avoid strenuous activity.
- Avoid afterload reduction.

Surgical

- Indications for surgery:
  - Presence of symptoms
  - Asymptomatic with high transvalvular gradient (> 50 mm Hg) and LVH or declining ejection fraction
  - Aortic valve area < 0.8 cm²
- Valvuloplasty produces only temporary improvement as rate of restenosis is very high.
- Valve replacement is definitive therapy.
  - Intra-annular and supra-annular placement of prosthesis (latter for small annulus).
  - *Ross procedure* for aortic valve replacement: Patient's own pulmonary valve is substituted (*autograft*), while a cryopreserved *homograft* (cadaveric) is used to replace the pulmonary valve. No need for anticoagulation, plus good durability (20-year failure rate of 15%).

PROGNOSIS

Ten-year survival after aortic valve replacement > 80% except in high-risk patients (e.g., severely impaired LV function, NYHA Class IV, pulmonary hypertension).

Aortic Regurgitation

ETIOLOGY

- Aortic root dilatation: Idiopathic (correlates with hypertension [HTN] and age), collagen vascular disease, Marfan syndrome
- Valvular disease: Rheumatic heart disease, endocarditis
- Proximal aortic root dissection: Cystic medial necrosis (Marfan syndrome again), syphilis, HTN, Ehlers–Danlos, Turner syndrome, third trimester

PATHOPHYSIOLOGY

Leads to LV dilation, eccentric hypertrophy, mitral insufficiency, cardiomegaly, CHF.

SIGNS AND SYMPTOMS

- Dyspnea, orthopnea, paroxysmal nocturnal dyspnea
- Angina (secondary to reduced diastolic coronary blood flow due to elevated LV end-diastolic pressure)
- Left ventricular failure (LVF)
- Wide pulse pressure
- Bounding "Corrigan" pulse, "pistol shot" femorals, pulsus bisferiens (dicrotic pulse with two palpable waves in systole)
- Duroziez sign: Presence of diastolic femoral bruit when femoral artery is compressed enough to hear a systolic bruit
- Hill's sign: Systolic pressure in the legs > 20 mm Hg higher than in the arms
- Quincke's sign: Alternating blushing and blanching of the fingernails when gentle pressure is applied
- De Musset's sign: Bobbing of head with heartbeat

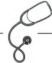

Other conditions with wide pulse pressure:
- Hyperthyroidism
- Anemia
- Wet beriberi
- Hypertrophic subaortic stenosis
- Hypertension

- High-pitched, blowing, decrescendo diastolic murmur best heard over second right interspace or third left interspace, accentuated by leaning forward.
- Austin Flint murmur: Observed in severe regurgitation, low-pitched diastolic rumble secondary to regurgitated blood striking the anterior mitral leaflet (similar sound to mitral regurgitation).
- A2 accentuated (due to high pulse pressure in the aorta at the beginning of ventricular diastole).
- Hyperdynamic down and laterally displaced PMI secondary to LV enlargement.
- ECG shows left ventricular hypertrophy.
- Echocardiography demonstrates regurgitant valve.

TREATMENT

Medical
- Treat LVF.
- Endocarditis prophylaxis.

Surgical
- Indications for surgery:
  - Presence of symptoms
  - Asymptomatic with first sign of declining LV function or rapid increase in cardiac size
- Valve *repair* may be suitable for pure aortic insufficiency (no stenosis and no other valves involved) and in cases of aortic root aneurysm.
- Valve *replacement* is necessary for severe cases and is the only definitive treatment.

PROGNOSIS

- See section on aortic stenosis.
- Valvular resection with annuloplasty: 10% reoperation rate at 2 years.

Tricuspid Stenosis

ETIOLOGY

Rheumatic heart disease, congenital, carcinoid.

SIGNS AND SYMPTOMS

- Peripheral edema
- Jugular venous distention (JVD)
- Hepatomegaly, ascites, jaundice

DIAGNOSIS

- Murmur is diastolic, rumbling, low pitched.
- Murmur accentuated with inspiration.
- Accentuated precordial thrust of right ventricle.
- Diastolic thrill at lower left sternal border.
- Best heard over left sternal border between fourth and fifth interspace.
- Echocardiography demonstrates diseased valve and quantifies transvalvular gradient

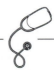

A rumbling diastolic murmur can be due to mitral stenosis or tricuspid stenosis. Tricuspid stenosis will increase with inspiration.

HIGH-YIELD FACTS

Cardiothoracic Surgery

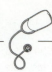

Heart block is a common complication in tricuspid valve replacement due to the close proximity of the conduction bundle to the tricuspid annulus.

Right-sided bacterial endocarditis is most frequently associated with nonsterile technique in IV drug abusers.

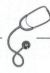

A holosystolic murmur can be due to mitral regurgitation, tricuspid regurgitation, or VSD.

TREATMENT

- Valve replacement for most cases
- Commissurotomy with annuloplasty used for commissural fusion

Tricuspid Regurgitation

ETIOLOGY

- Increased pulmonary artery pressure (e.g., from left-sided failure or mitral regurgitation/stenosis)
- Right ventricular dilation stretching the outflow tract (e.g., from right heart failure, infarction, or tricuspid regurgitation itself)
- Right papillary muscle rupture from infarction
- Tricuspid valvular lesions (e.g., from rheumatic heart disease or bacterial endocarditis)

SIGNS AND SYMPTOMS

Signs of right heart failure: Prominent JVD, pulsatile liver.

DIAGNOSIS

- Holosystolic, blowing, medium-pitched murmur heard best along the left sternal border in the fifth interspace, accentuated with inspiration.
- ECG shows right ventricular enlargement.
- Atrial fibrillation is common.
- Echocardiography demonstrates diseased valve.

TREATMENT

Medical
- Treat left heart failure if applicable.
- Diuresis to reduce volume load.

Surgical
- Seldom requires valve replacement; *annuloplasty* is preferred. *Total valve excision* is used in tricuspid endocarditis, sometimes with later valve replacement.

Types of Valve Prostheses

MECHANICAL PROSTHESES

- E.g., St. Jude
- Offer greater durability (15-year failure rate 5%), but need for lifelong anticoagulation (with associated risk of hemorrhagic complications)
- A better choice for the young

BIOPROSTHESES

- E.g., porcine or bovine xenografts.
- Fewer thromboembolic concerns (usually no need for anticoagulation) but less durable (15-year failure rate 50%).
- Better choice for the elderly.
- Calcification can complicate use in the young.

Types

- Small cell lung cancer:
  - Central location
  - Sensitive to chemotherapy
  - Surgery is not indicated.
  - Poor prognosis (2 to 4 months from diagnosis to death)
- Non–small cell lung cancer:
  - Includes squamous, large cell, and adenocarcinoma
  - Poor response to chemotherapy
  - Treated with surgery (debulking)
  - Prognosis varies with stage

EPIDEMIOLOGY

- Leading cause of cancer death in both men and women in the United States.
- Cases have been decreasing in men but increasing in women.
- Smoking is by far the most important causative factor in the development of lung cancer.

ETIOLOGY

- Smoking
- Passive smoke exposure
- Radon gas exposure
- Asbestos
- Arsenic
- Nickel

SIGNS AND SYMPTOMS

- Cough
- Hemoptysis
- Stridor
- Dyspnea
- Hoarseness (recurrent laryngeal nerve paralysis)
- Post-obstructive pneumonia
- Dysphagia
- Associated (paraneoplastic) syndromes (see Table 24-1)

DIAGNOSIS

See section on diagnostic evaluation of a lung mass below.

TREATMENT

The two main types of lung cancer, small cell and non–small cell cancer, have different responses to radiotherapy, chemotherapy, and surgery (see Table 24-2).

Diagnostic Evaluation of a Lung Mass

Plain Film
- Most malignant nodules seen by 0.8 to 1 cm in diameter (may be seen smaller) (see Figure 24-1).

Small cell lung cancer has a rapid mitotic rate, therefore is sensitive to chemotherapy. Surgery is not indicated.

Two types of cancer share a "s"entral location:
- Small cell
- Squamous cell

Bronchoalveolar cancer, a type of adenocarcinoma, is not linked to smoking, and is more common in women.

Chronic cough is the most common symptom of lung cancer.

HIGH-YIELD FACTS

Cardiothoracic Surgery

TABLE 24-1. Syndromes associated with lung cancer.

Horner syndrome	Sympathetic nerve paralysis produces enophthalmos, ptosis, miosis, ipsilateral anhidrosis.
Pancoast syndrome	Superior sulcus tumor injuring the eighth cervical nerve and the first and second thoracic nerves and ribs, causing shoulder pain radiating to arm.
Superior vena cava syndrome	Tumor causing obstruction of the superior vena cava and subsequent venous return, producing facial swelling, dyspnea, cough, headaches, epistaxis, syncope. Symptoms worsened with bending forward, and on awakening in the morning.
Syndrome of inappropriate antidiuretic hormone (SIADH)	Ectopic arginine vasopressin (AVP) release in the setting of plasma hyposmolality, producing hyponatremia without edema. Also caused by other lung diseases, central nervous system (CNS) trauma or infection, and certain medications.
Eaton–Lambert syndrome	Presynaptic nerve terminals attacked by antibodies, decreasing acetylcholine release, treated by plasmapheresis and immunosuppression. 40% associated with small cell lung cancer, 20% have other cancer, 40% have no cancer.
Trousseau syndrome	Venous thrombosis associated with metastatic cancer.

TABLE 24-2. Distinction between small and non–small cell lung cancer.

Characteristic	Small Cell Lung Cancer	Non–Small Cell Lung Cancer
Histology	Small dark nuclei Scant cytoplasm	Copious cytoplasm , pleomorphic nuclei
Ectopic peptide production	Gastrin, ACTH, AVP, calcitonin, ANF	PTH
Response to radiotherapy	80–90% will shrink	30–50% will shrink
Response to chemotherapy	Complete regression in 50%	Complete regression in 5%
Surgical resection	Not indicated	Stage I, II, IIIA
Included subtypes	Small cell only	Adenocarcinoma, squamous cell, large cell, bronchoalveolar
5-year survival rate—all stages	5%	11–83%

ACTH, adrenocorticotropic hormone; AVP, arginine vasopressin; ANF, atrial natriuretic factor; PTH, parathyroid hormone.

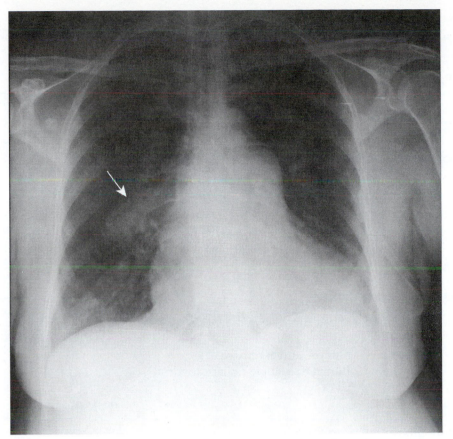

FIGURE 24-1. CXR demonstrating right middle lobe mass suspicious for malignancy.

- Comparison with previous films whenever possible.
- Those nodules stable for 2 years need no further evaluation.
- Those that are new in the last 2 months are unlikely to be malignant.
- Plain film may be the only imaging modality necessary if there is obvious bony metastasis or bulky, contralateral mediastinal adenopathy.
- Will more than likely need computed tomography (CT).

CT
- Provides better characterization and location of mass as well detecting mediastinal invasion
- Should be extended to include liver and adrenal glands as these are frequent sites of metastasis

Bronchoscopy
- Method of choice of centrally located masses (squamous cell and small cell).
- Specimens can be obtained via direct biopsy of visualized lesions, brushings, washings, or transbronchial needle aspiration (TBNA).
- The most important application of TBNA is staging of mediastinal lymph nodes.
- Risks of this procedure are respiratory arrest, pneumothorax, and bleeding.
- Although this method works well for centrally located lesions, it is poor when it comes to peripheral lung nodules.

Transthoracic Needle Biopsy (TNB)

- Method of choice for peripherally located nodules. Most are CT guided.
- Sensitivity: 70–100%

Thoracentesis

- Test of choice for patients with pleural effusion and suspected malignancy.

Solitary Pulmonary Nodule

- A single small (< 3 cm) intraparenchymal opacity that is reasonably well marginated
- Most will be benign.
- Benign: Granulomas, hamartomas, or intrapulmonary lymph nodes
- Malignant: Bronchogenic carcinoma

Small Cell Lung Cancer

- 70% metastatic at the time of diagnosis
- Generally considered inoperable for cure
- Two stages: Limited and extensive
- Limited: Confined to a single radiation portal
- Extensive: All others

Non–Small Cell Lung Cancer

- Need to determine resectability: Chest CT and search for distant metastases.
- Malignant pleural effusion precludes curative resection.
- Tumor, Nodes, Metastasis (TNM) Staging System

THORACIC AORTIC ANEURYSMS

DEFINITION

- **Aneurysm:** Ballooning defect in the vessel wall
- **Dissection:** Tear of the arterial intima

TYPES

- Degenerative:
  - Due to abnormal collagen metabolism
  - Seen with Marfan and Ehlers–Danlos syndromes
- Atherosclerotic:
  - Due to remodeling and dilatation of the aortic wall

ANATOMIC CLASSIFICATION

DeBakey Type I: Ascending and descending aorta
DeBakey Type II: Ascending aorta only
DeBakey Type III: Descending aorta only
Stanford A: Ascending aorta (same as DeBakey I/II)
Stanford B: Descending aorta (same as DeBakey III)

- Ascending aorta and aortic arch aneurysms are worse than descending aortic aneurysms.
- Expansion rate is ~0.56 cm/yr for arch aneurysms and ~0.42 cm/yr for descending aorta.

EPIDEMIOLOGY

- Six per 100,000 a year.
- Male-to-female ratio is 2:1.
- Familial clustering.
- Patients tend to be younger than those with abdominal aortic aneurysm (AAA).

SIGNS AND SYMPTOMS OF EXPANSION OR RUPTURE

- "Tearing" or "ripping" chest pain radiating to the back.
- Acute neurologic symptoms (syncope, coma, convulsions, hemiplegia).
- Palpable thrust may be seen in right second or third intercostal space.
- Pulsating sternoclavicular joint may be seen (secondary to swelling at the base of the aorta).
- Hoarseness.
- Stridor.
- Dysphagia.
- New aortic regurgitation murmur.
- Hemoptysis or hematemesis.
- Absent or diminished pulses.

DIAGNOSIS

CXR (Figure 24-2)
- Widened mediastinum
- Abnormal aortic contour
- "Calcium sign": Reflects separation of intimal calcification from the adventitial surface

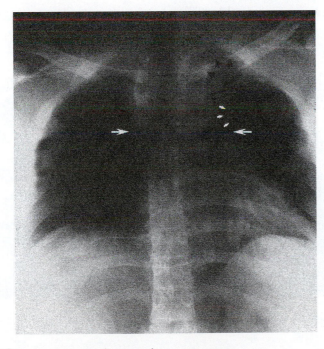

FIGURE 24-2. Thoracic aneurysm diagnosed on angiogram.

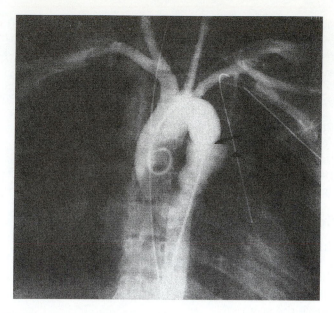

FIGURE 24-3. CXR demonstrating thoracic aneurysm.

Contrast CT (Figure 24-3)
- Two distinct lumens (true and false) separated by intimal flap
- Sensitivity 85–100%
- Specificity 100%

Magnetic Resonance Imaging (MRI)
- Excellent sensitivity and specificity
- Gives info about branch vessels that CT does not
- No need for contrast
- Limited to stable patients

Angiography (Figure 24-4)
- Requires contrast dye like CT
- Invasive

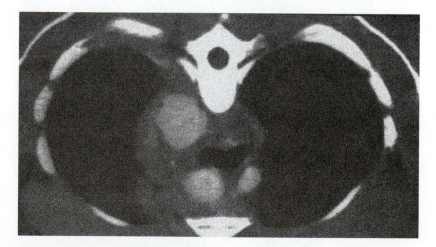

FIGURE 24-4. Thoracic aneurysm on CT.

Transesophageal Echocardiography (TEE)

- Presence of intimal flap separating the true from the false lumen
- Features of the false lumen: Larger in diameter, slower blood flow velocity
- Can be used in relatively unstable patients as well

Transthoracic Echocardiography (TTE)

- Available at bedside
- Noninvasive
- Suitable for unstable patients
- Requires operator expertise
- Moderate ability to detect ascending and arch dissections; poor for detecting descending arch dissection

TREATMENT AND PROGNOSIS

Medical

- Control hypertension with nitroprusside or labetalol.
- Parenteral analgesia.

Surgical

- For ruptured aneurysms, it is the only definitive therapy. Carries very high risk of mortality. Most patients die before reaching the operating room. Of those that reach the OR, less than 50% survive.
- Elective repair is considered for aneurysms > 7 cm or when aneurysm diameter is > 2.5× that of adjacent aorta. Mortality rate is 10–15%.
- For degenerative aneurysms, the entire aortic root must be replaced.
- Atherosclerotic aneurysms can be repaired either via open approach (median sternotomy approach for ascending arch and posterolateral thoracotomy for descending arch) or via endovascular technique.
- Ascending and descending arch aneurysms are repaired with patient under cardiopulmonary bypass, anticoagulation, and in mild-moderate hypothermia.
- Aortic arch aneurysms are repaired with patient in circulatory arrest and profound hypothermia.

COMPLICATIONS

- Hemorrhage
- Paraplegia
- Stroke
- MI
- Visceral ischemia

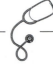

Major complication of any thoracic aneurysm repair is paraplegia. Key is to avoid perioperative hypotension.

THORACOABDOMINAL ANEURYSMS

CLASSIFICATION

Crawford classification:
- Type I: Most of descending thoracic aorta and abdominal aorta proximal to renal arteries
- Type II: Most of descending thoracic aorta and abdominal aorta distal to renal arteries

- Type III: Distal one-half of descending thoracic aorta and abdominal aorta proximal to renal arteries
- Type IV: Distal one-half of descending thoracic aorta and abdominal aorta distal to renal arteries

DIAGNOSIS

Made incidentally (routine physical exam or imaging for other reasons) or on postmortem exam (for ruptured ones).

TREATMENT

- Elective repair undertaken after weighing risk vs. benefit.
- Open surgical approach is used:
  - Type I: Thoracic incision
  - Types II and III: Incision from sixth intercostal space into abdomen
  - Type IV: Retroperitoneal incision from left flank to umbilicus

PROGNOSIS

Overall mortality < 10%.

COMPLICATIONS

Same as for thoracic aneurysm repair.

Vascular Surgery

Layers of Arterial Wall

- **Intima:** One layer of endothelial cells overlying a matrix of collagen and elastin
- **Media:** Thick layer of smooth muscle cells, collagen, and elastic fibers
- **Adventitia:** Collagen and elastin, important component to wall strength

Types of Arteries

- **Elastic:** Major vessels, including aorta, subclavian, carotid, pulmonary arteries
- **Muscular:** Branches from elastic arteries: Radial, femoral, coronary, cerebral
- **Arterioles:** Terminal branches to capillary beds

Venous Anatomy

- Also three layers, but adventitia is most prominent, and intima and media are generally thin.
- Valves prevent reflux.

Veins farther away from the heart have a greater number of valves.

VASCULAR PHYSICAL EXAM

Inspection

Signs of vascular insufficiency:
- Hairless, shiny skin
- Change of skin color—darkening, mottling, reddening, blanching
- Nail changes
- Presence of ulcers or gangrene

Auscultation

Auscultation for bruits: Carotid, abdomen, common femoral artery (CFA).

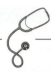

"Scoring" of pulses:
0 = no palpable pulse
1+ = present, but barely palpable
2+ = normal
3+ = normal, strong
4+ = hyperdynamic, abnormally strong

If you are not sure whether pulse is palpable, count out pulses with second person palpating an easier artery such as the radial artery. If pulsations are simultaneous, you are likely palpating pulse accurately.

Contrast contains iodine and is renally excreted. Therefore, you should use < 200 cc of dye, and use with caution in patients with renal dysfunction. Ask patients about iodine and shellfish allergies.

Palpation of Pulsatile Masses

- Pulsations of normal aorta are palpable in thin people.
- Examine abdomen with both hands around epigastrium and periumbilical area for AAA.
- Easily palpable pulses in either lower quadrant indicate distal aortic or common iliac aneurysm.

Palpation of Extremity Pulses

- Including: Brachial, radial, ulnar, femoral, popliteal, DP, posterior tibial.
- Patient should be reclining in supine position, with full exposure of abdomen and legs.
- Legs should be in gentle extension with feet supported.
- To examine pedal pulses, sit at foot of table facing patient.
- Common femoral artery: Found halfway from pubic tubercle to anterior superior iliac spine; look for pulse along course of external iliac artery toward inguinal ligament.
- Popliteal artery: Place both hands in the middle of the fossa, with fingertips parallel longways (fossa: area between pes anserinus tendon laterally medial head of gastrocnemius and biceps tendon medially, and biceps and lateral head of gastrocnemius laterally)
- Pedal pulses:
  - DP found between proximal first and second metatarsal (slight dorsiflexion may facilitate)
  - Posterior tibial found posterior to medial malleolus

DIAGNOSTIC TESTS

Doppler

Relates average flow velocity to frequency shift.

Duplex

Combines real-time ultrasound with Doppler analysis.

Plethysmography

Measures volume change in organ or body region:
- Pulse volume recording (PVR): Used with Doppler to assess perfusion of distal extremities, assuming change in volume corresponds to change in arterial pressure; useful to predict healing of ulcers and amputations
- Other types of plethysmography (seldom used):
  - Ocular plethysmography: Records change in eye volume caused by pulsatile flow of ophthalmic artery (representing carotid disease)
  - Impedance plethysmography: Measures volume changes in limb by changes in resistance (based on Ohm's law: voltage = current × resistance); excellent for identifying deep vein obstruction but does not allow diagnosis of specific cause
  - Photoplethysmography: Assesses venous congestion by measuring intensity of reflected light

Segmental Blood Pressure Measurement

- **Ankle–brachial index:**
  - ≥ 1: Normal
  - 0.5–0.7: Claudication
  - ≤ 0.3: Ischemic rest pain, gangrene
- **Penile–brachial index (PBI):** Used to help determine whether cause of impotence is vascular
  - PBI < 0.6 indicates likely vascular etiology.
- Misleading results associated with:
  - Diabetic patients, as calcification of vessels makes them less compressible, thereby elevating results falsely.
  - Collateral flow in long-standing insufficiency may artificially improve results.

A pseudoaneurysm does not contain all three layers of the arterial wall.

Arteriography

- Use of contrast dye with fluoroscopy to delineate arteries
- Risks: Hemorrhage, allergic reaction to dye, thrombosis of puncture site, embolization of clot, renal dysfunction
- Dose-independent reactions to dye: Asthma, laryngeal edema, spasm, cardiovascular (CV) collapse
- Complications:
  - Neurologic deficits secondary to emboli
  - Bleeding: Hematoma, hemorrhage at site
  - Decreased pulses compared to pre-angio: If resolves within 1 hour, may be due to spasm; otherwise, consider arterial injury, clot
- Post-procedure:
  - Maintain patient supine for at least 6 hours.
  - Check puncture site for hematoma or false aneurysm.
  - Follow neurologic exam, including mental status.
  - Maintain well-hydrated state.

Typical scenario: You are asked to see a patient with bleeding from an angiogram puncture site. She has an oozing, pulsatile expanding mass in her groin at the puncture site. *Think:* Expanding hematoma. Maintain direct pressure for 30 minutes. If bleeding continues, wound exploration may be indicated.

Digital Subtraction Angiography (DSA)

Dye is injected into vein or artery, and computerized fluoroscopy subtracts bone and soft tissue, so all that is visible is arterial system.

Spiral Computed Tomography (CT)

Especially useful for AAA.

Magnetic Resonance Angiography (MRA)

- Allows good visualization of patent distal vessels with minimal flow; also useful for evaluation of carotid bifurcation and abdominal aorta.
- Advantage: No contrast used.
- Gadolinium causes allergic reactions in fewer patients.

Arterial occlusion progresses to irreversible ischemia in 6 to 8 hours, depending on collateral circulation.

Given Poiseuille's law, in which the formula includes radius to the fourth power, note that radius is the most important determinant of flow.

The **six Ps** of acute arterial insufficiency:
Pain
Pulselessness
Pallor
Paresthesia
Paralysis
Poikilothermia

Typical scenario: You are asked to localize a lesion on a patient. You can palpate a femoral pulse but no popliteal or pedal pulses on the right side. Left-sided pulses are present. *Think:* Localize lesion to the vessel above site where pulse is first lost. The lesion is likely to be in the superficial femoral artery (SFA). Tissue ischemia will extend one joint level distal to segment of artery occluded.

PHYSIOLOGY OF ARTERIAL OBSTRUCTION

- Bernoulli's principle: In an ideal fluid system, energy lost as fluid moves through system is lost mainly as heat.
- Poiseuille's law: Flow = radius^4 × change in energy between 2 points/8 × distance between 2 points × viscosity.
- Critical stenosis: Narrowing that is enough to decrease pressure and flow significantly (when cross-sectional area is decreased by at least 75%).
- Autoregulation: Vascular muscle responds to chemical environment to attempt to maintain flow despite perfusion pressure.
- Exercise: Causes dilation of intramuscular arterioles, decreased resistance, increased flow.

SIGNS AND SYMPTOMS OF ACUTE ARTERIAL INSUFFICIENCY

- Paresthesia and paralysis are most important signs because nerves are most sensitive to ischemia. Secondarily, there will be loss of muscle function.
- Pain may not exist in diabetics with neuropathy or if rapidly progressive ischemia occurs with anesthesia.
- Earliest sign in lower extremity will be along distribution of peroneal nerve, with hypesthesia, no great toe dorsiflexion, foot drop.
- Progression in muscle damage: Muscles soft, then doughy, then stiff/hard.
- Once skin is mottled and no longer blanches, tissue ischemia is irreversible. Color change indicates extravasation of blood from capillaries into dermis.

ETIOLOGY

- Embolization: From heart or any proximal artery
- Trauma: Posterior knee dislocation, long-bone fracture, penetrating trauma
- Iatrogenic (catheter related)
- Thrombosis: Atherosclerosis, aneurysm

DIFFERENTIAL DIAGNOSIS

- Nerve root compression
- Deep venous thrombosis (DVT)
- Phlegmasia cerulea dolens
- Infection

DIAGNOSIS

- If diagnosis is certain (i.e., cold, newly pulseless, painful extremity), no further workup is required. Patient should be promptly taken to OR.
- Typically, ankle–brachial index (ABI) and/or angiography are performed to confirm the site of the lesion. Currently, on-table angiography is an option in some centers.

EMBOLISM

- Must find source of embolism, reason.
- Too large diameter artery: Usually of cardiac origin, to common femoral artery (CFA).
- Patient may have chronic atrial fibrillation, or history of MI or valvular disease (mitral stenosis, with valvular vegetation or mural thrombus).
- Atheroembolism: From aorta, iliac, or femoral vessels to distal vessels.
- "Blue toe" syndrome.
- Likely to have palpable pedal pulses anyway because at least one of proximal vessels is likely still patent.
- Suspect atheroembolism in patients with no history of peripheral vascular disease (PVD), with digital ischemia and palpable pulses.
- Treatment:
  - See below.
  - Address primary problem (i.e., atrial fibrillation).

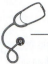

Sites commonly affected by embolism:
- **Lower extremity: 70% (CFA 34%, popliteal 14%)**
- **Upper extremity: 13%**
- **Cerebral circulation: 10%**
- **Visceral circulation: 5–10%**
- **Aorta: 9%**
- **Common iliac artery: 14%**

THROMBOSIS

- Usually underlying stenosis from atherosclerosis.
- May occur in hypercoagulable states, especially with repeated mild trauma.
- Effects of thrombus vary greatly from no symptoms to severe ischemia depending on extent of collateral circulation.
- All patients should have an angiogram unless ischemia is severe and rapidly progressive.
- Cause suggested by history of PVD, popliteal or aortic aneurysm.
- On exam, patient may have evidence of PVD such as skin changes or lack of distal pulses on contralateral side.

TREATMENT

- Thrombectomy or grafting (most common)
- Thrombolytic therapy
  - Success rate: 60–80%.
  - Mechanism: Activation of plasmin system causes fibrinolysis and clot dissolution.
  - Agents:
    - Streptokinase: Bacterial origin (antigenic), binds plasminogen to make plasmin, not often used
    - Urokinase: From renal parenchyma, directly activates plasminogen, not currently available in the United States
    - tPA: From vascular endothelium, directly activates plasminogen
    - Reteplase: Recombinant tPA, catalyzes cleavage of endogenous plasminogen to form plasmin
  - Indications: Acute occlusion of native vessel or graft
  - Contraindications: History of gastrointestinal (GI) or intracerebral lesion, pregnancy, any contraindication to angiography
  - Method: Catheter placed proximally, diagnostic angiogram performed, catheter advanced into clot, thrombolytic agent administered

Any patient with peripheral vascular disease is likely to have cardiac disease as well and will require appropriate preoperative or preprocedure medical stabilization and/or optimization.

COMPLICATIONS

- Intracerebral bleed, catheter site bleed (both infrequent).
- Patient may ultimately require operation to fix underlying problem.

Thrombolytic therapy for acute thrombotic occlusion is not done if severe ischemia is present, as it takes time to dissolve clot.

If chronic ischemia occurs at locations other than infrarenal aorta, iliacs, or SFA, the patient is likely to have a comorbid disease such as diabetes (increased risk at profunda femoris and tibial vessels) or an inflammatory disorder (increased risk at axillary arteries).

Presentation

- Claudication
- Rest pain
- Gangrene
- Most commonly affects infrarenal aorta, iliac arteries, SFA at adductor canal

Risk Factors

- Systolic hypertension (HTN)
- Cigarette smoking
- Hyperlipidemia
- Diabetes

Aortoiliac Disease

TYPES

- Localized disease of aorta and common iliac disease (10%)
- Localized disease of external iliac artery (25%)
- Multisegmental disease, including infrainguinal (65%)

DIFFERENTIAL DIAGNOSIS

Nerve root compression (lumbosacral) secondary to disc herniation or spinal stenosis.

DIAGNOSTIC TESTS

- Femoral–brachial pressure ratio
- Penile–brachial index
- Angiogram
  - Axillobifemoral has better patency rates and is often used for unilateral disease
  - Indicated when patient is extremely high risk for medical complications following intra-abdominal surgery or if graft from prior operation is infected

Leriche syndrome is indicative of aortoiliac disease and presents with claudication, impotence, and decreased (or absent) femoral pulses.

TREATMENT

- Aortofemoral bypass:
  - 5-year patency 90%, 10-year patency 75%
  - Better patency rates than aortoiliac bypass
- Aortoiliac endarterectomy: Acceptable for localized atherosclerotic disease when distal vessel is normal
- Extra-anatomic bypass:
  - Best option: Femoral–femoral bypass (5-year patency 50–75%)
  - Other options: Axillofemoral, axillobifemoral—used in high-risk patients for intra-abdominal surgery (elderly, hostile abdomen, abdominal infection)
- Percutaneous transluminal angioplasty (PTA): Indicated for short, nonoccluding lesions with less extensive atherosclerosis
  - Five-year patency rate is 90% with secondary interventions.

COMPLICATIONS

- Hemorrhage
- Thrombosis of reconstruction
- Distal embolization
- Ischemic colitis
- Paraplegia from lumbar vessel ischemia
- Sexual dysfunction (if operation involved abdominal aorta)

Infrainguinal Disease

- Most commonly affects SFA at adductor canal
- Patients have decreased life expectancy regardless of treatment and outcome
- Ulcers:
  - Arterial insufficiency: Lateral ankle and foot, pale, no granulation tissue
  - Venous insufficiency: Medial malleolus, pink, granulation tissue, other stigmata of venous disease

DIAGNOSTIC TESTS

- Doppler
- ABI
- PVRs
- Angiogram

Patients presenting with rest pain, ulcers, or gangrene most likely have multisegmental disease.

MANAGEMENT

- Nonoperative:
  - Smoking cessation, increase exercise tolerance, medication.
  - Pentoxifylline: Decreases viscosity, increases flow; unpredictable relief of symptoms but proven to increase microvascular flow.
  - Cilostazol: Type III phosphodiesterase inhibitor, reduces platelet aggregation and increases vasodilation. Can be more effective than pentoxifylline.
- Operative:
  - Revascularization requires adequate inflow, outflow, and conduit.
  - Bypass (femoral–popliteal): Uses PTFE or saphenous vein, reversed or in situ—RSVG best patency
  - Endarterectomy: Limited to short lesions of SFA at adductor canal or origin of profunda

ABI is likely to be artificially elevated in a diabetic patient because the vessels are generally less compressible than normal. PVRs are more useful because results are not affected by compressibility of vessels.

Upper Extremity Disease

- Compared to lower extremity, more often due to vasospasm or arteritis
- Palpate pulses: Axillary, radial, ulnar, brachial
- Subclavian steal syndrome
  - Nonhemispheric cerebrovascular symptoms with mild arm claudication due to decreased flow to posterior cerebral artery (PCA) when blood flows retrograde through vertebral artery to SCA.
  - If patient has neurologic symptoms, then carotid stenosis is present as well.
  - Cause is proximal SCA lesion.
  - Angiogram shows flow reversal in vertebral artery.

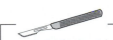

In situ bypass requires cutting of the valves so that blood flows from proximal to distal.

- Operate for:
  - Incapacitating claudication
  - Emboli to hand or to posterior cerebral circulation
  - Symptoms of subclavian steal (if also carotid symptoms, fix carotid first)

AMPUTATIONS

Indications

- Nonviable extremity that has become infected
- Irreparable vascular injury with irreversible ischemia (traumatic or atraumatic)
- Cancer
- Elderly patient with infection who is not a candidate for surgical revascularization

Types of Amputations

- **Toe:** For gangrene, or osteomyelitis distal to proximal interphalangeal joint (PIP) without proximal cellulitis, necrosis, or edema.
- **Transmetatarsal:** For necrosis between level of transmetatarsal incision and PIP, often interdigital crease necrosis.
- **Syme:** Amputation at base of tibia and fibula. For terminal arterial disease of distal foot—not done very often, requires palpable posterior tibialis pulse.
- **Below-knee amputation (BKA)** (most common level for nonviable foot): For ischemia up to malleoli.
  - Likely to adapt well to prosthesis
  - Contraindicated if gangrene more proximal than ankle, or if patient has hip or knee contractures
  - Likely to fail when there is no femoral pulse
- **Above-knee amputation (AKA):** For gangrene above BK level, for contractures at knee or hip, and for elderly nonambulatory patients.
  - Best chance of healing, particularly in PVD patients
- **Hip disarticulation:** For extensive lower extremity ischemia, proximal gangrene, tumor, extensive trauma.
  - Poor outcome when performed for PVD
- **Upper extremity amputations:** More commonly performed for trauma or tumor.
  - Digital, forearm, upper arm.
  - Leave as much as possible, unless for tumor.

Basic Principles

1. Patient should be medically stabilized first when possible.
2. Selecting level of amputation for PVD:
   - Use PVRs and ABI to help predict chance of healing.
   - At proposed level, infection is controlled, skin looks good, without proximal dependent rubor, proximal pain, and with a venous filling time < 20 seconds.
   - If for cancer, wide excision necessary.

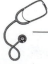

If patient has popliteal pulse, BKA has 90–97% success rate. Without palpable popliteal pulse, success rate is about 82%.

- If s/p trauma or for PVD, remaining tissue level must be acceptably healthy.
    - Consider length of stump re ease of fitting/using prosthesis
    - Consider overall condition of patient
3. Determination of closure:
    - Standard: Flaps constructed to close over bone.
    - Guillotine (in situation of sepsis): Level is lower than that eventually desired. Stump left open for dressing changes until sepsis is resolved, at which time completion amputation is performed.
4. Postoperative care:
    - Dressing left in place for at least 1 week unless patient becomes febrile or has profuse bleeding through dressing
    - Rehabilitation

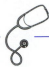

Longer stump is more functional. When patient is nonambulatory, AKA may be more appropriate given its higher primary healing rate and lower rate of contracture compared to BKA.

CHRONIC VENOUS DISEASE: OBSTRUCTION AND INCOMPETENCE

Basics

- Postphlebitic syndrome: After DVT, many patients (50%) get chronic venous insufficiency due to valvular incompetence of recanalized veins.
- Up to 50% of patients with signs and symptoms of venous insufficiency have no documented history of DVT.
- Presentation:
    - Pain and swelling in affected leg.
    - Findings on exam include induration, swelling, skin darkening, and possibly ulcers.

Treatment Goals

- Alleviate symptoms.
- Heal any ulcers that exist.
- Prevent development of new ulcers.

When the patient is compliant and therapy is properly done, 85% of ulcers heal, but may recur.

Nonoperative Treatment

- Compression stockings
- Leg elevation
- Ulcer treatment: Bed rest, antibiotics when cellulitis present, thromboembolism deterrents (TEDs), Unna's boots, Profore dressings
- Generalized skin care, with antifungal creams when appropriate, moisturizer for eczema

Operative Therapy

- Indications: Severe symptoms, failure of conservative measurements, recurrent ulcers
- Options:
    - **Ligation** of responsible perforators (usually around medial malleolus)
    - **Valvuloplasty** (leads to symptomatic improvement in 60–80%)
    - **Venous reconstruction** with grafting (not popular)

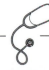

Unna's boots: Similar to a cast, this is a wrap soaked usually in Calamine lotion and applied to the leg; it lasts until the patient takes a shower.

Definition

An irreversible dilatation of an artery to at least 1.5 times its normal caliber.
- True aneurysm: Involves all layers of arterial wall
- False aneurysm: Involves only a portion of wall, or involves surrounding tissue

Varieties of Aneurysm

- **Degenerative**—due to atherosclerosis, the most common type of aneurysm:
  - Intima replaced by fibrin
  - Media fragmented with decreased elasticity
  - Imbalance in elastin metabolism, between elastase and alpha-1-antithrombin.
- **Traumatic**—due to iatrogenic, catheter-related injury, or to penetrating trauma:
  - Results in focal defect in wall, hemorrhage controlled by surrounding tissue
  - Formation of fibrous capsule
- **Poststenotic**—from Bernoulli's principle, occurs distal to cervical rib in thoracic outlet syndrome, distal to coarctation of aorta, or to aortic or pulmonary valvular stenosis
- **Dissecting**—blood travels through an intimal defect, creating a false passageway between the intima and the inner two thirds of the media:
  - If ruptures externally, patient exsanguinates
  - Risk factors: HTN, Marfan syndrome, Ehlers–Danlos, cystic medial necrosis, blunt trauma, cannulation during CP bypass
- **Mycotic**—infected
- **Anastomotic**—separation between graft and native artery, with formation of sac and fibrous capsule, often in CFA s/p aortofemoral bypass:
  - Painless, pulsatile, groin mass.
  - Diagnose with duplex for peripheral aneurysms, and CT for abdominal aneurysms, or angiogram.

Abdominal Aortic Aneurysm (AAA)

- Fusiform dilatation of abdominal aorta more than 1.5 times its normal diameter
- Incidence: 2% of elderly population (9 times more common in males than females)
- Relative risk of AAA: 11.6% in patients with first-degree relative with known AAA (ultrasound screening recommended)
- 75% asymptomatic at diagnosis
- Risk factors for rupture: Diastolic hypertension, initially large size at diagnosis, chronic obstructive pulmonary disease (COPD)

INDICATIONS FOR REPAIR

- Size at which the risk of rupture exceeds the risk of mortality from the operation (generally about 2–5%).
- Increasing size.

AAA risk of rupture in 5 years:
< 4 cm: 9.5%
4 to 7 cm: 25%

Size at which AAA is considered for surgical repair: 5 cm

- Consider factors that increase risk of rupture (diastolic hypertension, COPD).
- Pain over AAA site.

DIAGNOSIS

- Exam: Periumbilical palpable pulsatile mass
- CT: Provides information about character, wall thickness, location with respect to renal arteries, presence of leak or rupture
- Magnetic resonance imaging (MRI): Provides more details than CT or ultrasound about the lumen, surface anatomy, neck, relationship to renal arteries
- Ultrasound: Used more frequently to follow aneurysm size over time than to assess in acute phase (see Figure 25-1)
- Angiogram: Defines vascular anatomy and is especially important in cases of mesenteric ischemia, HTN, renal dysfunction, horseshoe kidney, claudication

PREOPERATIVE ASSESSMENT

Includes assessment of carotid disease and cardiac, pulmonary, renal, and hepatic systems.

Cardiac Workup and Optimization
- No history of CAD: 1–3% chance of MI, pulmonary edema, or cardiac death perioperatively
- Known CAD, risks increase to 5–10%
- Steps to minimize risk:
    - No cardiac history, normal electrocardiogram (ECG): No further workup
    - Known but stable CAD: Echocardiogram/dipyridimole or thallium
        - If abnormal, consider preoperative revascularization.
    - Clinically severe CAD: Definite need for revascularization
        - If percutaneous, may proceed immediately with AAA repair.
- If coronary artery bypass graft (CABG), wait 4 to 6 weeks.

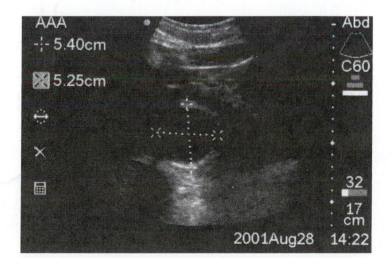

FIGURE 25-1. AAA on ultrasonography. Aortic diameter is 5.40 cm.

Graft is placed within the lumen of the aorta, and the vessels walls are closed around it. The aneurysm is not resected.

- Mortality for ruptured AAA is 90%.
- Of those who reach the hospital alive, mortality is still 50%.
- Mortality is further increased in patients with history of CAD, hypotension on arrival, and renal insufficiency, and is also increased by inexperienced surgical team.

Typical scenario: You are called to the emergency department to see a 65-year-old male with a history of AAA, for which he is followed by the vascular service. He now complains of abdominal pain and reports syncope at home. *Think:* Syncope and abdominal pain or hypotension in a patient with known AAA is presumed to be rupture unless proven otherwise. Notify the OR and mobilize your team.

OPERATIVE PLAN (ELECTIVE)

Open Repair

- Approach: Transperitoneal or retroperitoneal
- Retroperitoneal approach: Avoids formation of intra-abdominal adhesions, does not interfere with any GI or genitourinary (GU) stoma that may exist, is better tolerated in COPD patients, and provides better suprarenal exposure

Endovascular Repair

- Endovascular system consists of the graft, stents, and a delivery mechanism.
- Problems include immediate thrombosis and leakage at anatomic sites.
- Should be considered in patients who are elderly and/or have high operative risk due to a multitude of medical comorbidities.

EMERGENT REPAIR OF RUPTURED AAA

- Higher-risk operation
- Signs and symptoms: Abdominal pain, severe back or flank pain, cardiovascular collapse
- Differential diagnosis: Perforated peptic ulcer, renal or biliary colic, ruptured intervertebral disc
- Treatment:
  - In an unstable patient with known AAA: Proceed to OR immediately—"mobilize the team."
  - In a stable patient, without history of AAA: CT first, then OR as needed.
- OR:
  1. Team scrubs and preps/drapes.
  2. Only then is anesthesia induced, as surgeon has knife in hand. (Anesthesia causes vasodilatation, which may worsen hypotension.)
  3. Right angle retractor used to compress supraceliac aorta against vertebrae so patient can be resuscitated by anesthesia.
  4. Retractor replaced with supraceliac clamp.
  5. AAA repaired.

COMPLICATIONS OF AAA REPAIR

- Renal failure: 6% elective, 75% ruptured—ATN (ruptured) or atheroemboli (elective)
- Ischemic colitis (5%): Bloody diarrhea, elevated white blood count (WBC), peritonitis
- Spinal cord ischemia: Disruption of artery of Adamkiewicz

Other Aneurysms

ILIAC ARTERY

- 90% common iliac artery, 10% hypogastric artery.
- Hypogastric artery aneurysms may cause a pulsatile mass palpable on digital rectal examination.
- Resection indicated when > 3 cm, otherwise 6-month follow-up indicated.
- Common iliac artery (CIA) aneurysm is treated with interposition graft.

POPLITEAL ARTERY

- Most common peripheral aneurysm.
- 50–75% of cases, bilateral aneurysms.
- Untreated, 60% will lead to thrombosis or distal embolization, and 20% to amputation.
- Diagnosis established on exam, and using ultrasound and angiography.
- Operation indicated if no serious comorbidity: Excision and interposition graft with RSVG or ligation and bypass.

FEMORAL ARTERY

- Uncommon
- On exam, mass, local pain, venous obstruction, embolism, thrombosis
- Whether symptomatic or not, resection and graft indicated once larger than 2.5 cm

DIABETIC DISEASE

Location

- Usually spares aortoiliac vessels.
- Affects distal profunda femoris, popliteal, tibial, and digital arteries of the foot.
- Small vessels affected: Microangiopathy occurs with intimal and basement membrane thickening.
- Large vessels affected with atherosclerosis and calcification of media.

Problems

- Diabetic neuropathy: Causes motor and sensory deficits as well as high arch deformity in the foot that increases pressure on tarsal heads (atrophy of intrinsic muscles)
- Arteriopathy
- Infection: Likely to be worse—gram negatives, gram positives, and anaerobes all potential culprits, in particular *Peptococcus*, *Proteus*, *Bacteroides*

Treatment

Revascularization indicated when ulcers occur if there are significant vessels to use in repair. (See above information for further details that apply to diabetic and nondiabetic patients.)

VENOUS THROMBOTIC DISEASE

Anatomy

- Superficial: Greater and lesser saphenous veins
- Deep: Veins follow arteries and have same names (popliteal, SFV, DFV, CFV, external iliac vein [EIV])
- Perforators: Connect deep and superficial

In pregnant women, iliac artery aneurysms are associated with fibromuscular dysplasia.

External iliac artery is *never* involved when the cause is atherosclerosis.

One third of patients with unilateral popliteal artery aneurysms will have AAAs.

Patients with bilateral popliteal artery aneurysms have a 50% chance of concurrent AAA.

ABI in a diabetic patient may be falsely elevated secondary to vessel calcification.

The diabetic patient may be unaware of skin or other minor injuries. Classic site of infection: Over metatarsal heads on plantar aspect of foot.

Perforators adjacent to medial malleolus are responsible for stasis ulcers when they become incompetent.

The superficial femoral vein is actually a deep vein.

About one third of apparently healthy patients with DVTs of unknown cause will be diagnosed with a malignancy within 2 years.

Central line placement is responsible for one third of upper extremity DVTs.

Physiology

- Systemic veins contain two thirds of circulating volume.
- Further from heart, there are more valves.
- Venous return depends on respiration: Inspiration causes descent of diaphragm, increased intra-abdominal pressure, and decreased venous return.
- Venous return generated by the relationship among contraction of the heart, static filling pressure, and gravity.
- Virchow's triad: Stasis, blood abnormality, vessel endothelium injury (factors allowing thrombosis to occur).

Deep Venous Thrombosis

- Stasis leads to thrombin formation, which leads to platelet aggregation.
- Endothelial injury and/or a hypercoagulable state may contribute.
- Screening warranted for younger patients or those with repeated occurrences.
- Check PT, PTT, WBC, hematocrit (Hct), erythrocyte sedimentation rate (ESR), platelets.
- For extremely high-risk patients, also check homocysteine level, APL Ab, proteins C and S, AT III, APC-r, platelet aggregation, mutant factor V Leiden, prothrombin gene mutation (factor II).
- Also check CT scan of the chest, abdomen, and pelvis to look for malignancy if patient has no other risk factors for DVT.

Risk Factors

Acquired
- Central venous line placement
- Congestive heart failure (CHF) and MI (20–40%): Passive congestion and increased blood viscosity
- Joint replacement operation (15–30%): Femoral vein trauma, long OR, postop immobility
- Fractures of hip, pelvis, proximal femur (35–60%): Endothelial damage
- Laparoscopic surgery (7–10%): Intra-abdominal pressure > pressure of venous return from legs
- Prior DVT (5 times): Scarring, valvular damage, decreased muscle pumping, stasis
- Hormone replacement therapy (HRT) (2 to 6 times): Increases coagulation factors, and decreases protein S, antithrombin III (AT III), and fibrinolytic activity
- Other: Trauma patients, malignancy, obesity, pregnancy, sepsis, prolonged immobility

Congenital
- Antiphospholipid antibody syndrome (APS): Antibodies change normal endothelial function.
- AT III deficiency.
- Plasminogen deficiency: Decreased fibrinolysis.
- Dysfibrinogenemia: Fibrin resistance to plasmin proteolysis, abnormal fibrinogen, defective thrombin binding, increased blood viscosity.
- Factor V Leiden/activated protein C resistance (APC-r): Factor Va resistant to degradation by APC; hyperviscosity syndrome.
- Lupus anticoagulant: Exact mechanism unknown.

- Protein C and S deficiency: Factors V and VIII are not appropriately inactivated.
- Prothrombin gene mutation (factor II).

DIAGNOSIS

- Exam: Calf tenderness, swelling, Homan's sign (not very reliable)
- Duplex: Demonstrates thrombus, assesses compressibility of veins, analyzes venous flow

PROPHYLAXIS

- TEDs (compression stockings): Increase velocity of venous flow, reduce venous wall distention, and enhance valvular function
- Should apply 18 mm Hg
- Sequential compression devices: Reduce incidence of DVT by up to 75% when used properly
- Pharmacologic: SQ heparin, low-molecular-weight heparin

TREATMENT

- Bed rest until pain and swelling subside.
- Lower extremity elevation.
- Anticoagulation (period of 6 months for first DVT).
- Elastic stockings once ambulating.
- Consider fibinolytics for large thrombi.

LONG-TERM OUTCOME

Recurrent DVT: 18% at 2 years, 30% at 8 years.

POSTPHLEBITIC SYNDROME

- Occurs in 24%
- Risk of recurrent DVT then increased 6 times
- Symptoms: Edema, pain, aches, fatigue, skin discoloration, scarring, ulcers

SUPERFICIAL VENOUS THROMBOSIS (SVT)

- Usually a noninfected, localized inflammatory reaction.
- Signs and symptoms: Swelling, pain, erythema, tenderness.
- Diagnosis: Duplex ultrasonography to rule out associated DVT.
- Treat with nonsteroidal anti-inflammatory drugs (NSAIDs) as needed until symptoms resolve (about 2 to 3 weeks).
- Use elastic stockings.
- Consider anticoagulation for involvement of saphenofemoral junction.

VASCULAR TRAUMA

Clues to Vascular Injury in the Trauma Patient

- Pulsatile or expanding hematoma
- Pulsatile bleeding
- Bruit/thrill
- End-organ ischemia

HIGH-YIELD FACTS

Vascular Surgery

- Unexplained shock
- Likely location
- Injury to adjacent nerve
- Extremity fractures with weak or absent pulses

A Few Facts

- Carotid artery injury with hematoma can affect cranial nerves IX, X, XI, and XII.
- *All* zones in neck injury are likely to have vascular injury.
- Limb loss secondary to arterial injury associated with lower extremity fracture > 40%.
- Twenty percent of patients with penetrating abdominal trauma will have major vascular injury.

Transplant

DEFINITIONS

Autograft: Donor and recipient are same individual, or of same genetic makeup.
Allograft: Donor and recipient belong to same species but have different genetic makeup.
Xenograft: Donor and recipient are of different species.
Orthotopic: Transplant graft placed into its anatomic position
Heterotopic: Transplant graft placed at different site

DONORS

Donor Qualification

- Exclusions:
  - Age over 70 (flexible)
  - Active sepsis
  - History of cancer except for primary brain tumor or basal cell carcinoma
  - History of transmissible disease
- High risk donors (careful assessment required):
  - Sexually active gay men
  - History of IV, IM, or SQ recreational drug use within 5 years
  - History of hemophilia or any other clotting disorder requiring previous transfusion of human-derived clotting factors
  - Prostitution within 5 years
  - Solicitor of sex for money within 5 years, suspicion of HIV, exposure to HIV within 2 months, inmates of prison

In the United States, there are extensive organ donor networks to contact with questions regarding eligibility. They usually recommend allowing their trained staff to first approach family members to discuss the possibility of organ donation.

Adult Criteria

1. No cerebral function: Patient is in a deep coma, unresponsive to stimuli.
2. No brain stem function: No evidence on exam of cranial nerve function; lack of reflexes (papillary, corneal, cold water calorics, Doll's eyes, gag).
3. No spontaneous breathing: Apnea test.
   - Requirements: Normothermia, no central nervous system (CNS) depressants or neuromuscular blockers in effect
   - Suggestions: Electroencephalogram (EEG), though not legally required; 6-hour observation period prior to performing brain death examination

Pediatric Criteria

1. 7 days to 2 months: Two clinical exams, apnea tests, and EEGs at least 48 hours apart
2. 2 months to 1 year: As above, but 24 hours apart
3. Over 1 year: Two clinical exams and apnea tests 12 hours apart

Non–Heart-Beating Donors

Applies to patients with cardiac arrest near hospital, and to patients requesting removal of life support or in whom death is expected.

Donor Management

Goal: To optimize organ function
Issues:
1. Temperature: Maintain normothermia.
2. Hypoxia: Attempt to maintain $PaO_2 > 100$ on 40% FIO_2 with positive end-expiratory pressure (PEEP) 5.
3. Hypotension: Be generous with colloid and crystalloid to maintain central venous pressure (CVP) 5–10.
4. Low urine output: Assess hydration status; once assured that donor is well hydrated, give furosemide or mannitol; if in diabetes insipidus (DI), give desmopressin (DDAVP).
5. Frequent assessment via chemistries, complete blood count (CBC), arterial blood gas (ABG), chest x-ray (CXR), electrocardiogram (ECG).
6. If patient has been hospitalized over 3 days, start broad-spectrum antibiotics after sending blood and urine cultures.

If the patient does not qualify for organ donation, cornea, skin, bone, and heart valves may still be used.

Basics

Major histocompatibility complexes (MHCs) present antigens to T cells and are the major target of activated lymphocytes.

HIGH-YIELD FACTS

Transplant

MHC I
- Found on all nucleated cells
- Consists of heavy and light chains, and beta-2 microglobulin
- Encodes cell surface transplant antigens
- Primary target for CD8 T cells in graft rejection
- Gene loci: A, B, C

MHC II
- Found on hematopoietic cells
- Composed of alpha and beta chains
- Primary target for T-helper cells
- Gene loci: DR, DQ, DP

MHC III
- Encodes complement proteins
- Not addressed here

B cells are responsible for antibody-mediated hyperacute rejection when the transplant contains an antigen that the recipient B cells have seen before.

Tissue Typing
- Determination of MHC alleles in an individual to minimize differences in histocompatibility.
- Of above alleles, only A, B, and DR are used in tissue typing.
- Of these three genes, DR is most important to match, followed by B and then A, as evidenced by United Network for Organ Sharing (UNOS) data regarding graft survival.

Crossmatch
- Test for preformed cytotoxic antibody in serum of potential recipient.
- Donor lymphocytes are cultured with recipient serum in the presence of complement and dye.
- Lymphocyte destruction is evidenced by uptake of dye, indicating a positive crossmatch.
- A positive crossmatch is generally a contraindication to transplant as hyperacute rejection is likely.

Graft survival is improved with matching for kidney, pancreas, and heart transplants, but is not improved, and in fact, may be *worsened* for liver transplants. (Human leukocyte antigen [HLA] presents viral peptides to T cells and compatibility may potentiate the inflammatory phase of viral reinfection after transplant, thereby increasing chance of recurrence of original disease.)

IMMUNOSUPPRESSION

Steroids
- Most commonly, prednisone (PO) or methylprednisolone (IV)
- Used as maintenance therapy to prevent rejection and at higher doses to treat rejection
- Binds to intracellular receptor, is transported into nucleus where it is a DNA-binding protein that works to limit, ultimately, the inflammatory response by blocking NF-B, interleukin-1 (IL-1), tumor necrosis factor-alpha (TNF-α), interferon, and phospholipase A_2, as well as histamine and prostacyclin.
- Side effects: Impaired glucose tolerance, impaired wound healing, fluid retention, insomnia, depression, nervousness, psychosis

- Chronic effects: Cushing syndrome, increased risk for peptic ulcer disease, osteoporosis

CsA (Cyclosporine)

- Used as maintenance immunosuppression only.
- Calcineurin inhibitor: CsA binds to cyclophilin and, together, they bind to calcineurin–calmodulin complex, blocking calcium-dependent phosphorylation and activation of NF-AT, thereby preventing transcription of several genes needed for T-cell activation, including IL-2.
- P_{450} metabolism: Levels are increased by P_{450} inhibitors such as ketoconazole, erythromycin, calcium channel blockers, and decreased by P_{450} inducers like rifampin, phenobarbital, and dilantin.
- Side effects: Nephrotoxicity (dose related, based on vasoconstriction of proximal renal arterioles), hemolytic uremic syndrome (uncommon), hypertension, tremors, headache, paresthesia, depression, confusion, seizures (rare), hypertrichosis, gingival hyperplasia, hepatotoxicity

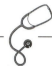

Azathioprine is not generally used in liver transplant because it is likely to cause hepatotoxicity.

MMF (Mycophenolate Mofetil)

- Cellcept
- Noncompetitive reversible inhibitor of inosine monophosphate dehydrogenase: Thereby halts purine metabolism, blocks proliferation of T and B cells, suppresses B-cell memory, and inhibits antibody formation
- Side effects: Mild diarrhea or nausea
- Maintenance therapy or treatment of rejection
- Very effective

Azathioprine

- Inhibits DNA synthesis by alkylating DNA precursors and depleting cell of adenosine
- Used for maintenance therapy only
- Side effects: Leukopenia, hepatotoxicity

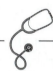

FK-506 and CsA have an additive immunosuppressive effect, but the toxicity may be too much.

FK-506 (Tacrolimus)

- Used for maintenance immunosuppression, and is drug of choice for liver transplant
- Calcineurin inhibitor: Works in similar fashion to CsA, but binds initially to FK-binding protein
- 100 times more potent than CsA
- Side effects as for CsA, though more neurotoxic and diabetogenic, and fewer cosmetic effects

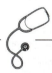

Some studies have found up to 40% incidence of post-transplant lymphoproliferative disorder with tacrolimus, and therefore, this drug is used with extreme caution in children.

ATG (Antithymocyte Globulin)

- Usually used for treatment of steroid-resistant rejection, but may also be used for induction therapy.
- Polyclonal antihuman gamma globulin extracted from horse sera of horses immunized with thymus lymphocytes.

- Side effects include fever and chills (20%), thrombocytopenia, leukocytopenia, rash (15%).
- Cautions: Must be given through central line or dialysis catheter; required monitoring of white blood count (WBC) during treatment; inquire about horse serum allergy.

OKT3

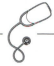

- Monoclonal antibody to CD3, a signal transducer on human T cells, thereby prevents transduction of antigen binding; also downregulates T-cell receptor
- Used as rescue agent for steroid-resistant rejection and also for induction
- Side effects: Hypotension, pulmonary edema, cardiac depression

Patients who are to receive OKT3 must be pre-treated with steroids.

Rapamycin (New/Use Not Yet Standard)

- Similar to tacrolimus.
- Interacts with FK-binding protein but inhibits binding to calcineurin complex. It then impairs IL-2 receptor signal transduction by interacting with and inhibiting one of the kinases in the cascade. End result is prevention of T cells from entering S-phase.
- May be synergistic with cyclosporine and steroids.
- Side effects: Hypertriglyceridemia.

Risk of Malignancy

- Overall incidence in kidney transplant recipients: 6%—lymphoma, skin cancer, genital neoplasms
- PTLD (post-transplant lymphoproliferative disease): Caused by Epstein–Barr virus (EBV), leads ultimately to monoclonal B-cell lymphoma/treatment to lower or stop immunosuppression and restore immunity

REJECTION

Hyperacute

- Cause: Presensitization of recipient to donor antigen.
- Timing: Immediately following graft reperfusion.
- Mechanism: Antibody binds to donor tissue, initiating complement-mediated lysis, which has a procoagulant effect. End result is thrombosis of graft.
- Prevention: ABO typing and negative crossmatch prevent hyperacute rejection in > 99% of patients.
- Variant: Delayed vascular rejection.
  - Mediated by humoral immunity
  - Occurs when preformed antibodies at levels too low to be detected by usual assays
  - Deterioration of graft function, postoperative day (POD) 3
- Treatment: None.
- Outcome: Graft failure/loss.

Presensitization of the recipient to a donor antigen can result from prior pregnancy, transfusion, or transplant.

Forty to 50% of kidney transplant recipients and 70–80% of pancreas transplant recipients will have at least one episode of acute rejection.

Typical scenario: A kidney transplant recipient is seen in the ER for nausea and abdominal pain, fever, and elevated creatinine. *Think:* Acute rejection. Diagnosis may be confirmed by ultrasound-guided biopsy. Pulse steroid treatment is indicated.

Treatment of acute rejection of a kidney transplant (with pulse steroids or OKT3 for SRR) is effective in 90% of cases.

Warm ischemia time should be minimized because it leads to rapid decline in adenosine triphosphate (ATP) and therefore decrease in biosynthetic reactions, a redistribution of electrolytes across cell membranes, and continuation of biodegradation reactions leading to acidosis and ultimately loss of organ viability.

Acute

- Cause: Normal T-cell activity (would ultimately affect every allograft were it not for immunosuppression).
- Timing: Between POD 5 and postoperative month 6.
- Mechanism: T cells bind antigens in one of two ways—directly through T-cell receptor (TCR) or after phagocytosis and presentation of donor tissue, resulting in T-cell infiltration of graft with organ destruction.
- Diagnosis: Generally by decreased graft function and by biopsy.
- Histology: Lymphocytic infiltrate and/or graft necrosis. Liver rejection also characterized by eosinophilic infiltrate.
- Prevention: Minimize mismatch of MHC; usual immunosuppression; monitor for organ dysfunction as signs of rejection that may otherwise be asymptomatic.
- Treatment: Kidney—high-dose steroids; OKT3 or antithymocyte globulin (ATG) when steroid-resistant rejection (SRR) after 2 days.
- Outcome: Ninety to 95% of transplants are salvaged with treatment.

Chronic

- Cause: Cumulative effect of recognition of MHC by recipient immune system
- Timing: Insidious onset over months and years
- Mechanism: Recipient's immune system recognizes donor MHC; other factors not yet understood
- Diagnosis: Biopsy
- Histology: Parenchymal replacement with fibrous tissue, some lymphocytic infiltrate, endothelial destruction
- Prevention: None known
- Treatment: None
- Outcome: Graft failure/loss

ORGAN PRESERVATION

Optimum and Maximum Times for Each Organ

- Heart and lungs: 4 to 6 hours; preferred within 5 hours
- Pancreas: Up to 30 hours, preferred by 10 to 20 hours
- Liver: 24 hours, preferred 6 to 12 hours
- Kidney: 48 hours

Principles

- Maintenance of donor's hemodynamic state.
- Minimize warm ischemia time.
- Hypothermia: Rapid cooling of organ, in situ or on table, and maintenance around 4°C (slows metabolism).
- Organ preservation solution: Flush blood out of organ at pressure of 60 to 100 cm H_2O, and of appropriate volume:
  - Liver: 2 to 3 L
  - Kidney: 200 to 500 mL
  - Pancreas: 200 to 500 mL

- Appropriate solution contains impermeable molecules to suppress cell swelling induced by hypothermia, and is an appropriate biochemical environment.

Alternative: Perfusion

- **Continuous perfusion:** Perfusion fluid, similar in nature to cold storage solution, is pumped continuously through organ, delivering oxygen and substrates, thereby allowing the continuation of metabolism, including synthetic reactions.
- **Pulsatile perfusion:** Allows the pharmacologic manipulation of the perfusate during storage and a pretransplant assessment of the donor kidney.
- Has been found to improve graft function at 1 and 2 years (Polyak et al., 2000)

KIDNEY TRANSPLANTATION

Background

- Most common solid organ transplanted
- 30,000 patients awaiting kidneys on UNOS list
- 4,000 to 5,000 donors per year

Causes of End-Stage Renal Disease (ESRD)

Adults
1. Diabetes
2. Hypertension
3. Glomerular nephritis
4. Congenital anomalies
5. Urologic abnormalities
6. Dysplasia
7. Focal segmental glomerular sclerosis

Children
1. Congenital urologic anomalies
2. Other congenital renal anomalies
3. Focal segmental glomerular sclerosis
4. Congenital renal dysplasia
5. Glomerular nephritis
6. Diabetes
7. Hypertension

Types of Donors

CADAVERIC

- **Ideal donor:** Young brain dead patient without other disease who remains normotensive, and in whom warm ischemia time is short
- **Marginal donor:** Used now because of extreme shortage of kidneys; older patients, perhaps with nonrenal disease, even mild renal dysfunction or prolonged warm ischemia time

Continuous Perfusion
Results in decreased delayed graft function compared to simple cold storage: Approximately 25% versus less than 10%

Morbidity and mortality associated with dialysis: A 49 year old with ESRD on dialysis has an expected duration of life of 7 years, compared to 30 years for a healthy 49 year old.

Decreased quality of life in ESRD is associated with time commitment for dialysis and increased number of hospital days.

Cardiovascular disease is responsible for 50% of dialysis patients' deaths, and infection accounts for 15–30%.

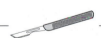

The left kidney is preferred by surgeons because of its longer renal vein, but preoperative imaging studies in the potential donor can identify variants of normal anatomy (like multiple arteries) that may make the right kidney a better choice.

- May be related or unrelated
- Decreased warm ischemia time
- Associated with less delayed graft function and better outcome
- Shorter waiting period
- Donor mortality: 1/10,000
- Donor morbidity up to 10%
- Living donor evaluation: Rule out potential donors with:
  - Diabetes, hypertension, malignancy, chronic obstructive pulmonary disease (COPD), renal disease
  - Age over 65 (flexible)
  - Genitourinary (GU) anomalies assessed by proteinuria > 250 mg/24 hr or creatinine clearance rate (CCr) < 80 mL/min, computed tomography (CT) of urinary tract

Appropriate Recipient

- General health assessment:
  - Identify comorbidities such as heart disease, COPD, and diabetes.
  - Assess ability to handle immunosuppression and compliance.
  - Laboratory evaluation consisting of chemistries, CBC, urinalysis, serologies for hepatitis B and C, cytomegalovirus (CMV), and human immunodeficiency virus (HIV).
- Conduct ECG and CXR.
- Further cardiac workup based on need.
- Metastatic workup if history of any cancer.
- Thorough evaluation: Esophagogastroduodenoscopy (EGD) when indicated; pancreatic ultrasound (US) or CT and workup for hyperparathyroidism if history of pancreatitis; colonoscopy when history of diverticulosis
- May require cholecystectomy if symptomatic gallbladder disease or diabetic with documented gallstones; elective colon resection for diverticulosis; bilateral nephrectomy if needed because of recurrent urinary tract infection (UTI) with reflux, or polycystic kidney disease (PCKD)
- Appropriate time for referral: Ideally prior to beginning dialysis.
- Psychosocial evaluation regarding compliance.
- See Table 26-1 for contraindications to kidney transplantation.

Operation

DONOR NEPHRECTOMY

- Flank incision, retroperitoneal approach.
- Left kidney used preferentially because renal vein is longer.
- Use kidney with fewer arteries if multiple renal arteries are present.
- Mannitol and furosemide, and possibly heparin, generally given prior to clamping vessels.
- In cadaveric donors, kidney is usually retrieved through multiorgan procurement.
- Phentolamine is given to prevent vasospasm.
- Furosemide and mannitol used here as well for diuresis prior to removal.

TABLE 26-1. Contraindications to kidney transplantation.

Absolute Contraindications	Relative Contraindications
Cancer (other than SCC or BCC of skin)	Obesity
Infection (HIV, tuberculosis)	Likely to be noncompliant
Cirrhosis (chronic active)	Ischemic heart disease severe, without possibility of CABG or angioplasty
Ongoing drug use	Sickle cell disease

RECIPIENT OPERATION

- Anesthesia:
  - Invasive monitoring where indicated—if older patient, hypertensive, cardiac disease, diabetes, previous coronary artery bypass graft (CABG)—consider Swan or CVP line.
  - Atracurium is the preferred muscle relaxant.
  - Inhalational agents preferable.
  - Fluids given assuming delayed graft function.
- Right side preferred site for transplanted kidney because iliac artery and vein are more superficial here than on the left side.
- Anastomosis: End-to-side with common or external iliac artery or end-to-end with hypogastric artery
- Renal vein anastomosis to common or external iliac vein or to distal inferior vena cava (IVC)
- Ureteral anastomosis typically to bladder, but may do ureteroureterostomy

POSTOPERATIVE CARE

- Routine care.
- Expect diuresis with functioning transplant; replace lost fluid.
- Expect moderate hypertension due to preexisting hypertension as well as due to aggravation by prednisone, CsA, and FK-506, all of which may elevate blood pressure.
- Immunosuppression: See section on immunosuppression.

Complications Specific to Kidney Transplantation

EARLY COMPLICATIONS

- **Delayed graft function:**
  - Evidenced by oliguria or anuria (assess volume status, ensure that Foley is working; once checked, but still anuric/oliguric, Doppler ultrasound indicated to assess blood flow). If blood flow adequate, look for urine leak or obstruction at ureterovesicular junction (UVJ) with US or renal scan. Once all workup negative, diagnosis is delayed graft function.
  - Management may include dialysis in postoperative period.
  - Occurs in 25% of cadaveric transplants.
- **Graft thrombosis:**
  - Requires immediate reoperation to save transplant.
  - Diagnosis indicated by abrupt cessation of urine output.
  - May assess with Doppler ultrasound.

- **Urine leak:**
    - Usually at UVJ.
    - Technical failure: Ureteral anastomosis too loose or too tight or due to less than watertight bladder closure.
    - Also due to distal ureteral sloughing secondary to inadequate blood supply.
    - Ureteral length should not be excessive.
    - Diagnosis: Decreased urine output, lower abdominal pain, scrotal or labial edema, rising creatinine
    - Tests: Ultrasound with fluid aspiration and analysis, renal scan with extravasation of radioisotope.
    - Treatment: Reexploration and repair.
- **Bleeding:** May be due to bleeding of small vessels that were in spasm at time of operation or to dysfunctional platelets in a uremic patient.
    - Present with hypotension, graft tenderness, and swelling
    - If patient stable, may confirm diagnosis with CT
    - Reoperation required for significant bleeding
- **Wound infections: See chapter on wounds.**

Late Complications

- **Lymphocele:** Perinephric fluid collection
    - Incidence 5%
    - Due to excessive iliac dissection and failure to ligate overlying lymphatics
    - Presents with swelling over transplant and unilateral leg edema due to compression of iliac vein, creatinine increased because ureter is compressed as well
    - Diagnosis: Ultrasound with aspiration and/or Doppler venous ultrasound of iliac veins
    - Treatment: If asymptomatic, may leave/otherwise must drain.
- **Ureteral stricture:**
    - Rising creatinine and hydronephrosis on ultrasound
    - Distal stricture result of rejection or ischemia; antegrade pyelogram best diagnostic tool
    - Treatment: Balloon dilatation; longer ones require surgical repair
- **Renal artery stenosis:**
    - 10% of renal transplants within first 6 months
    - Presentation: Hypertension, fluid retention
    - Diagnosis: Angiogram, US, magnetic resonance angiography (MRA)
    - If distal to anastomosis, may be secondary to rejection, atherosclerosis, clamp or other iatrogenic injury. Occurs more frequently with end-to-end anastomoses
    - Treatment: > 80% correctible with angioplasty; others require surgical repair
- **Donor complications:** UTI, wound infection, pneumothorax

Outcome

- 5-year survival (graft)
- Cadaveric: < 60%
- Living related: 70–80%, depending on donor source
- Common causes of death: Cardiovascular or infectious disease, malignancy

- Morbidities: Hepatic dysfunction, osteopenia, hyperglycemia
- Causes of graft loss: Chronic rejection, recurrent disease (2%)

Pediatric Transplantation

- Workup similar but less need for comorbidity evaluation
- Minimum age 1 year
- 1-year graft survival for cadaveric—80%; for living related donor—90%

PANCREAS TRANSPLANTATION

Indications

- Type I insulin-dependent diabetes mellitus and age < 45

Exclusions

- Significant coronary artery disease (CAD)
- Severe peripheral vascular disease (PVD) resulting in amputations
- Severe visual impairment
- Untreated malignancy
- Active infection
- HIV

Timing of Operation

Pancreas Transplant (5%)
- For the nonuremic diabetic patient with minimal or no evident nephropathy

Pancreas Transplant After Kidney Transplant (PAK) (7%)
- For the uremic diabetic patient with potentially reversible secondary effects, with suitable living related kidney donor available

Simultaneous Pancreas and Kidney Transplants (SPK) (87%)
- For the diabetic uremic patient with potentially reversible secondary effects, lacking a suitable living related kidney donor

Operations

DONOR OPERATION

- Pancreatic graft is harvested en bloc with liver and 10- to 12-cm duodenal segment.
- Pancreatic blood supply is reconstructed with donor iliac artery graft.

RECIPIENT OPERATION

- Intra-abdominal placement of graft—pancreas in the right iliac fossa, kidney in the left iliac fossa.
- Portal vein of pancreas graft is anastomosed to IVC or iliac vein.
- Arterial anastomosis is made from the reconstructed donor iliac artery graft and common iliac artery.

Alternatives to whole-organ pancreas transplant is use of insulin pump and islet of Langerhans transplant.

The pancreas transplant is placed in the abdominal cavity rather than in the retroperitoneal space because of a lower incidence of peripancreatic fluid collections and lymphocele.

Pancreas transplant:
- Delayed graft reperfusion minimizes edema and blood loss.
- Intraoperatively, mannitol and albumin are given to limit reperfusion injury and tissue edema.
- Expect euglycemia within 12 hours of operation; no postop insulin should be required.

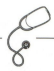

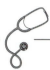

DRAINAGE OPTIONS

- **Bladder drainage:**
  - Advantage: Urinary amylase may be used as a sign of rejection.
  - Up to 25% may require conversion to enteric drainage.
- **Enteric drainage:**
  - Avoidance of postop GU complications that affect 30% of bladder drained patients
  - Avoidance of chronic dehydration
  - No need for bicarbonate replacement
  - Equal efficacy, graft survival, morbidity

Postoperative Management

- Immunosuppression: Quadruple drug regimen: ATG or OKT3/MMF, CsA or FK-506 and steroids
- Expect rejection: Treatment is high-dose steroids for 2 days. If no response, treat with OKT3 or ATG; 90% resolve.
  - Signs: Early decrease in exocrine function (decrease in urinary amylase).
  - Confirm with biopsy (ultrasound-guided percutaneous, or duodenal needle biopsy).
  - In SPK, rejection usually involves pancreas and kidney. May diagnose by creatinine and renal biopsy.

Complications

- Gross hematuria
- Urinary leak
- UTI
- Urethritis
- Hyperamylasemia
- Peripancreatic fluid collections on CT and US. Drain if suspect infection

Outcomes

- Graft loss: Most commonly due to rejection.
- 1-year patient survival > 90%.
- 1-year graft survival > 75%.
- SPK has the highest graft survival and lowest technical failure rate (compared to percutaneous transluminal angioplasty [PTA] and PAK)
- 1-year graft function rate:
  - SPK: 78
  - PAK: 56
  - PTA: 55
- By 5 years out, no difference in enteric and bladder drained in terms of patient or graft survival.
- In terms of diabetic secondary effects: Reversal of neuropathy, prevention of nephropathy, improvement or stabilization of retinopathy.

Indications

Irreversible liver failure:

Chronic (More Common)
- Cirrhosis (posthepatic, alcoholic)
- Primary and secondary biliary cirrhosis
- Primary sclerosing cholangitis
- Metabolic defects (alpha-1-antitrypsin deficiency, amyloidosis, hemochromatosis, sarcoidosis, tyrosinemia, ornithine transcarbinase deficiency)
- Malignancy (hepatocellular carcinoma [HCC] or cholangiocarcinoma)
- Biliary atresia
- Polycystic liver disease
- Budd–Chiari
- Cystic fibrosis
- Crigler–Najjar
- Histiocytosis X

Acute or Fulminant
- Viral or alcoholic hepatitis
- Wilson's disease
- Hepatotoxic drugs (e.g., acetaminophen overdose)

Contraindications

- Multisystem organ failure
- Severe cardiopulmonary disease
- Sepsis secondary to nonhepatic source
- Widespread cancer
- Noncompliance with medical therapy
- Severely impaired neurologic status

Evaluation

- Assessment of signs and symptoms of liver failure: Jaundice, bleeding abnormality/coagulopathy, encephalopathy, ascites, malnutrition, infection, hepatorenal syndrome
- CT or magnetic resonance imaging (MRI) head
- Laboratory: Increased bilirubin, decreased hematocrit, elevated coags, thrombocytopenia, hypoalbuminemia, elevated ammonia, elevated creatinine
- Preoperative control of:
  - Variceal bleeding: Transjugular intrahepatic portosystemic shunt (TIPS) when needed
  - Ascites: Diuretics and/or paracentesis

Types of Liver Transplants

- Living donor
- Cadaveric

Liver transplant outcome is generally better for chronic liver failure patients.

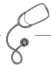

Cancer and alcohol abuse remain controversial indications for liver transplant:
- Alcoholic liver disease accounts for 75% of liver failure in the United States. Patients have excellent outcome, with low rate of recidivism. Pretransplant abstinence, evidence of support system, and lack of other alcohol-related comorbidities are required.
- Patients transplanted for liver cancer have worse outcome than patients transplanted for other reasons, but survival is improved compared to cancer patients who are not transplanted (40% 5-year survival).

HIGH-YIELD FACTS

Transplant

Operation

1. Native hepatectomy
2. Implantation of donor liver: On venovenous bypass, or using technique in which three principal hepatic veins are anastomosed to donor suprahepatic IVC, allowing restoration of IVC flow after suprahepatic caval anastomosis
3. Reconstruction of common bile duct, end-to-end

Postoperative Management

- Avoid vasoconstrictors, which reduce blood flow to liver.
- Diuretics as needed to mobilize fluid.
- Tacrolimus immunosuppression.

Complications

- Graft failure: Usually secondary to primary nonfunction, recurrence of disease, biliary or vascular complications (not generally due to rejection).
- Rejection occurs in first 3 months post-transplant with 50% incidence, but is well-treated with steroids or antilymphocyte therapy (indicated by elevated liver function tests [LFTs], particularly gammaglutamyl transpeptidase [GGTP])

Outcome

- Patient survival:
  - 2-year: 69–83%
  - 5-year: 37–58%
  - 2-year graft survival: 64–74%
- Above numbers are based on UNOS data from 1988–1996 (Nair et al., 2002). Ranges represent difference in outcome by race stratification: Significantly improved patient and graft survival for white and Hispanic patients compared to African-American and Asian patients.

SMALL BOWEL TRANSPLANTATION

Indications

- Adults: Short bowel syndrome, due to Crohn's disease, mesenteric thrombosis, trauma
- Children: Short bowel syndrome, due to necrotizing enterocolitis, intestinal pseudo-obstruction, gastroschisis, volvulus, intestinal atresia

Operation

- Isolated intestinal failure: Isolated intestinal transplant
- With liver failure: Liver–intestine combined transplant
- Sometimes, multivisceral transplant: Liver, stomach, pancreas, duodenum, small intestine, possibly large bowel

- Stoma usually placed for monitoring and biopsies
- Postop: Early feeding

Complications

- Graft versus host disease (GVHD): Prevent with immunosuppression, and/or pretreatment of donor.
- Rejection: More difficult to treat than in other organs; newer agents may prove to be more useful than older ones (tacrolimus-based).
- Diagnosed by fever, abdominal pain, elevated white count, ileus, gastrointestinal (GI) bleed, positive blood cultures; also by biopsy showing cryptitis, villi shortening, mononuclear infiltrate.

Outcome

- 1-year graft survival: Approximately 65% intestine ± liver, and approximately 50% for multivisceral transplants
- 3-year: 29–37%

CARDIAC TRANSPLANTATION

Background

- Approximately 150 donor hearts become available each month. Twenty-eight hundred patients are waiting on the UNOS list, with 300 new patients added to that list each month.
- Cause of disease in patients receiving transplants: Cardiomyopathy (50%), CAD (38%), congenital disease (6%), valvular disease (2%)

Indications

- Severe cardiac disability on maximal medical therapy (multiple hospitalizations for congestive heart failure [CHF], New York Hospital Association class III [NYHA III] or IV, or peak oxygen consumption < 15 mL/kg/min)
- Symptomatic ischemia or recurrent ventricular arrhythmias refractory to usual therapy, with left ventricular ejection fraction (LVEF) < 30%, or with unstable angina and not a candidate for CABG or percutaneous transluminal coronary angioplasty (PTCA)
- All surgical alternatives already excluded

Contraindications

- Irreversible, severe, pulmonary, renal, or hepatic dysfunction
- Unstaged, or incompletely staged, cancer
- Psychiatric illness
- Severe systemic disease
- Age > 60 (varies from center to center)

Evaluation

- UNOS status:
  - I: Patients in intensive care unit (ICU) requiring inotropic or mechanical support
  - II: All others
- Matching/compatibility based on:
  1. ABO compatibility
  2. Body size
  3. Donor weight/recipient weight
  4. Phosphoribosylamine (PRA) (if PRA > 5%, crossmatch is done)

Operation

DONOR OPERATION

- Aorta and pulmonary artery (PA) dissected
- Superior vena cava (SVC) mobilized
- IVC dissected from pericardial reflection
- Cardioplege and heparin administered
- SVC and IVC ligated
- Ascending aorta clamped distal to perfusion cannula and hyperkalemic cardioplege rapidly infused
- Heart elevated from pericardial wall, pulmonary veins divided, and organ passed off for preservation (in cold crystalloid cardioplege)

RECIPIENT OPERATION

- Median sternotomy
- Pericardium opened
- Aorta, SVC, IVC cannulated
- Bypass initiated
- Ascending aorta cross-clamped, plege is infused into aortic roof, causing diastolic arrest
- Aorta and pulmonary arteries divided
- Atria transected, leaving atrial cuffs (heart passed off)
- Left and then right atrial cuffs of donor and recipient anastomosed
- Patient rewarmed and caval snares released
- Aorta anastomosed
- Air in ascending aorta vented with needle
- Patient is decannulated
- Temporary atrial pacers placed
- Chest closed

Postoperative Management

- ICU management.
- Wean to extubate once awake.
- Swan–Ganz if pulmonary hypertension.
- Immunosuppression: CsA, azathioprine, prednisone.
- Expect transient sinus node dysfunction (up to 20%), requiring temporary pacing or isoproterenol, afterload reduction, and renal dose dopamine.

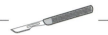

Cardiac transplant: Cold ischemic time up to 6 hours may be tolerated, though 3 to 4 is ideal (2 hours maximum for patients with pulmonary hypertension).

Denervated (transplanted) heart has higher resting heart rate, no sinus arrhythmia or carotid reflex bradycardia.

Transplanted heart has increased sensitivity to catecholamines, with increased density of adrenergic receptors with loss of norepinephrine uptake; cardiac output and index remain at low normal, with adequate but abnormal exercise response (increase in heart rate is usually delayed).

- Keep urine output > 0.5 mL/kg/hr. Cardiac output (CO) is adequate with this urine output without diuretics and with warm lower extremities.
- Expect return to normal cardiac function after 3 to 4 days, at which time pressors and afterload reducers may be weaned.
- Remove chest tubes when drainage < 25 cc/hr.
- Remove atrial pacers POD 7 to 10.

Transplanted heart has normal vasodilatation with increased oxygen demand but abnormal vasodilatory reserve is in rejection, hypertrophy, or wall abnormalities.

Complications

The most common cause of perioperative death is infection (50%). Other common causes are pulmonary hypertension and nonspecific graft failure.
- Infection:
    - Peak incidence: Early postoperative period.
    - Eighty-five percent will have an infection at some point in the first 5 postoperative years.
    - See Table 26-2 for causes of infection in the cardiac transplant patient.
- Rejection:
    - At least 75% incidence in first 3 post-transplant months
    - Diagnosis confirmed by endomyocardial biopsy (via right IJ)
    - Histology: Lymphocyte infiltration and/or myocytic necrosis
    - Treatment: Pulse steroids if early on (later in course, mild rejection treated by 3-day increased dose of oral prednisone); refractory rejection treated with ATG or OKT3.

TABLE 26-2. Causes of infection in the cardiac transplant patient.

Early Infection	Organisms
Pneumonia	GNB
Mediastinitis	*Staphylococcus epidermidis, S. aureus,* GNB
Catheter-related	*S. epidermidis, S. aureus,* GNB, *Candida*
UTI	GNB, *Enterococcus, Candida*
Skin	Herpes simplex virus
Late Infection	
Viral	Cytomegalovirus, herpes simplex virus, varicella-zoster virus, hepatitis C virus
Bacterial	*Listeria, Nocardia, Legionella, Mycobacteria*
Fungal	*Aspergillus, Cryptococcus, Candida, Mucor*
Protozoan	PCP, toxoplasmosis

CMV occurs at 75–100% incidence in cardiac transplant patients and has been identified as trigger for graft-related atherosclerosis (treated with ganciclovir and hyperimmune globulin).

- Chronic rejection: Concentric intimal proliferation with smooth muscle hyperplasia yielding atherosclerosis more diffuse than in non-transplanted hearts
  - Prevalence of CAD: 25% at 1 year and 80% at 5 years
  - Yearly angiogram recommended
  - PTCA and CABG as indicated for discrete proximal lesions
- Cancer:
  - Increased risk, with immunosuppression, of skin, vulvar, or anal cancer; B-cell lymphoproliferative disorder (BLPD), and cervical intraepithelial neoplasia (CIN).
  - BLPD: Incidence is increased 350 times.
    - Possible relationship to EBV infection.
    - Diagnose via lymph node biopsy.
    - Treat with decreased immunosuppression and antiviral therapy.
    - Thirty to 40% response rate.

Outcome

Overall survival:
- 1 year: 82%
- 5 year: 61%
- 10 years: 41%

Pediatric Cardiac Transplant

- Usual indications: Congenital heart disease or dilated cardiomyopathy.
- Contraindications as in adults.
- Most important matching considerations: Blood type and donor size.
- Similar immunosuppression, with faster steroid taper.
- Signs and symptoms of acute rejection: Fever, tachycardia, anorexia, restlessness, echo abnormalities.
- Graft CAD occurs as in adults.
- Survival: 75% (1 year), 60% (5 year), 50% (10 year), with most at functional NYHA I.

LUNG TRANSPLANTATION

Types of Operations and Indications

- Single lung for fibrotic lung disease: Pulmonary fibrosis, emphysema, bronchopulmonary dysplasia, primary pulmonary hypertension (without cardiac dysfunction), post-transplant obliterative bronchiolitis
- Bilateral single lung for septic lung disease: Cystic fibrosis, bronchiectasis, COPD
- Heart–lung for pulmonary vascular disease, end-stage lung disease with cardiac dysfunction
- Lobar lung, to increase donor pool from living related and cadaveric donors

Contraindications

- Old age (definition varies)
- Significant systemic disease, including hepatic or renal disease
- Active infection
- Malignancy
- Psychiatric illness/noncompliance
- Current smoking

Evaluation

- ABO-compatible.
- Infection-free donor and recipient.
- Donor: Good pulmonary gas exchange, no significant smoking history, similar lung volume, where possible.
- Workup includes: PRA, ABO testing, serologies, CXR clear, $PaO_2 > 300$ on FiO_2 of 100% with positive end-expiratory pressure (PEEP) of 5, bronchoscopy.
- CIT (cold ischemic time) up to 6 hours is tolerated.

Postoperative Management

- ICU management, intubated.
- Swan–Ganz catheter, arterial line, end tidal carbon dioxide ($ETCO_2$) monitor.
- Limit peak airway pressures to < 40 cm H_2O.
- Aggressive pulmonary toilet.
- Careful fluid and loop diuretic use to minimize early graft edema (due to inadequate preservation).
- Wean to extubate once fully awake, usually by POD 3.
- Immunosuppression as for cardiac transplantation.

Complications

- Acute rejection:
    - Sixty to 70% incidence in first postoperative month.
    - Diagnosed by clinical parameters: Fever, dyspnea, decreased PaO_2, decreased forced expiratory volume in 1 second (FEV_1), CXR with interstitial infiltrate.
    - Confirm with biopsy via bronchoscopy.
    - Histology: Lymphocytic infiltrate to varying degrees.
- Chronic rejection:
    - Presents as obliterative bronchiolitis.
    - 20–50% of long-term survivors
    - Lumen obliterated by eosinophilic submucosal scar tissue
    - Increased in patients with CMV, exposure to toxic fumes, chronic foreign body, and immunologic reasons
    - No treatment
- Infection:
    - Early, predominance of GNB (Gram-negative bacillus) infection
- Viral: CMV, treated with ganciclovir, also EBV
- Fungal: *Candida, Aspergillus*
- Protozoan: Pneumocystis carinii pneumonia (PCP)

Outcome

- 1-year survival: 70%
- 2-year survival: 60%

Pediatric Transplantation

- Indications similar, operation similar
- Outcome:
  - 1-year survival: 55%
  - 2-year survival: 41%

The Genitourinary System

ANATOMY OF THE GU SYSTEM

Penis

- Made up of three cylindrical bodies:
  - Two corpora cavernosa covered by tunica albigunea
  - One corpus spongiosum, which surrounds the urethra
- Blood supply: Internal pudendal artery.
- Lymphatic drainage: Deep and superficial inguinal nodes.

Scrotum

- Made up of smooth muscle, elastic tissue layers of Darto's fascia, and the combined layers of Camper and Scarpa fascia continued from the abdominal wall
- Blood supply: Femoral and internal pudendal artery
- Lymphatic drainage: Inguinal and femoral nodes

Undescended testes increase risk for cancer.

Testes

- Lie in the scrotum, usually vertically
- 4 to 5 cm × 3 cm × 3 cm.
- Encased in tunica albigunea except posteriolaterally, where it is attached to the epididymis. This anchors the testes to the posterior wall.
- Inferiorly, it is anchored by scrotal ligaments.
- Potential space exists between visceral tunica vaginalis and anterior tunica vaginalis.
- Appendix testes: Vestigial structure of müllerian duct origin, usually situated in the uppermost portion of the testes.
- Blood supply:
  - Internal spermatic artery
  - Differential artery
  - External spermatic artery
  - All three travel in the spermatic cord
- Venous return:
  - Internal spermatic
  - Epigastric

Lack of proper fixation increases risk for torsion.

Torsion of the appendix can cause extreme pain mimicking torsion of the testes.

- Internal circumflex
- Scrotal
- Lymphatic drainage: External, common iliac, and periaortic nodes.

Epididymis

- Tubular structure
- 4 to 5 meters in length compressed to an area about 5 cm
- Promote sperm maturation and motility

Vas Deferens

Muscular tube within the scrotal sac, which extends in the spermatic cord traveling in the inguinal canal and crossing medially behind the bladder over the ureters to form the ampulla of vas. It joins the seminal vesicles to form the paired ejaculatory ducts in the prostatic urethra.

Prostate

- Originates from the urogenital sinus
- Enlarges as a man matures
- Posterior surface easily palpable on rectal exam

HEMATURIA

- Presence of blood in the urine.
- Can be gross and microscopic.
- Microscopic hematuria can be detected with a dipstick if hemoglobin concentration is > 0.003 mg/L (which is equal to 1 to 2 red blood cells per high-power field of spun urine)

Causes

- 0 to 20 years: Acute urinary tract infection (UTI), glomerulonephritis, congenital urinary tract abnormality
- 20 to 60 years: Acute UTI, bladder cancer, renal stones
- > 60 years: Benign prostatic hypertrophy (men)

Other Causes

- Coagulopathy
- Anticoagulation
- Sickle cell disease
- Collagen vascular disease
- Renal disease—glomerulonephritis, vascular abnormalities, pyelonephritis, polycystic kidney, granulomatous disease, interstitial nephritis, neoplasm
- Postrenal causes: Urethritis, stones, cystitis, prostatitis, epididymitis

ACUTE SCROTAL MASS

DIFFERENTIAL DIAGNOSIS

- Testicular torsion
- Epididymitis
- Testicular tumor
- Torsion of testicular appendage
- Orchitis
- Trauma to scrotum
- Acute hernia
- Acute hydrocele

The major challenge to the diagnosis of acute scrotal mass is to differentiate which of these are an acute medical emergency. Of note, the extreme urgency associated with the process of testicular torsion requires immediate recognition.

The diagnosis of an acute scrotal mass will depend largely on the history and physical examination. For instance, acute hernia and hydrocele are both reasonable considerations in the differential diagnosis of acute scrotal mass. However, careful physical exam should elucidate the different processes.

SIGNS AND SYMPTOMS

The physical exam in a patient with acute scrotal pain is generally difficult because of the extreme pain, which permits limited physical examination. Nevertheless, it should include a search for:

- Lateralization of swelling.
- Erythema of scrotal skin.
- Position of the testicle.
- Localization of testicular mass and pain.
- Presence of hydrocele by transillumination.
- Presence or absence of cremateric reflex.
- Prehn's sign—relief of pain by elevation of the testicle; may be indicative of epididymitis.
- Urethral discharge should be searched for as well as inguinal node.
- Cremasteric reflex.
- Fever.
- Previous history of trauma.
- Previous history of similar pain.
- Acute vs. subacute onset.
- Previous history of urethral discharge or unprotected sex.

TESTICULAR TORSION

- Two peak periods—the first year of life and at puberty
- 10 times more likely in an undescended testis
- Salvage rate of 80–100% if pain is < 6 hours
- Frequently preceded by strenuous activity or athletic event
- Usually develops acutely

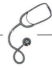

Torsion and epididymitis cause 60–70% of scrotal/testicular masses.

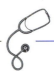

A hydrocele is typically nonpainful depending on the underlying process.

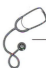

Transillumination can easily distinguish a hydrocele from other testicular masses.

Cremasteric reflex retraction of the testicle as the medial aspect of the thigh is stroked.

Always suspect torsion in a patient with inguinal pain and an empty scrotum.

HIGH-YIELD FACTS

The Genitourinary System

Typical scenario: An adolescent presents with acute testicular pain and swelling immediately after a sporting event. He is ill-appearing, writhing in pain. On further questioning, he has had similar episodes of this in the past. *Think:* Testicular torsion.

PATHOPHYSIOLOGY

- The testicle twists on its spermatic cord, causing obstruction of venous return leading to swelling. If obstruction persists, venous thrombosis occurs, followed by arterial thrombosis. Infarction develops promptly when arterial thrombosis occurs.
- Torsion results from maldevelopment of fixation between the enveloping tunica vaginalis and the posterior scrotal wall.
- This maldevelopment is usually bilateral. However, torsion generally occurs unilaterally.

SIGNS AND SYMPTOMS

- Acute onset of severe pain in testicle, lower abdomen, or the inguinal canal.
- Pain may be constant or intermittent and not positional.
- May be accompanied by nausea or vomiting.
- Scrotum is swollen and tender.
- Classic sign: High-riding testis with a horizontal lie. However, this is often difficult to distinguish because of the degree of swelling in the scrotum.
- Presence of a reactive hydrocele.
- Loss of cremateric reflex.

DIAGNOSIS

Since epididymitis is most commonly confused with testicular torsion, several tests may aid in distinguishing the two entities. In torsion:

- Urinalysis (UA) and complete blood count (CBC) will be unremarkable.
- Most will be afebrile.

Since the ability to salvage the affected testis is dependent on how quickly the testis becomes detorsed, time is of the essence. If the diagnosis is thought to be torsion, surgical exploration is the test of choice. Any procedure that delays surgical repair is not wise.

If the clinical diagnosis is uncertain, color Doppler ultrasound has become the test of choice in most hospitals. It has a sensitivity of 85–100% and specificity of 100%, similar to radioisotope scans, and has the advantage of being more rapid and readily available than radioisotope scans.

TREATMENT

- Surgical repair is the definitive treatment.
- Manual detorsion should be attempted while awaiting surgical repair. It is a temporizing procedure, not curative.
- Most testes torse medially; one can manually twist the testis laterally, unless the cord appears to be shortened and worsening the torsion, in which case detorsion in the opposite direction should be attempted.

TESTICULAR TUMOR

DEFINITION AND EPIDEMIOLOGY

- The most common malignancy to affect young men.
- There is a peak frequency in early childhood, and a larger peak incidence between 20 and 35 years of age.

- Uncommon after age 40.
- Occurs in whites more than African-Americans.

RISK FACTORS

- Men with cryptorchid (undescended) testes (intra-abdominal testes with the highest risk. Both the affected testis and the normally descended testis are at risk.)
- History of mumps orchitis.
- Inguinal hernia in childhood.
- Testicular cancer in the contralateral testis.

SIGNS AND SYMPTOMS

Symptoms are varied and may range from asymptomatic nodule to symptoms of massive metastasis:

- Asymptomatic nodule or presence of mass.
- Swelling.
- Sensation of heaviness.
- Most are painless but may be painful if there is hemorrhage into the tumor.
- Back or abdominal pain secondary to retroperitoneal adenopathy.
- Weight loss.
- Dyspnea secondary to pulmonary metastasis.
- Gynecomastia.

DIAGNOSIS

- Testicular sonogram
- Magnetic resonance imaging (MRI)
- Tumor markers—alpha fetoprotein (AFP) and human chorionic gonadotropin (HCG)

CLASSIFICATION AND PATHOLOGY

- Most widely used classification is the Mostofi and is based on the cell type from which the tumor is derived, germinal or stromal.
- Germinal cell tumors comprise 95% of all testicular tumors:
  - Seminomas (pure single-cell tumors)
  - Nonseminomas
  - Combination tumors
- Tumors of gonadal stroma (1–2%):
  - Leydig cell
  - Sertoli cell
  - Primitive gonadal structures
- Gonadoblastomas (germinal cell + stromal cell):
  - The distinction between seminomas and nonseminomas is important because the staging evaluation and subsequent management in the two differs as a consequence of the relative radioresponsiveness of seminomas compared with the radioresistance of nonseminomas.
  - Pure seminomas: Radiation therapy (XRT) is the mainstay of treatment.
  - Nonseminomas: Retroperitoneal lymph node dissection ± chemotherapy.

- To determine whether the cancer is:
  - Localized to the testis
  - Regional lymphatics
  - Widely metastasized
- For pure seminomas:
  - Abdominal and pelvic computed tomography (CT) scan to determine the presence of adenopathy or visceral involvement
  - Chest x-ray (CXR) ± chest CT
  - Biologic markers—AFP and HCG
- If AFP is elevated, the patient should be treated as having nonseminomas.
- If HCG is elevated, a search should be made for syncytiotrophoblastic giant cells. Otherwise, there may be an occult foci of nonseminomatous component producing the HCG.
- If the workup does not reveal metastatic disease, serum HCG level should be followed after orchiectomy. If it does not decline as predicted, the presence of occult metastatic cancer should be considered.
- **Nonseminomas:** The staging workup for nonseminomas is similar to that described for seminomas.
- **Stage I:** No clinical, radiographic, or marker evidence of tumor presence beyond the confines of the testis.
- **Stage II:**
  - *Early:* Nonpalpable, small, retroperitoneal adenopathy on CT scan (< 4 to 5 cm).
  - *Advanced:* Retroperitoneal adenopathy > 5 cm on CT scan or palpable retroperitoneal adenopathy with disease limited to lymphatic below the diaphragm.
- **Stage III:** Visceral involvement of the cancer.
- Conceptually, patients have either early or advanced. Early disease is stage I and early stage II. Advanced disease is advanced stage II or any form of stage III.

TREATMENT

- Operative approach: High radical inguinal orchiectomy.
- Trans-scrotal biopsy of the testis or a trans-scrotal orchiectomy should not be performed if the diagnosis of testicular cancer is likely because the lymphatic drainage of the testes is different from that of the scrotum; a scrotal incision in the presence of testicular cancer may cause local recurrence and metastasis.
- **Early seminoma:** Orchiectomy + XRT.
- **Advanced seminoma:** Combination chemotherapy followed by restaging.
- **Stage I nonseminoma:** Orchiectomy + retroperitoneal lymph node dissection (RPLND) or surveillance.
- **Stage II nonseminoma:** The optimal management of this group of patients is controversial. RPLND can be curative but have a high relapse rate. If relapse occurs, chemotherapy can be given as adjunctive therapy. Alternatively, chemotherapy can be given prior to RPLND.
- **Advanced stage nonseminoma:** Chemotherapy ± tumor reductive surgery.
- Commonly used chemotherapeutic regimens:
  - BEP—etoposide, bleomycin, cisplatin
  - PVB—vinblastine, bleomycin, cisplatin

- VAB-6—vinblastine, bleomycin, cisplatin, cyclophosphamide, actinomycin D

Following appropriate therapy, patients need to undergo continuous surveillance for at least 18 to 24 months via tumor markers and/or radiographs for regression of disease or for relapses.

Most relapses occur within 24 months but later relapses do occur.

UROLITHIASIS

DEFINITION AND EPIDEMIOLOGY

Also called kidney stone, renal stone, nephrolithiasis.
- One of the most common diseases of the urinary tract.
- Two to 5% of the population will form a urinary stone at some point in their lives.
- Majority of stones form between the ages of 20 and 50.
- Male-to-female ratio of 3:1.
- Familial tendency in stone formation.
- Tendency for recurrence: Thirty-six percent of patients with a first stone will have another stone within one year, and 50% will recur within years.

ETIOLOGY

- Seventy-five percent of stones are composed of calcium oxalate or a mixture of calcium oxalate and calcium phosphate.
- Fifteen percent are magnesium–ammonium–phosphate stones (struvite)—occurs exclusively in patients with UTI.
- Ten percent are uric acid stones.
- Less than 1% are cystine stones.

RISK FACTORS

- Dietary history: Large calcium and alkali intake
- Prolonged immobilization
- Residence in hot climate
- History of UTI
- History of calculus in the past and in family members
- Drug ingestion (analgesics, alkalis, uricosuric agents, protease inhibitors)
- Prior history of gout
- Underlying gastrointestinal disease (Crohn's, ulcerative colitis, peptic ulcer disease [PUD])

SIGNS AND SYMPTOMS

- Severe, abrupt onset of colicky pain, which begins in the flank and may radiate toward the groin. In male, the pain may radiate toward the testicle. In female, it may radiate toward the labium majoris.
- Nausea and vomiting are almost universal with acute renal colic.
- Abdominal distention from an ileus.
- Gross hematuria.

Typical scenario: A 40-year-old man presents with sudden onset left-sided flank pain that he rates a 10/10. He is writhing, unable to stay still or find a comfortable position. *Think:* Renal colic. Check a urine dip for blood and consider imaging.

- Urinalysis:
  - Vast majority of patients (about 85%) will have RBCs in the urine. However, its absence does not rule out renal stones.
  - Urinary pH can aid in differentiating the type of stone present. Normal urinary pH is about 5.85. If the pH is > 6, one should suspect the presence of urea-splitting organisms (*Proteus*). A low urine pH (≤ 5) suggests uric acid stones.
  - WBCs or bacteria may suggest underlying UTI and should be aggressively treated.
- Laboratory studies (serum):
  - WBC may be slightly elevated.
  - Blood urea nitrogen (BUN) and creatinine should be measured.
  - Uric acid, calcium, and phosphate levels should be measured.
- Radiographic studies:
  - **Plain abdominal film (KUB):**
    - Often standard initial study.
    - Only radiopaque stones will be seen (60–70% specific in the diagnosis of a calculus).
    - However, it is a cheap and quick test to do, and is useful in combination with other studies.
  - **Renal ultrasound:**
    - Fast, easy, and relatively inexpensive.
    - No IV contrast is needed.
    - Good for detecting hydronephrosis (85–95% sensitive, 100% specific).
    - Cannot assess renal function.
    - Not very good for detecting small stones (64% sensitivity).
    - Cannot discriminate between radiolucent and opaque stones, so both types of stones will be seen.
    - Good way to follow known stones.
    - Good for shedding light on alternative diagnoses such as abdominal aortic aneurysm or cholelithiasis, which can confuse the clinical picture.
  - **Noncontrast abdominal/pelvic CT** (Figure 27-1):
    - Fast, requires no IV contrast.
    - Most useful to diagnose small stones (95% sensitivity), hydronephrosis, hydroureter, and perinephric stranding.
    - However, in the absence of hydronephrosis, it cannot reliably distinguish between ureteral stones and pelvic calcification.
    - Cannot assess renal function.
    - Useful for revealing other abdominal/pelvic pathology.
  - **Intravenous pyelogram:**
    - **Clearly outlines the entire urinary system, making it easy to see hydronephrosis and the presence of any type of stones.**
    - Can assess renal function and allow for verification that the opposite kidney is functioning properly.
    - Typically, if a ureteral stone exists, the IVP will show a delayed nephrogram and columnization of dye, indicating obstruction. In a normally functioning kidney without obstruction, the entire ureter is not visualized on a single film because of the peristaltic movement of dye through the ureter.
    - IVP is generally preferred by the urologist because of its better orientation of the stone and demonstration of its size and shape.

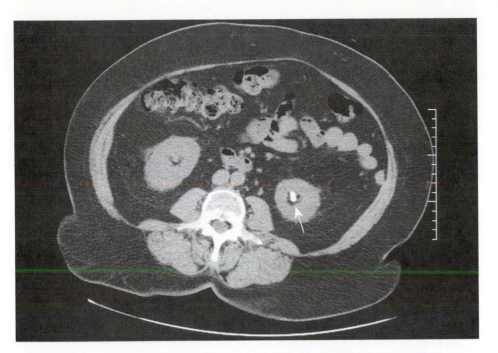

FIGURE 27-1. Noncontrast abdominal CT demonstrating nephrolithiasis (arrow) in the right kidney, which shows up as radiopaque (white).

- Disadvantages: Time consuming due to need for delayed films; requires IV contrast.
- **Retrograde pyelogram:**
  - Most precise method of determining the anatomy of the ureter and renal pelvis as diagnosing renal calculi.
  - Done under anesthesia in the cystoscopy suite where a contrast dye is injected into the ureter via a ureteral catheter inserted into the uretheral orifice in the bladder.
  - Because of the invasive nature of the procedure, this is done only when a precise diagnosis cannot be made by other means or when there is a clear need for an endoscopic surgical procedure.

MANAGEMENT

- Analgesia with nonsteroidal anti-inflammatory drugs (NSAIDs) and/or opiates.
- IV or PO hydration.
- During passage of a stone, there are five sites where the passage is likely to become arrested:
  - Calyx of the kidney
  - Ureteropelvic junction
  - Pelvic brim where the ureter arched over the iliac vessels
  - Ureterovesical junction
  - Vesicle orifice

These sites correspond to the narrowest points of the urinary system. If impaction occurs and hydronephrosis develops, surgical decompression of the affected kidney may be necessary to preserve kidney function.

- For stones unlikely to pass spontaneously:
  - Extracorporeal shockwave lithotripsy (ESWL) has been effective for stone located in the kidney with 85% success rate.

- Percutaneous nephrolithotomy, which establishes a tract from the skin to the collecting system, is used when stones are too large or too hard for lithotripsy.

BENIGN PROSTATIC HYPERTROPHY

DEFINITION

- Development of prostatic hypertrophy is almost universal in men as they get older.
- The prostate enlarges during puberty when it undergoes androgen-mediated growth. It remains stable in size until about the fifth or sixth decade, when its size increases again.

PATHOPHYSIOLOGY

- Hyperplasia begins in the periuretheral area, then progresses to the remainder of the gland; hence, the most common initial symptoms are those of obstructive in nature.
- Histologically, the hyperplastic tissue is comprised of glandular epithelium, stroma, and smooth muscle.
- As hyperplasia increases with increasing obstruction, frank obstruction can occur or may be precipitated by extrinsic etiologies, such as infection, anticholinergic drugs, or alcohol.

SIGNS AND SYMPTOMS

- Early symptoms:
  - Hesitancy in initiating voiding
  - Postvoid dribbling
  - Sensation of incomplete emptying
- As the amount of residual urine increase:
  - Nocturia
  - Overflow incontinence
  - Palpable bladder
  - Frank obstruction

DIAGNOSIS

- Clinical history
- Digital rectal exam—in hyperplasia, the prostate will be smooth, firm, but enlarged.
- Measurement of postvoid residual urine volume.

MANAGEMENT

- Many patients without treatment show no progression of symptoms.
- In patients with advanced symptoms, several options exist.
- Medical:
  - Luteinizing hormone-releasing hormone (LHRH) analogues shrink prostatic hyperplasia.
  - Alpha-adrenergic antagonists decrease urethral resistance.
- Surgical:
  - Transurethral prostatectomy (TURP) is usually the procedure of choice.
  - Open prostatectomy

DEFINITION

- The most common malignancy in men in the United States.
- Only about one third of the cases identified at autopsy were manifested clinically.
- Rare before age 50.

CLASSIFICATION

- Ninety-five percent are adenocarcinoma, which has a predilection to start in the periphery.
- Generally multifocal.
- The remaining 5% are squamous, transitional cell, carcinosarcoma, and occasional metastatic tumors.

SIGNS AND SYMPTOMS

- Most patients are asymptomatic at the time of diagnosis; about 80% of patients have stage C or D disease at the time of diagnosis.
- In symptomatic patients, common complaints include:
  - Dysuria
  - Difficulty in voiding
  - Urinary frequency
  - Urinary retention
  - Back or hip pain
  - Hematuria
- Symptoms in advanced disease may include spinal cord compression, deep venous thrombosis and pulmonary emboli, myelophthisis.

DIAGNOSIS

- The most important physical exam is the digital rectal exam. The carcinoma begins most often on the posterior surfaces of the lateral lobes where it can be easily palpated on digital exam. Carcinoma is usually hard, nodular, and irregular. The typical middle raphe of the prostate may be obscured by either a malignant or a benign process.
- Biochemical markers such as the prostate-specific antigen (PSA) is the most sensitive test for early detection of prostatic cancer. Following diagnosis, PSA is used to follow progression of disease and response to treatment. However, the PSA is not a specific test. PSA can be elevated in prostatic hyperplasia or prostatitis.
- Imaging studies:
  - Transrectal sonography is a sensitive test to detect prostate cancer. Carcinomas appear as hypoechoic densities in the peripheral zone.
  - MRI or CT may also be helpful in defining the extent of the tumor but is used with less frequency.
- Biopsy: Essential in establishing the diagnosis of prostate cancer. It should be done when an abnormality is detected on rectal exam or elevation of PSA level, and/or when lower urinary symptoms occur in men without known causes of obstruction.

STAGING

- Metastatic spread occurs via:
  - Direct extension

Typical scenario: An 87-year-old man with a history of prostate cancer presents with low back pain. *Think:* Bony metastases and possibly cord compression.

- Lymphatics
- Hematogenous
- Direct extension can occur upward into the seminal vesicles and bladder floor.
- Lymphatic spread is to obturator, internal iliac, common iliac, presacral, and periaortic nodes.
- Hematogenous spread occurs to bone more frequently than viscera.

Standard staging scheme used is the **Whitmore.**
- **Stage A:** Cancer not detectable by physical exam but incidentally on surgical specimen.
- **Stage B:** Palpable but confined to the prostate.
  - **B1:** Involves only a single nodule surrounded by normal tissue.
  - **B2:** Involves the gland more diffusely.
- **Stage C:** Palpable tumor extends beyond the prostate but no distant metastasis.
- **Stage D:** Distant metastases are present.
  - **D1:** To pelvic nodes only
  - **D2:** Widespread metastasis

Bony metastasis can contain both osteoblastic and osteolytic components. Pelvis and lumbar vertebrae are most commonly affected. Skeletal survey has a low sensitivity for detecting bony metastasis. Radionuclide bone scan has a much higher sensitivity and is also useful in monitoring progression and response to therapy.

To assess lymph node involvement, either lymphangiography or pelvic CT can be employed. Alternatively, operative staging may be employed.

TREATMENT

- **Radical prostatectomy:**
  - Most clearly indicated in Stage B disease. In men with 1- to 2-cm nodules involving only one lobe of the prostate, this group has the highest cure rate.
  - Not indicated in most Stage A1 disease since the disease is usually cured definitively by the simple prostatectomy at which the diagnosis is made.
  - For locally advanced disease, the effectiveness of surgery is uncertain. With the renewed interest in androgen ablation therapy, there may be a role for radical prostatectomy in advanced disease.
  - There is a definite role for surgery in reducing morbidity such as bladder outlet obstruction, hematuria, and ureteral obstruction.
- **Radiation:**
  - For Stage A and B disease: 50% survival in 10 years
  - For Stage C disease: 30% survival in 10 years
  - For stage D disease: 55% survival in 5 years
- **Androgen deprivation:**
  - Since growth of the normal prostate is dependent on testicular androgens, deprivation of androgens would arrest the development of prostate cancer. Androgen deprivation can be achieved via:
    - Surgical castration (bilateral orchiectomy results in 90% reduction in testosterone)
    - Luteinizing hormone–releasing hormone (LHRH) analogue therapy
    - Estrogen administration

Each of the aforementioned therapies still leaves a small amount of circulating androgen. To achieve androgen depletion beyond the level of surgical castration, adrenalectomy is needed. This can be achieved by antiandrogen drugs (e.g., flutamide). Various clinical trials comparing the different combinations of androgen ablation therapy has yielded inconsistent results. However, the current trend is to treat advanced disease with combination androgen ablation therapy.

RENAL CELL CARCINOMA

ETIOLOGY

- Eighty-five percent of all primary renal neoplasms.
- Peak incidence between 55 and 60 years.
- Male-to-female ratio is 2:1.
- Environmental factors:
  - Cigarette smoking
  - Exposure to cadmium
- Hereditary link: Genetic defect linked to translocations between chromosome 3 and 8, and 3 and 11

SIGNS AND SYMPTOMS

- Classic triad (seen in < 10% of cases)
  - Gross hematuria
  - Flank pain
  - Palpable abdominal mass
- The most common presenting abnormality is **hematuria.**
- Most often diagnosed via its systemic symptoms:
  - Fatigability
  - Weight loss and cachexia
  - Intermittent fever
  - Anemia
- Other symptoms may relate to the production of hormones and hormone-like substances:
  - Hypercalcemia (parathyroid hormone)
  - Galactorrhea (prolactin)
  - Cushing syndrome (glucocorticoid)

DIAGNOSIS

- IVP with nephrotomography is the primary method for evaluating renal masses.
- It is most important to differentiate cystic from solid lesions.
- Ultrasound has improved the ability to differentiate a solid from a cystic lesion.
- In combination, ultrasound and IVP approach 97% accuracy in diagnosing a benign cyst. If the diagnosis of benign cyst is questionable on ultrasound, a CT scan should be done.
- CT is the method of choice for diagnosis and staging of renal cell carcinoma.

STAGING

- **Stage I:** Tumor confined within the kidney capsule
- **Stage II:** Invasion through the kidney capsule but confined within the Gerota's fascia

- **Stage III:** Involvement of regional lymph nodes, ipsilateral renal vein, or vena cava
- **Stage IV:** Distant metastasis

TREATMENT

- Radical nephrectomy is the treatment of choice if there is no evidence of metastasis.
- There are no standard chemotherapeutic regimens or hormonal therapy for metastatic disease, and have been employed with limited success.

PROGNOSIS

Five-year survival rates:
- Stage I: 60–75%
- Stage II: 45–65%
- Stage III: 25–50% (without regional node involvement); 5–15% (with regional node involvement)
- Stage IV: < 5%

BLADDER CANCER

DEFINITION AND EPIDEMIOLOGY

- Approximately 50,000 cases of bladder cancer are diagnosed annually.
- Men are affected 3 times more than women.
- Peak incidence occurs between the ages of 60 and 70.

The lining of the urinary system from the renal pelvis to the urethra is made up of transitional cells. This entire lining is subject to carcinomatous changes. However, the bladder is involved most frequently.

Squamous cell and adenocarcinomas have a worse prognosis compared to transitional cell carcinoma.

RISK FACTORS

- Environmental:
  - Cigarette smoking
  - Workers in dye or chemical industries
- Chronic UTI
- Recurrent nephrolithiasis

SIGNS AND SYMPTOMS

- Gross and microscopic hematuria are the most common complaints.
- Dysuria.
- Urinary frequency.
- Urgency.
- Ureteral obstruction.

DIAGNOSIS AND STAGING

- Urine cytology
- IVP—ureteral obstruction with hydronephrosis or filling defect
- Cystoscopy with tumor biopsy

Additional staging may be obtained via CT of abdomen and pelvis and endoscopic resection of a bladder neoplasm.

Superficial
Stage 0: Carcinoma in situ, mucosal involvement
Stage A: Submucosal involvement

Invasive
Stage B: Involvement of bladder muscularis
Stage C: Involvement of perivesical fat

Metastatic
Stage D1: Metastasis to lymph nodes
Stage D2: Metastasis to bone or other viscera

TREATMENT

- Superficial carcinoma can be treated with endoscopic resection with repeat cystoscopy every 3 to 6 months. However, 50–70% of these patients will have superficial recurrence within 3 years. These patients can be treated with:
  - Intravesical therapeutic agents, the most effective of which is BCG (bacillus Calmette–Guérin).
  - Laser therapy.
- Approximately 10% of those with initially superficial disease will develop invasive disease.
  - Mainstay of treatment is simple or radical cystectomy.
  - Five-year survival is about 50% with such treatment.
  - Majority of patients die of metastatic disease rather than local recurrence.
- In patients with metastatic disease, chemotherapy has shown good result; however, it is short lasting. Chemotherapuetic agents used are:
  - Cisplatin
  - Methotrexate
  - Doxorubicin
  - Cyclophosphamide
  - Vinblastine

PROGNOSIS

- The survival rate of patients with metastatic disease is generally < 2 years.

Orthopedics

SPRAINS

- Occur due to microfailure of collagen fibers when ligaments are subjected to stress which exceed their physiologic capacity

SEVERITY OF LIGAMENT INJURY

- **First-degree sprain:** Minimal pain, no detectable joint instability.
  - Treat symptomatically and return to full activity within a few days.
- **Second-degree sprain:** Severe pain, minimal joint instability, and progressive failure of collagen fibers. Partial ligament rupture, 50% decrease in ligament strength and stiffness.
  - Treated with rehabilitative exercise, brace for support and avoidance of physical activity.
- **Third-degree sprain:** Severe pain during course of injury and minimal pain afterward, joint is completely unstable. Ligament may appear continuous since a few collagen fibers are still intact, but cannot support any load—putting load results in high stress on the articular cartilage.
  - Treated surgically unless there is a specific contraindication.

STRAINS

- Injury to muscle or its tendinous attachment to the bone as a result of excessive stretching or violent contraction
- Occurs when a nonconditioned muscle is overstressed

Severity of Injury

- **First-degree strain:** Minor tearing of the musculotendinous fibers with slight loss of function, swelling, and local tenderness.
  - Treat with few days of rest, application of ice, and frequent analgesics.
- **Second-degree strain:** More tearing of fibers with marked loss of strength, swelling, and ecchymosis.
  - Treated similarly as first-degree strain along with avoiding aggravating activity.

- **Third-degree strain:** Muscle or tendon is totally interrupted resulting in muscle–muscle, muscle–tendon, or tendon–bone separation.
  - Initially treated with rest, ice, analgesia, and elevation and immobilization. Surgical intervention depends on patient's age, occupation, activity level, and muscle affected.

SPLINTING

DEFINITION

Method of short-term immobilization of fractures, dislocations, and soft-tissue injuries.

MATERIALS

Plaster or fiberglass.

INDICATIONS

- Fractures and sprains
- Acute arthritis
- Contusions and abrasions
- Skin laceration that crosses joint
- Lacerated tendons
- Tenosynovitis
- Puncture wounds
- Animal bites
- Deep space and joint infections

ADVANTAGES

Prevents further soft-tissue injury, prevents closed fractures from becoming open, relieves pain, lowers incidence of clinical fat embolism and shock, reduces risk of ischemic injury, facilitates patient transportation and radiographic studies, and allows patient to temporarily remove it for bathing, wound care, and exercising the injured part.

DISADVANTAGES

Not as stable as a circular cast and loosens rapidly with time.

COMPLICATIONS

- *Ischemia:* Can lead to a compartment syndrome and to Volkmann's ischemic contracture.
- *Heat injury:* Drying plaster can cause second-degree burns. Patients with vascular insufficiency and sensory deficits are high risk for plaster burns.
- *Others:* Pressure sores, infection, dermatitis, joint stiffness.

FRACTURES

- Categorized by anatomical location (proximal or middle third of shaft), direction of fracture line (transverse, oblique, spiral), and whether it's linear or comminuted.

- Patient presents with loss of function, pain, tenderness, swelling, abnormal motion, and often deformity.

Open Fractures

- Fracture communicates with the external environment due to a breach of the overlying soft tissue.
- **True orthopedic emergency:** Almost always results in bacterial contamination of soft tissues and bone.
- Prognosis dependent on extent of soft-tissue injury and by type/level of bacterial contamination.
- Treatment plan: Prevent infection, restore soft tissues, achieve bone union, avoid malunion, and institute early joint motion and muscle rehabilitation.

Pathologic Fracture

- Occurs due to minimal trauma on a bone weakened by preexisting disease.
- *Predisposing conditions:* Primary or metastatic carcinoma, cysts, enchondroma, giant cell tumors, osteomalacia, osteogenesis imperfecta, scurvy, rickets, and Paget's disease.
- Orthopedic surgeon must not only treat the broken bone but should also diagnose and treat the underlying condition.

Stress or Fatigue Fracture

- A complete fracture resulting from repetitive application of minor trauma.
- Most stress fractures occur in the lower extremities and commonly affect individuals involved in sports and military recruits ("march fracture").
- Pathophysiology of stress fractures is unclear but possibly due to inability of the fatigued muscle to protect bone from strain.
- If the patient is seen within first 2 weeks of onset of symptoms, the plain radiograph is likely to be normal.
- Patients usually complain of pain only with activity.
- Treatment: Decrease physical activity.

Comminuted Fracture

- Fracture in which the bone is divided into more than two fragments by fracture lines.

SALTER–HARRIS FRACTURE

- Fracture involving the physis. Occur irregularly through the weak zone of hypertrophic cartilage (Figure 28-1).
- *Salter–Harris Types I and II:* Fracture is transverse and does not travel vertically across the germinal cell layer. Prognosis for normal healing is good.
- *Salter–Harris Types III and IV:* Fracture traverses the growth plate in a vertical fashion often causing angular deformity from continued growth. Surgical intervention necessary.
- *Salter–Harris Type V:* Crush injury to the physis such that metaphysis and epiphysis are impacted on one another. No visible fracture line. Poor prognosis with high risk of growth plate arrest.

Osteoporosis is the most common pathologic condition associated with pathologic fractures.

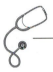

Suspect violence or battering if fracture occurs on normal bone and history reveals trivial trauma.

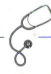

Incidence of stress fractures by site:
Metatarsals: > 50% stress fractures
Calcaneus: 25%
Tibia: ~20%
Tarsal navicular: Basketball players

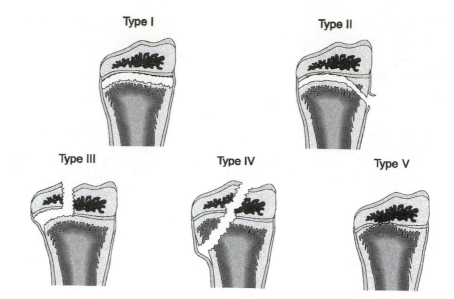

FIGURE 28-1. Salter Harris classification of fractures. (Reproduced, with permission, Stead L: BRS Emergency Medicine. Copyright ©2001 Lippincott Williams & Wilkins.)

Greenstick Fracture

- An incomplete and angulated fracture of the long bones. A transverse crack that hangs on to its connection.
- Very common in children, rarely seen in adults.
- Since kids have "softer" less brittle bone and thicker (leathery) periosteal membrane, they get incomplete fractures with unique patterns.

TORUS FRACTURE

- An incomplete fracture characterized by buckling or wrinkling of cortex due to compression.
- Typically occurs in the metaphyseal areas in children, especially at the distal radius.
- Heals in 2 to 3 weeks with simple immobilization.

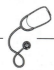

Greenstick fracture: Think of a young, moist twig, which would break without snapping apart!

Torus fracture: In Greek architecture, a torus is a bump at the base of a column, which is what the fracture looks like at the end of long bones.

FAT EMBOLISM SYNDROME

DEFINITION

An acute respiratory distress syndrome caused by release of fat droplets from the marrow as may occur following a long bone fracture.

CAUSES

- Long bone fracture
- Hemoglobinopathy
- Collagen disease
- Diabetes
- Burns
- Severe infection
- Inhalation anesthesia
- Metabolic disorders
- Neoplasms

- Osteomyelitis
- Blood transfusion
- Cardiopulmonary bypass
- Renal infarction
- Decompression sickness
- Renal homotransplantations

PATHOPHYSIOLOGY

- Microdroplets of fat are released into the circulation at the site of fracture, occluding pulmonary circulation causing ischemic and hemorrhagic changes.
- Another theory: Release of free fatty acids from the marrow have toxic effects in all tissues, especially the lung.

SIGNS AND SYMPTOMS

- Symptoms may occur immediately or 2 to 3 days after trauma.
- Shortness of breath with respiratory rate above 30.
- Confusion, restlessness, disorientation, stupor, or coma.
- Fleeting petechial rash on chest, axilla, neck, and conjunctiva.
- Fever, tachycardia.

DIAGNOSIS

- *Hallmark finding:* Arterial hypoxemia. Arterial PO_2 < 60 mm Hg is suggestive.
- Chest x-ray: Progressive snowstorm-like infiltration.
- Cryostat—frozen section of clotted blood reveals presence of fat.
- Absence of fat globules in urine makes diagnosis unlikely; however, their presence is not specific for fat embolism.

TREATMENT

- Administer oxygen to decrease hypoxemia and monitor PO_2 to maintain it over 90 mm Hg.
- In severe hypoxemia: Mechanical ventilatory support.
- Use of ethanol, heparin, hypertonic glucose, or steroids has been suggested but their effectiveness is questionable.
- Prevent fat embolism syndrome by careful stabilization of fractures and effective treatment of shock.

PROGNOSIS

- Mortality from fat embolism thought to be as high as 50% following multiple fractures

Classic triad for fat embolism:
- Confusion
- Dyspnea
- Petechiae

Typical scenario: A 25-year-old male complains of difficulty breathing. His family notes he is acting a little confused, and that he has a spotty purplish rash. Two days ago, he sustained a femur fracture after a high-speed motor vehicle collison. *Think:* Fat embolism syndrome.

	Anterior Dislocation	Posterior Dislocation	Inferior Dislocation (Luxatio Erecta)
Features	High risk of recurrence 70% occur in patients younger than 30 years of age	Diagnosis missed in 60% of cases Often precipitated by a convulsion, seizure, electrical shock, and falls	< 1% of all shoulder dislocations
Types	Subcoracoid (most common), subclavicular, subglenoid	Subacromial (most common), subglenoid, subspinous	
Mechanism of injury	Abduction and external rotation of the arm causes strain on anterior capsule and glenohumeral ligaments	Internal rotation and adduction (when one falls on an arm that is forwardly flexed and internally rotated)	Hyperabduction always results in detachment of rotator cuff
Signs and symptoms	■ Arms held to the side ■ Patient resists medial rotation and adduction ■ Prominent acromion ■ Loss of normal rounded shoulder contour	■ Patient holds arm medially rotated and to the side ■ Abduction limited ■ External rotation limited ■ Prominence of the coracoid process and posterior part of shoulder ■ Flattening of anterior aspect of shoulder	■ Patient in severe pain ■ Arm held in 180° elevation ■ Arm appears shorter compared to opposite side ■ Humeral head often felt along the lateral chest wall

COMPLICATIONS COMMON TO ALL DISLOCATIONS

Axillary artery injury (more common with luxatio erecta), venous injury, injury to nerves of brachial plexus (most common being axillary nerve):
- Palpate radial pulse to check axillary artery.
- Check motor component of axillary nerve by assessing strength of the deltoid muscle.
- Check sensory component of axillary nerve by assessing sensation over the lateral part of upper arm.
- Do a neurologic exam to evaluate all brachial nerve lesions.

COMPLICATIONS SPECIFIC TO TYPE OF DISLOCATION

Anterior Dislocation	Posterior Dislocation	Inferior Dislocation
■ Rotator cuff tear ■ Glenoid labral lesions ■ Coracoid fractures ■ Greater tuberosity fractures (seems to decrease recurrence) ■ Hill–Sachs deformity (compression fracture of humeral head)	■ Fractures of the lesser tuberosity ■ Fractures of posterior glenoid rim and proximal humerus	■ Rotator cuff tear ■ Fractures of greater tuberosity

RADIOGRAPH

Anterior Dislocation	Posterior Dislocation	Inferior Dislocation
■ Obtain anterior, posterior, and axillary views ■ Look for Hill–Sachs deformity in the posterolateral portion of humeral head (occurs in 50%)	■ Look for loss of the normal elliptical pattern produced by the overlap of humeral head and posterior glenoid rim ■ Look for the greater tuberosity rotated internally	■ Top of humerus is displaced downward

TREATMENT

Anterior Dislocation	Posterior Dislocation	Inferior Dislocation
■ Reduction (Hennipen technique, Stimson technique, traction and countertraction and lateral traction) ■ Immobilize shoulder ■ Surgery if needed	■ Apply longitudinal traction (Stimson technique) ■ Surgery if needed, although neurovascular complications are rare	■ Rotate arm inferiorly while applying traction longitudinally along the humerus with countertraction in the supraclavicular region ■ Surgical repair of rotator cuff

DEFINITION

- A group of conditions in which increased pressure within a limited space compromises the circulation and function of tissues within that closed space
- Theories of tissue ischemia:
  - Arterial spasms due to increased pressure.
  - Increased pressure leads to decreased transmural pressure, causing arterioles to close.
  - A decrease in arteriovenous gradient for flow due to collapse of veins.

CAUSES

- Fractures
- Soft-tissue crush injuries
- Vascular injuries
- Drug overdose with prolonged limb compression
- Burn injuries
- Trauma
- Muscle hypertrophy and nephrotic syndrome

SIGNS AND SYMPTOMS

- Clinical presentation often indefinite and confusing.
- Hallmark finding: Pain in a conscious and fully oriented person that is out of proportion to injury or findings.
- **Pain:** Deep, unremitting, and poorly localized. Pain increases with passive stretching of involved muscle.
- **Pallor:** Not necessary for diagnosis, may not be present.
- **Paresthesias:** Of cutaneous distribution supplied by the compressed nerve is an early sign.
- **Paralysis:** Occurs after ischemia is well established.
- **Pulselessness:** Shown to occur late at times. Pulse may be present.
- Compartment may get tense on palpation.

DIAGNOSIS

- Measure pressure within compartment with commercially available monitors.
- Pressure < 30 mm Hg will not produce a compartment syndrome.
- Pressure > 30 mm Hg is an indication for fasciotomy.

TREATMENT

Complete fasciotomy: Goal is to decompress all tight compartments and salvage a viable extremity.

VOLKMANN'S ISCHEMIC CONTRACTURE

- A consequence of untreated or inadequately treated compartment syndrome involving the forearm.
- Due to fibrous replacement of necrotic muscle tissue.
- Has different degrees of tissue injury, with flexor digitorum involvement being the earliest.
- Early warning symptom: Deep, persistent pain in the forearm along with pallor and paresthesias distally.

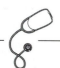

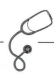

DO NOT DELAY treatment of compartment syndrome! Elevation of pressure to > 30 mm Hg for more than 8 hours leads to irreversible tissue death.

Most common etiology for Volkman's ischemis contracture: Compression of anterior aspect of elbow and upper forearm after a supracondylar fracture in childhood.

HIGH-YIELD FACTS

Orthopedics

- Diagnose by estimating intracompartmental pressure with needling, use of Doppler stethoscope, and arteriography.
- Urgent treatment: Remove constricting cast and fasciotomy.

OSTEOMYELITIS

Acute

EPIDEMIOLOGY

Mainly affects children.

PATHOPHYSIOLOGY

- Bacteria lodge in end artery of metaphysis and multiply.
- Local increase in serum and white blood cells (WBCs).
- Decrease in blood flow and pressure necrosis.
- Pus moves to haversian and medullary canals.
- Goes beneath the periosteum.

CAUSE

- Route of infection is mainly hematogenous, rarely trauma.
- Most cases of acute hematogenous osteomyelitis caused by *Staphylococcus aureus*.

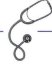

Most common site for acute osteomyelitis is the metaphyseal end of a single long bone (especially around the knee).

SIGNS AND SYMPTOMS

- History of infection (e.g., skin or throat) or trauma
- Significant pain in the affected area, anorexia, fever, irritability, nausea, malaise, rapid pulse
- Limited joint motion, tenderness, swelling of soft tissue, and guarding apparent on physical exam

DIAGNOSIS

- Elevated WBC, erythrocyte sedimentation rate (ESR), and C-reactive protein; ± anemia
- Deep circumferential soft-tissue swelling with obliteration of muscular planes

DIFFERENTIAL DIAGNOSIS

- *Septic arthritis:* Swelling and tenderness directly on the joint with intense pain on joint movement, high WBC, and positive culture.
- *Rheumatic fever:* More insidious onset, less local and constitutional symptoms.
- *Ewing's sarcoma:* Early symptoms are more insidious and less intense and present with bone destruction.

TREATMENT

- Medical: Infection must be diagnosed early. Intravenous antibiotics (usually oxacillin or cloxacillin 8 to 16 g adult) started soon after obtaining specimen for culture. Monitor temperature, swelling, pain, WBC, and joint mobility.

- Surgical: Open drainage of abscess if antibiotics fail or signs of abscess appear. After surgical drainage, wound is left open to heal by secondary intention.

Chronic

EPIDEMIOLOGY

Often seen in lower extremities of a diabetic patient.

PATHOPHYSIOLOGY

- Untreated acute osteomyelitis results in a cavity walled off by an involucrum containing granulation tissue, sequestrum, and bacteria.
- Drainage of pus into surrounding soft tissue and skin via sinus tracts.
- Persistent drainage can lead to carcinoma.
- Bone fragments and exudates unreachable by antibiotics.
- Result is severely deformed bone and pathologic fracture.

CAUSE

- Usually an end result of untreated or treatment failed acute osteomyelitis. Occasionally due to trauma or surgery.
- Cause is usually polymicrobial—difficult to eradicate.

SIGNS AND SYMPTOMS

- Characterized by persistent drainage following an episode of acute osteomyelitis or onset of inflammation and cellulitis following an open fracture.
- Fever, pain, mild systemic symptoms, tenderness.
- Easy to diagnose when drainage is present and x-ray shows bone destruction and deformity. In cases with absence of drainage, radionuclide imaging studies very helpful.

DIAGNOSIS

Radiographic findings:
- Areas of radiolucency within an irregular sclerotic bone.
- Irregular areas of destruction present. Often periosteal thickening can be seen.

DIFFERENTIAL DIAGNOSIS

- Acute suppurative arthritis.
- Rheumatic fever: Examine synovial fluid.
- Cellulitis: Absence of soft-tissue swelling on radiographs.

TREATMENT

- Varies from open drainage of abscess or sequestrectomy to amputation
- Most effective: Extensive debridement of all necrotic and granulation tissue along with reconstruction of bone and soft-tissue defects with concomitant antibiotics
- Excellent adjunct: Temporary placement of polymethylmethacrylate beads in the wound for a depot administration of antibiotics

COMPLICATIONS

- Soft-tissue abscess
- Septic arthritis due to extension to adjacent joint
- Metastatic infections to other areas
- Pathologic fractures
- If significant spinal involvement, paraplegia

BRODIE'S ABSCESS

- Subacute pyogenic osteomyelitis in the metaphysis
- Roentgenographic finding: Lucent lesions surrounded by sclerotic bone
- Usually caused by *Staphylococcus aureus* and *S. albus*

SEPTIC BURSITIS

- Infection of the superficial bursa commonly affecting the bunion, olecranon, and prepatellar bursa.
- Most common offending organism is *S. aureus*.
- Clinically presents with painful bursal swelling, often along with intense cellulitis. Systemic signs of sepsis often present along with regional lymphadenopathy.
- Treatment: Aspirate bursa for culture and sensitivity. Give broad-spectrum antibiotic. Take care not to aspirate the joint since passing the needle through the area of cellulitis might spread it to the joint!

LOW BACK PAIN

EPIDEMIOLOGY

- Four out of five people suffer from low back pain sometime in life.
- Incidence 15–20%, males > females.
- Most patients with low back pain have no systemic disorder.
- Often, back pain is a symptom of a systemic illness such as primary or metastatic neoplasm, infectious disease, or an inflammatory disorder.

Low back pain is the leading cause of an orthopedic visit.

HISTORY

- Very important, although often the only presenting complaint is pain that is poorly localized.
- Character of pain needs to be described: *What is the pain like? Does it radiate? When does it occur? How does it interfere with sitting, standing, walking? What factors make the pain better or worse? How many episodes have you had? Any other symptoms along with back pain?*
- Give patient a diagram and ask patient to mark areas of pain.
- History of pain development and how it affects everyday life.
- History of weight loss, malaise, fever, gastrointestinal (GI) or genitourinary (GU) illnesses.
- Psychological assessment in patients with chronic pain.

PHYSICAL EXAMINATION

- Straight leg-raising test: Positive in nerve root irritation.
- Check for reflexes and motor and sensory deficits.
- Check presence of nonorganic signs (Waddell's signs) when patient responds to axial loading, local touch, and simulated rotation.
- Check spine for range of motion.
- Bowel and bladder symptoms are suggestive of cauda equina syndrome.
- Leg and buttock pain are suggestive of herniated disk.

DIAGNOSIS

- X-rays of lumbar spine especially if patient is over 50 years of age and has history of other medical illnesses or trauma.
- Magnetic resonance imaging (MRI) of the lumbar spine if x-rays are negative: Great for assessing neural tissue.
- Computed tomography (CT) scan if MRI not helpful.
- Technetium bone scan and gallium scan can be done if an infection of the spine is suspected.

TREATMENT

- Rule out a serious pathologic condition.
- Goal is early return to normal activities.
- Patients with acute low back pain should avoid sitting or lifting and use mild analgesics and anti-inflammatory drugs.
- Physical and occupational therapy programs prove to be helpful.
- Antidepressants often help those with pain persistent for 3 months.
- Other questionable treatments: Transcutaneous electrical nerve stimulation (TENS), traction, manipulation with radicular signs, biofeedback, acupuncture, trigger point injections, and muscle relaxants.

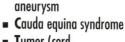

Emergency causes of low back pain: FACTOID
- **F**racture
- **A**bdominal aortic aneurysm
- **C**auda equina syndrome
- **T**umor (cord compression)
- **O**ther (osteoarthritis [OA], severe musculoskeletal pain, other neurological syndromes)
- **I**nfection (e.g., epidural abscess)
- **D**isk herniation/rupture

BONE TUMORS

- Occur due to uncontrolled cellular proliferation of a single clone of cells whose regulatory mechanisms are defective.
- Benign tumors are 200 times more likely to occur than malignant ones.
- A careful history and physical is very crucial and will reveal the duration of the mass, onset of pain, other associated symptoms, and the chronological sequence of these symptoms.
- A thorough physical exam consists of evaluation of patient's general health status. The mass should be noted for size, location, consistency, mobility, tenderness, local temperature, and change with position. Note any muscular atrophy.

RADIOGRAPHY FOR BONE TUMORS

- Never diagnose a bone tumor without an x-ray (best way to judge whether biopsy samples are truly from the lesion).
- Bone reacts to a benign or malignant tumor by bone production or destruction.
- An x-ray appearance shows a combination of bone production and bone destruction.

- Three patterns of x-ray appearance:
  - *Permeative:* Implies a rapidly spreading intramedullary tumor; tumor replaces marrow and fat.
  - *Moth eaten:* Implies a poorly circumscribed, slow-growing malignant tumor.
  - *Geographic:* Implies a well-circumscribed slow-growing tumor, therefore bone has time to react and results in sclerotic margins.

BENIGN BONE TUMORS

- Patient is usually asymptomatic, and the x-ray shows a well-defined lesion with sclerotic margins.

Osteoid Osteoma

SIGNS AND SYMPTOMS

- Most common osteoid-forming benign tumor (10%)
- Male-to-female ratio is 2:1 to 3:1, three fourths of cases between ages 5 and 25.
- Most common sites: Diaphysis of long tubular bones, especially the proximal femur.
- Local tenderness and dull aching pain that is localizable, tends to be more severe at night and relieved by nonsteroidal anti-inflammatory drugs (NSAIDs).
- Pain can radiate and mimic other diseases (sciatica if present in vertebra).

RADIOGRAPHY

Localized area of bone sclerosis with a central radiolucent nidus. Little sclerosis seen if it is present in cancellous bone.

HISTOLOGY

Usually measures < 1 cm. Circumscribed, highly vascular nidus made of fibroconnective tissue and woven bone.

STAGING

Most lesions are Stage I.

Staging for Benign Tumors
Stage I: Latent, usually asymptomatic
Stage II: Active and less well demarcated but resolve
Stage III: Aggressive lesion with extensive destruction

TREATMENT AND PROGNOSIS

Mostly treated symptomatically with aspirin or NSAIDs. If this fails, surgical intervention to remove the nidus. Prognosis is excellent.

Osteoblastoma

EPIDEMIOLOGY

- One percent of benign bone tumors. Larger than osteoid osteomas.
- Male > female, most patients between ages 10 and 35 years.
- Most common sites: Mostly axial skeleton, less common in jaw, hands, and feet. One third to one-half of cases are in the vertebral column.

SIGNS AND SYMPTOMS

Pain is the major complaint. Tenderness and swelling may be present over the lesion.

RADIOGRAPHY

Nonspecific x-ray findings, which may be interpreted as osteoid osteomas, aneurysmal bone cysts, or malignant tumors.

HISTOLOGY

Histologically similar to osteoid osteoma.

TREATMENT AND PROGNOSIS

- Vigorous curettement of the lesion. Prognosis is generally good except occasionally can become locally aggressive or recur locally if they are not adequately excised.
- Have potential to undergo malignant transformation and metastasize.

OSTEOCHONDROMA

- An outgrowth of bone capped by cartilage.
- Most common benign tumor of the bone (45%) with most patients in their first two decades of life.
- Usually solitary. Originates in childhood from growing epiphyseal cartilage plate. Mostly Stage I lesions.
- Most common sites: Metaphysis of long bones of extremities; rarely in flat bones, vertebrae, or clavicle.

SIGNS AND SYMPTOMS

May be asymptomatic; patient may complain of pain, mass, or impingement syndromes.

RADIOGRAPHY

Shows a mushroom-like bony prominence.

HISTOLOGY

Trabecular, cancellous bone continuous with the marrow cavity and covered by hyaline cartilage cap.

Multiple hereditary osteochondroma is an autosomal dominant disorder in which multiple bones have osteochondromas (1% risk of malignant transformation).

TREATMENT AND PROGNOSIS

- Surgical excision if the patient complains of pain or if it enlarges after puberty
- Rarely undergo malignant transformation to chondrosarcoma (< 1%)

ENCHONDROMA

- Neoplasm consisting of mature hyaline cartilage (chondroma).
- A centrally located chondroma. Can be single or multiple.
- ~10% of benign tumors. Peak incidence in ages 20 to 50 years.
- Most common sites: Tubular bones of hands and feet.
- Chondromas can arise close to cortex or periosteum (ecchondroma) or in relation with synovium, tendons, or joints (synovial chondroma).
- Stage I or Stage II lesions.

SIGNS AND SYMPTOMS

Asymptomatic until a pathologic fracture brings attention to it

RADIOGRAPHY

Geographic lysis in a well-circumscribed area with spotty calcifications.

HISTOLOGY

- Consists of hyaline cartilage often with active nuclei. Interpretation depends on size, location, and growth.

TREATMENT AND PROGNOSIS

- No treatment if patient is asymptomatic. If pathologic fracture occurs, then allow fracture to heal. Perform a simple excision and bone grafting procedure.

GIANT CELL TUMOR

- Thought to arise from mesenchymal stromal cells supporting the bone marrow
- Five to 10% of benign bone tumors. Peak incidence in 30s.
- Female-to-male ratio is 3:2.
- Most common sites: Around the knee (distal femur, proximal tibia), distal radius, and sacrum.
- Mostly, Stage II or III lesions

SIGNS AND SYMPTOMS

- Pain, swelling, and local tenderness; often presents with arthritis or joint effusions due to proximity to the joint
- May also present with a pathologic fracture

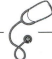

Ollier's disease:
Enchondromas in multiple bones. More likely for malignant transformation. Can result in bowing and shortening of long bones.

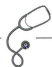

Factors that predispose to malignancy:
- Size (> 4.5 cm)
- Location (long and axial bones)
- Growth (active and painful)

HIGH-YIELD FACTS

Orthopedics

RADIOGRAPHY

- A radiolucent lesion occupying the epiphysis and extending into the metaphysis; asymmetrical with bone destruction
- Occasional "soap bubble" appearance due to a thin subperiosteal bone shell

HISTOLOGY

Abundant mononuclear stromal cells interspersed with a lot of giant cells with numerous nuclei.

TREATMENT AND PROGNOSIS

- Curettage and bone grafting (recurrence rate > 50%)
- Aggressive curettage with adjuvant phenol, hydrogen peroxide, or liquid nitrogen (recurrence rate 10–25%)
- Important to obtain chest x-ray every 6 months for 2 to 3 years for monitoring
- Often recurs after incomplete removal

MALIGNANT TUMORS

Metastatic tumors are much more common than primary tumors.

Osteosarcoma

Osteosarcoma can occur secondary to Paget's disease.

- Tumor made of a malignant spindle cell stroma producing osteoid
- Many subtypes of osteoid forming sarcomas
- Peak incidence in ages between 10 and 30 years, male > female
- Most common sites: Around the knee (distal femur, proximal tibia), proximal humerus, rarely mandible

SIGNS AND SYMPTOMS

- Pain associated with a tender mass.
- Dilated veins may be visible on the skin over the mass.
- Constitutional symptoms may be present.

RADIOGRAPHY

- X-ray shows a poorly defined lesion in the metaphysis with areas of bone destruction and formation.
- *Codman's triangle:* Due to new bone formation under the corners of the raised periosteum.
- *Sun-ray appearance:* Occurs when the bone spicules are formed perpendicular to the surface of the bone.

HISTOLOGY

Spindle-shaped tumors cells with odd, hyperchromatic nuclei showing a high mitotic rate. Giant cells may be present.
- High-dose methotrexate, doxorubicin, cisplatin, and ifosfamide along with surgical intervention.
- Tumors hematogenously metastasize to the lung.

- Surgery plus chemotherapy: Five-year survival is about 60%.
- Better prognosis if the tumor is in a small bone.

Chondrosarcoma

- Low-grade malignant tumor that derives from cartilage cells
- 7–12% of primary bone tumors; male > female
- Peak incidence between ages 30 and 60 years
- Most common sites: Pelvis, femur, flat bones, proximal humerus, scapula, upper tibia, and fibula

SIGNS AND SYMPTOMS

Pain and swelling over months or years.

RADIOGRAPHY

- Central chondrosarcomas show well-defined radiolucent areas with small, irregular calcifications to ill-defined areas breaking through the cortex.
- Peripheral chondrosarcomas look like large, lobulated masses hanging from the surface of a long bone with calcification.

HISTOLOGY

Varies from well-differentiated hyaline cartilage with little nuclear atypia to highly anaplastic spindle cell tumor with little cartilaginous differentiation.

TREATMENT AND PROGNOSIS

- Surgical resection of the tumor
- *Do not* respond to radiation or chemotherapy.
- Prognosis better than osteosarcoma since chondrosarcoma grows slowly and metastasizes late

Ewing's Tumor

- Tumor of small round cells arising in the medullary cavity
- 7% of primary bone tumors
- 90% of cases between ages 5 and 25 years; male > female
- Most common sites: Diaphysis or metaphysis of long bones, pelvis, and scapula; potential to occur anywhere in the body

SIGNS AND SYMPTOMS

- Pain that increases with time and is more severe at night
- Local swelling and a tender mass
- Malaise, fever, leukocytosis, mild anemia, increased ESR
- Often mimic subacute osteomyelitis, syphlitic osteoperiostitis, or other tumors

RADIOGRAPHY

- Shows lytic bone lesions with a permeative pattern.
- Elevations and permeations of the periosteum give rise to lamellated "onion skin" appearance.

Ewing's sarcoma is the most lethal of all bone tumors.

Ewing's sarcoma usually occurs after age 5. If patient < 5 years of age, *think* metastatic neuroblastoma instead.

HISTOLOGY

Area contains densely packed small round cells containing glycogen with little intercellular stroma arranged in sheets, cords, or nests.

TREATMENT AND PROGNOSIS

- Vincristine, cyclophosphamide, actinomycin D, and adriamycin along with surgery.
- Advanced metastatic disease: Five-year survival is 30%.
- Surgically resectable lesion treated with drugs and surgery has a 70% chance of 5-year survival.
- Males have worse prognosis.

Multiple Myeloma

- A malignant plasma cell tumor with multiple site involvement
- Most common primary malignant tumor of the bone (45%)
- 90% of cases in patients over the age of 40 years; male > female
- Most common sites: Vertebral column, ribs, skull, pelvis, femur, clavicle and scapula; can occur anywhere in the body

SIGNS AND SYMPTOMS

- Bone pain
- Weight loss, weakness, neurologic impairment if pathologic fractures in the vertebrae present
- Pathologic fractures or deformities
- Susceptibility to infections
- Amyloidosis
- Kidney damage due to protein plugging of renal tubules

LABS

- Increased serum calcium due to bone reabsorption
- Elevated uric acid due to increased cell turnover
- Monoclonal gammopathy, Bence Jones proteinuria, increased ESR, and rouleaux formation
- Anemia due to marrow suppression

RADIOGRAPHY

Classically shows sharply punched out lesions giving a soap-bubble appearance or often shows diffuse demineralization

HISTOLOGY

Marrow aspirate shows larger-than-normal plasma cells with many nuclei, a nucleoli, and showing mitotic activity.

TREATMENT AND PROGNOSIS

- Chemotherapy with Melphalan, often with prednisone.
- Biphosphonates and other bone absorption–reducing agents help in reducing pathologic fractures.
- Untreated cases rarely survive more than 6 to 12 months.
- Chemotherapy induces remission in about 50–70% of cases.
- Poor prognosis with 90% of patients dying within 2 to 3 years

Classic triad for multiple myeloma: **PAM**
- **"Punched out" lytic lesions**
- **Atypical plasma cells**
- **Monoclonal gammopathy**

Two percent of myeloma cases will present with **POEMS:**
- **Polyneuropathy**
- **Organomegaly**
- **Endocrinopathy**
- **M-component spike**
- **Skin changes and Sclerosis of bone**

- Metastatic tumors comprise 95%, primary bone tumors 5%.
- Spread via direct extension, lymphatics, vascular system, or intraspinal seeding.
- In children: Bone metastasis most likely from a neuroblastoma.
- Most common sites: Vertebral column, ribs, pelvis, upper ends of femur and humerus.

Most likely site of origin for metastatic tumors:

BLT with Kosher		Pickle
Breast	**Kidney**	**Prostate**
Lung		
Thyroid		

SIGNS AND SYMPTOMS

- Pain (most common symptom).
- Spine involvement: Neurologic symptoms due to pressure on nerve roots or spinal cord.
- Hypercalcemia and anemia.
- Pathologic fractures are common.
- Increased acid phosphatase in prostatic metastasis.

DIAGNOSTIC WORKUP

- Order complete blood count (CBC), ESR, liver and renal panels, alkaline phosphatase, and serum protein electrophoresis.
- Plain chest x-ray, x-ray of most commonly involved bones.
- Staging bone scan (more sensitive than x-ray).

RADIOGRAPHY

- Lesions may be multiple or solitary (kidney), well or poorly circumscribed, osteoblastic or osteolytic (majority).
- Osteoblastic: Breast and prostate.

HISTOLOGY

Generally, primary tumors produce matrix for the tumor stroma, whereas epithelial tumors form clusters in fibrous tissue.

TREATMENT AND PROGNOSIS

- Radiation as palliative treatment along with chemotherapy.
- Surgical intervention aims at relieving pain and prevents pathologic fractures.
- Radioactive iodine for thyroid carcinoma metastasis.
- Tamoxifen for metastatic carcinoma of the breast.
- Bilateral orchiectomy, estrogens or antiandrogens for metastatic prostate tumors.
- Poor prognosis with average survival time being 19 months after suffering a pathologic fracture.

The Hand

ANATOMY

Muscles

- Intrinsic muscles of the hand have their origin and insertion in the hand. See Table 29-1.
- Extrinsic muscles of the hand have their muscle bellies in the forearm and their tendon insertions in the hand. See Table 29-2.

Bones of the Hand

- There are 27 bones in the hand: 5 metacarpals, 14 phalanges, and 8 carpals.
- Each finger has one metacarpal.
- Each finger or digit has three phalanges: A proximal, middle, and distal.
- The thumb has only two phalanges: A proximal phalanx and a distal one.
- The joints between the phalanges are the metacarpophalangeal (MCP), proximal interphalangeal (PIP), and distal interphalangeal (DIP).
- The thumb has only MCP and DIP joints.
- Carpal bones (see Figure 29-1):
  - Scaphoid
  - Lunate
  - Triquetrum
  - Pisiform
  - Trapezium
  - Trapezoid
  - Capitate
  - Hamate

The wrist bones are easily remembered by the saying: **Some Lovers Try Positions That They Can't Handle.**

Nerves

- **Sensory:**
  - Radial: Sensory to lateral aspect of dorsum of hand and lateral 3.5 fingers
  - Median: Sensory to skin on lateral half of palm

The radial nerve does not innervate any of the intrinsic muscles of the hand. See Table 29-3 for clinical maneuvers to test function of the hand.

TABLE 29-1. Intrinsic muscles of the hand.

Muscle	Innervation	Function
Thenar Group		
Abductor pollicis brevis	Median	Abduction of thumb
Adductor pollicis brevis	Median	Adduction of thumb
Flexor pollicis brevis	Median	Flexes thumb MCP joint
Opponens pollicis	Ulnar (deep branch)	Opposes—pulls thumb medially and forward across palm
Remainder of Hand		
Palmar interossei	Median	▪ Adduct finger toward center of third digit ▪ Flex MCP, extend PIP and DIP
Dorsal interossei	Median	▪ Abduct finger from center of third digit ▪ Flex MCP, extend PIP and DIP
Lumbricals	First and second: Median Third and fourth: Ulnar (deep branch)	Flex MCP, extend PIP and DIP
Palmaris brevis	Ulnar (superficial branch)	Aids with hand grip
Hypothenar Group		
Abductor digiti minimi	Ulnar (deep branch)	Abducts little finger
Flexor digiti minimi	Ulnar (deep branch)	Flexes little finger
Opponens digiti minimi	Ulnar (deep branch)	Aids little finger with cupping motion of hand

- Ulnar: Sensory to skin on medial aspect of dorsum of hand, hypothenar eminence, and medial 1.5 fingers
- **Motor:** See Tables 29-1 and 29-2 for muscles innervated by the radial, median, and ulnar nerves.

Tendons

ZONES OF THE HAND

- Two main groups: Flexors and extensors.
- Extensor tendon lacerations can usually be repaired in the emergency department.
- Flexor tendons are more difficult and usually require operative repair.
- The flexor and extensor tendons are grouped into zones (see Figures 29-2 and 29-3).
- Flexor tendon injury repair timetable by zone:
  - Zones I and II: 1 to 3 weeks.
  - Zones III–V: Immediate.

TABLE 29-2. Extrinsic muscles of the hand.

Muscle	Compartment	Innervation	Function
Flexor carpi radialis	Anterior	Median	Flexes and abducts hand at wrist
Palmaris longus	Anterior	Median	Flexes hand
Flexor carpi ulnaris (humeral and ulnar heads)	Anterior	Ulnar	Flexes and aducts hand at wrist
Flexor digitorum superficialis (humeroulnar and radial heads)	Anterior	Median	■ Flexes middle phalanx ■ Assists with flexion of proximal phalanx and hand
Flexor digitorum profundis	Anterior	Median and ulnar nerves	■ Flexes distal phalanx ■ Assists in flexion of middle and proximal phalanx and wrist
Extensor carpi radialis longus	Lateral	Radial	Extends and abducts hand at wrist
Extensor carpi radialis brevis	Posterior	Radial	Extends and abducts hand at wrist
Extensor digitorum	Posterior	Radial	Extends fingers and hand
Extensor digiti minimi	Posterior	Radial	Extends little finger MCP joint
Extensor carpi ulnaris	Posterior	Radial	Extends and adducts hand at wrist
Abductor pollicis longus	Posterior	Radial	Abducts and extends thumb
Extensor pollicis longus	Posterior	Radial	Extends distal phalanx of thumb
Extensor pollicis brevis	Posterior	Radial	Extends thumb MCP joint
Extensor indici	Posterior	Radial	Extends index finger MCP joint

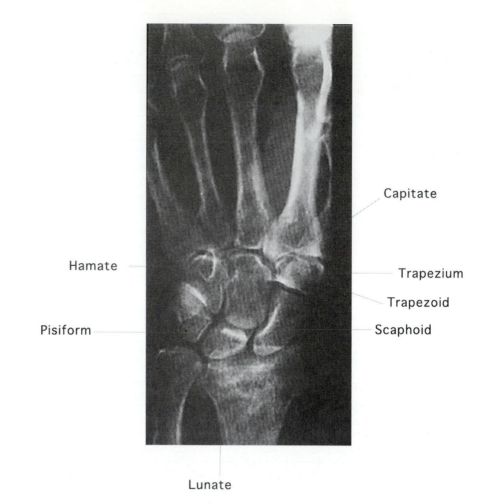

FIGURE 29-1. Bones of the wrist on AP radiograph.

A flexor tendon injury will present with a straight finger (unopposed extensors).

- Zone IV injuries are technically difficult because tendons lie within the carpal tunnel.
- Zone V tendon injuries are relatively easy to fix, but functional outcome is often poor due to associated nerve injury.

HISTORY

Focused hand history:
- Hand dominance
- Time of injury
- Status of tetanus immunization
- Occupation
- Cause and mechanism of injury

PHYSICAL EXAMINATION

See Figure 29-4.
1. Sensibility:
   - Pinprick (two-point discrimination): Normal is < 6 mm when the points are static and < 3 mm when the points are moving. Abnormal values seen with underlying nerve injury.

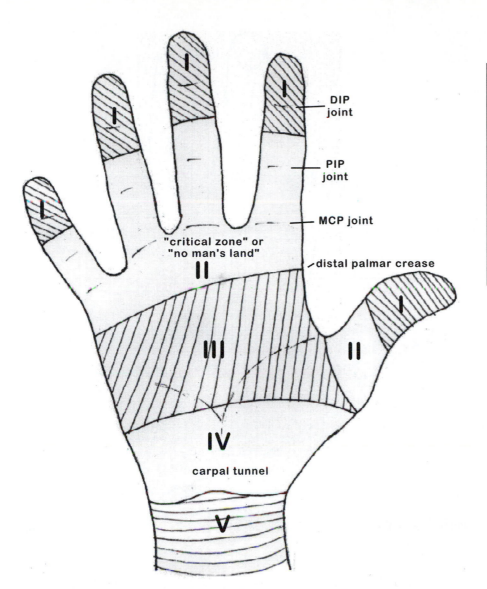

FIGURE 29-2. Flexor tendon zones of the hand. (Artwork by Elizabeth N. Jacobson, Mayo Medical School.)

- Immersion test: Skin on palm of hand should wrinkle within 10 minutes when immersed in water. Failure to do so suggests underlying nerve injury.
2. Strength:
   - Test grip
   - Fromment's sign
3. Vascular:
   - Capillary refill: Normal is < 2 seconds.
   - Allen test:
     - Patient makes a tight fist for 20 seconds.
     - Examiner occludes both ulnar and radial arteries by holding direct pressure.
     - Examiner releases ulnar artery—a normal (patent) radial artery will perfuse the hand within 5 to 7 seconds (color returns).
     - Test is repeated with the radial artery released to check ulnar flow.

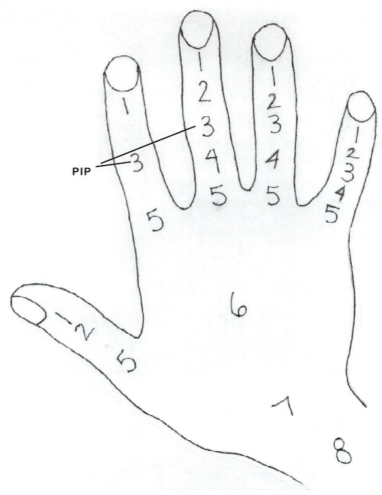

FIGURE 29-3. Extensor tendon zones of the hand. (Artwork by Elizabeth N. Jacobson, Mayo Medical School.)

4. Motor and sensory function:
   - See section under Nerves for which nerves supply which muscles and sensory areas.
   - See Table 29-3.

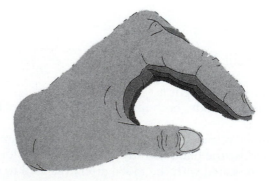

FIGURE 29-4. "Safe" position of hand.

490

TABLE 29-3. Clinical maneuvers for testing muscles of the hand.

Patient Maneuver	Muscle Tested
Making a fist	
Bending the tip of the thumb	Flexor pollicis longus
Bending each individual fingertip against resistance while PIPs are stabilized by examiner	Flexor digitorum profundus
Bending each individual fingertip against resistance while DIPs are stabilized by examiner	Flexor digitorum superficialis
Bring thumb out to side and back	Extensor pollicis brevis and abductor pollicis longus
Flexing and extending a fist at the wrist	Extensor carpi radialis longus and brevis
Raising thumb only while rest of hand is laid flat	Extensor pollicis longus
Making a fist with little finger extended alone	Extensor digiti minimi

NERVE BLOCKS

- Used to anesthesize a portion of the hand innervated by certain nerve(s) (see Figure 29-4)
- Advantages over local anesthesia:
  - Does not distort area you want to examine/suture
  - Eliminates need for multiple injections

INFECTIONS OF THE HAND

Felon

DEFINITION

Infection of the pulp space of any of the distal phalanges (see Figure 29-5).

ETIOLOGY

Caused by minor trauma to the dermis over the finger pad.

COMPLICATIONS

Results in increased pressure within the septal compartments and may lead to cellulitis, flexor tendon sheath infection, or osteomyelitis if not effectively treated.

TREATMENT

- Using a digital block, perform incision and drainage with longitudinal incision over the area of greatest induration but not over the flexor crease of the DIP.

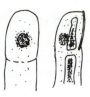

FIGURE 29-5. Felon (infection of pulp space). (Reproduced, with permission, from DeGowin RL, Brown DD. *DeGowin's Diagnostic Examination,* 7th ed. New York: McGraw-Hill, 2000: 703.)

- Drain may be placed and wound checked in 2 days.
- Antibiotics: Usually first-generation cephalosporin or anti-*Staphylococcus* penicillin

Paronychia

DEFINITION

Infection of the lateral nail fold (see Figure 29-6)

ETIOLOGY

Caused by minor trauma such as nail biting or manicures.

TREATMENT

- Without fluctuance, this may be treated with a 7-day course of antibiotics, warm soaks, and retraction of the skin edges from the nail margin.
- For more extensive infections, unroll the skin at the base of the nail and at the lateral nail or incision and drainage (I&D) at area of most fluctuans using a digital block. Pus below the nailbed may require partial or total removal of the nail. Warm soaks and wound check in 2 days. Antibiotics are usually not necessary unless area is cellulitic.

Tenosynovitis

ETIOLOGY

This is a surgical emergency requiring prompt identification. Infection of the flexor tendon and sheath is caused by penetrating trauma and dirty wounds (e.g., dog bite). Infection spreads along the tendon sheath, allowing involvement of other digits and even the entire hand causing significant disability.

Kanavel signs of tenosynovitis: **STEP**
Symmetrical swelling of finger.
Tenderness over flexor tendon sheath.
Extension (passive) of digit is painful.
Posture of digit at rest is flexed.

FIGURE 29-6. Paronychia. (Reproduced, with permission, from DeGowin RL, Brown DD. *DeGowin's Diagnostic Examination,* 7th ed. New York: McGraw-Hill, 2000: 703.)

ORGANISMS

- Polymicrobial
- *Staphylococcus* most common
- *Neisseria gonorrhoeae* with history of sexually transmitted disease (STD)

TREATMENT

- Immobilize and elevate hand.
- Immediate consultation with hand surgeon.
- Parenteral antibiotics; first-generation cephalosporin and penicillin, or beta-lactamase inhibitor

GAMEKEEPER'S THUMB

DEFINITION

Avulsion of ulnar collateral ligament of first MCP joint.

ETIOLOGY

- Forced abduction of the thumb
- Can be associated with an avulsion fracture of the metacarpal base

SIGNS AND SYMPTOMS

- Inability to pinch.

DIAGNOSIS

- Application of valgus stress to thumb while MCP joint is flexed will demonstrate laxity of ulnar collateral ligament.

TREATMENT

- Rest, ice, elevation, analgesia
- Thumb spica cast for 3 to 6 weeks for partial tears
- Surgical repair for complete tears

Gamekeeper's thumb is commonly associated with ski pole injury (see Figure 29-7).

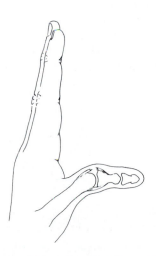

FIGURE 29-7. Gamekeeper's thumb. (Reproduced, with permission, from Scaletta TA et al. *Emergent Management of Trauma.* New York: McGraw-Hill, 1996: 220.)

Carpal tunnel syndrome is the most common entrapment neuropathy.

Typical scenario: A 37-year-old female presents with pain in her right wrist and fingers, accompanied by a tingling sensation. The pain awakens her from sleep, and she is unable to perform her duties as a word processor. *Think:* Carpal tunnel syndrome.

DEFINITION

Compression of the median nerve resulting in pain along the distribution of the nerve (see Figure 29-8).

ETIOLOGY

- Tumor (fibroma, lipoma)
- Ganglion cyst
- Tenosynovitis of flexor tendons secondary to rheumatoid arthritis or trauma
- Edema due to pregnancy, thyroid or amyloid disease
- Trauma to carpal bones
- Gout

RISK FACTORS

Repetitive hand movements.

EPIDEMIOLOGY

More common in women 3:1.

SIGNS AND SYMPTOMS

- Pain and paresthesia of volar aspect of thumb, digits 2 and 3, and half of digit 4.
- Activity and palmar flexion aggravate symptoms.
- Thenar atrophy: Uncommon but irreversible and indicates severe long-standing compression
- Sensory deficit (two-point discrimination > 5 mm)

DIAGNOSIS

- **Tinel's test:** Tapping over median nerve at wrist produces pain and paresthesia.

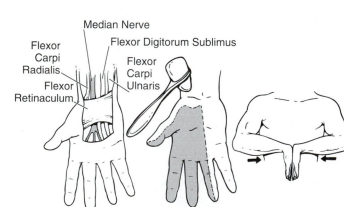

FIGURE 29-8. Carpal tunnel syndrome. (Reproduced, with permission, from DeGowin RL, Brown DD. *DeGowin's Diagnostic Examination*, 7th ed. New York: McGraw-Hill, 2000: 720.)

- One minute of maximal palmar flexion produces pain and paresthesia.
- Consider erythrocyte sedimentation rate (ESR), thyroid function tests (TFTs), serum glucose, and uric acid level to look for underlying cause.

TREATMENT

- Treat underlying condition.
- Rest and splint.
- Nonsteroidal anti-inflammatory drugs (NSAIDs) for analgesia
- Surgery for crippling pain, thenar atrophy and failure of nonoperative management

Twenty to 50% of the population normally have a positive Phalen's and Tinel's test.

GANGLION CYST

DEFINITION

A synovial cyst, usually present on radial aspect of wrist.

ETIOLOGY

Idiopathic.

SIGNS AND SYMPTOMS

- Presence of mass that patient cannot account for
- May or may not be painful
- Pain aggravated by extreme flexion or extension
- Size of ganglia increases with increased use of wrist
- Compression of median or ulnar nerve may occur (not common)

DIAGNOSIS

- Radiographs to ascertain diagnosis; since a ganglion cyst is a soft tissue problem only, no radiographic changes should be noted.

Differential diagnosis includes bone tumor, arthritis, and intraosseus ganglion.

TREATMENT

- Reassurance for most cases
- Wrist immobilization for moderate pain
- Aspiration of cyst for severe pain
- Surgical excision for cases involving median nerve compression and cosmetically unacceptable ganglia

MALLET FINGER

DEFINITION

Rupture of extensor tendon at its insertion into base of distal phalanx (see Figure 29-9).

ETIOLOGY

- Avulsion fracture of distal phalanx
- Other trauma

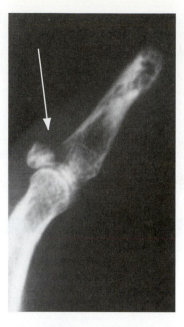

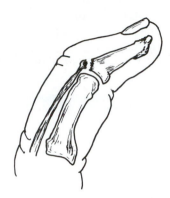

FIGURE 29-9. Mallet finger. (Reproduced, with permission, from Schwartz DT, Reisdorf EJ. *Emergency Radiology.* New York: McGraw-Hill, 2000: 40.)

SIGNS AND SYMPTOMS

Inability to extend DIP joint.

TREATMENT

- Splint finger in extension for 6 to 8 weeks.
- Surgery may be required for large avulsions of distal phalanx and for injuries that were not splinted early.

TRIGGER FINGER

DEFINITION

Stenosis of tendon sheath flexor digitorum, leading to nodule formation within the sheath (see Figure 29-10).

RISK FACTORS

- Rheumatoid arthritis
- Middle-aged women
- Congenital

FIGURE 29-10. Trigger finger. (Reproduced, with permission, from DeGowin RL, Brown DD. *DeGowin's Diagnostic Examination,* 7th ed. New York: McGraw-Hill, 2000: 701.)

> Left untreated, mallet finger results in permanent boutonniere deformity.

SIGNS AND SYMPTOMS

Snapping sensation or click when flexing and extending the digit.

TREATMENT

- Splinting of MP joint in extension
- Injection of corticosteroid into tendon sheath
- Surgical repair if above fail

AMPUTATION INJURIES

Prognosis is best for:
- Sharp vs. crush or avulsion amputations
- Children vs. adults
- Clean vs. dirty

INDICATIONS

- Amputations with good prognosis as listed above.
- Thumb amputations (unlike other single digits, amputation of the thumb leaves a significant deficit in function of the hand)
- Multiple digit amputations

CONTRAINDICATIONS

- Amputations in smokers (poor healing). This is especially true if patient cannot commit to abstain from smoking for a 3-month period post reimplantation
- Severe crush or avulsion injury
- Grossly contaminated injuries
- Amputations at multiple levels along the amputated limb

COMPLICATIONS

- Stiffness.
- Cold intolerance.
- Decreased sensibility.
- Patients often require long-term hand therapy following surgery.

PREOPERATIVE MANAGEMENT

- IV antibiotics.
- Tetanus prophylaxis.
- NPO for possible surgery.
- Gentle cleansing of wound site and amputated part with saline or lactated Ringer's.
- Wrap amputated part in sterile gauze.
- X-ray both limb and amputated part.

HIGH-PRESSURE INJECTION INJURIES

- Commonly associated with grease guns, spray guns, and diesel fuel injectors
- Usually occurs to index finger of nondominant hand, index finger

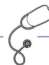

Do not be fooled by how insignificant a high-pressure injection injury to the hand appears on initial presentation.

HIGH-YIELD FACTS

The Hand

- Seemingly innocuous puncture wound at initial presentation
- Edema and minimal pain progress to more severe pain, discoloration, and swelling, then to intense tissue necrosis within 24 hours

DIAGNOSIS

- Hand radiograph may reveal path of injectate if radiopaque.

TREATMENT

- IV antibiotics
- I&D—often operative; obtain hand surgery consult
- Amputation may be necessary if part not salvageable
- Physical therapy after acute management

OTHER COMMON HAND AND WRIST INJURIES

- Please see Table 29-4.

TABLE 29-4. Common hand and wrist injuries.

Injury	Description	Treatment
Boxer's fracture	Fracture of neck of fifth metacarpal sustained in a closed fist injury	■ Thumb spica cast for 3–6 weeks for partial tears ■ Surgical repair for: ■ Any rotational deformity 　■ Angulation of fourth/fifth metacarpal > 40° 　■ Angulation of second/third metacarpal > 10–15°
Bennet fracture	Fracture–dislocation of base of thumb	■ Initially immobilization in thumb spica cast ■ Definitive treatment is with surgical fixation
Rolando fracture	Comminuted fracture of the base of the thumb	■ Initially immobilization in thumb spica cast ■ Definitive treatment is surgical fixation
Scaphoid fracture	■ Most commonly caused by fall on outstretched hand ■ Snuffbox tenderness is classic	■ Immobilization in thumb spica cast with wrist in neutral position for 12 weeks ■ May take up to 2 weeks to be seen on radiographs
Colles' fracture	■ Distal radius fracture with dorsal angulation ■ Most commonly caused by fall on outstretched hand ■ "Dinner fork deformity" is classic	■ Short arm cast for 4–6 weeks with volar flexion and ulnar deviation ■ Surgical repair for: 　■ Open fracture 　■ Comminuted fracture 　■ Intra-articular displaced fracture > 5 mm

(continues)

TABLE 29-4. Common hand and wrist injuries. (continued)

Injury	Description	Treatment
Smith fracture	■ Distal radius fracture with volar angulation ■ Most commonly caused by direct trauma to dorsal forearm	■ Surgical repair needed for most cases
Galeazzi fracture	■ Distal one-third radial fracture with dislocation of distal radioulnar joint ■ Commonly caused by fall on outstretched hand with forearm in forced pronation or direct blow to back of wrist	■ Surgical repair needed for most cases
Monteggia fracture	■ Proximal one-third ulnar fracture with dislocation of the radial head ■ Commonly caused by fall on outstretched hand with forearm in forced pronation or direct blow to posterior ulna ■ May note injury of radial nerve	■ Surgical repair for adults ■ Closed reduction for children (children can tolerate a greater degree of displacement)
Nightstick fracture	■ Isolated fracture of the ulnar shaft	■ Long arm cast for 3–6 weeks ■ Surgical repair for: 　■ Angulation > 10° 　■ Displacement > 50%

HIGH-YIELD FACTS

The Hand

Classified Awards for Surgery

GENERAL AND ONCOLOGY

American Association for the Surgery of Trauma

The AAST has a program whereby up to five interested medical students per year can attend the AAST Annual Meeting. Students must be nominated by a department of surgery or orthopedics at their home institution, and will be selected by the AAST scholarship committee. The scholarship covers conference registration, meals, and lodging, plus an additional $25/day for incidentals. It is the responsibility of the sponsoring institution to cover transportation costs. Deadline is June 1. Contact: *www.aast.org*

American Medical Association Education and Research Foundation

Open to third- and fourth-year medical students who have completed the required clerkships in medicine, surgery, and pediatrics. The program consists of 4- to 6-week clerkships in general, pediatric, and surgical nutrition. Scholarships are only for students who do not have clinical nutrition clerkships available at their own schools. Students accepted into the program will receive a $700 award to defray living and traveling costs. Deadline: August 1 for December–June clerkships; February 1 for June–December clerkships. Contact: *www.ama-assn.org*

American College of Chest Surgeons—Alfred A. Richman International Essay & Research Contest

This contest is offered to encourage and stimulate medical students to explore and investigate problems relating to the disciplines of respiration and circulation. The author of the best research paper will receive $1,000. Deadline: May 31. Contact: American College of Chest Physicians, 300 Dundee Rd, Northbrook, IL 60062-2348. Phone: (800) 343-2227. Web site: *www.chestnet.org*

Society for Clinical Vascular Surgery Allastair Karmody Essay Contest

Medical students should submit an essay based on experimental or clinical analysis and review of previously published data on the anatomy, physiology, pathology, biochemistry, or genetics of the vascular system and its diseases. There is a $1,000 award plus transportation and accommodations at the Society's Annual Meeting. Deadline: January 15.

Lehigh Valley Hospital Internships

Twelve-week practical learning experience shaped to the student's knowledge and experience. Over 40 positions in a variety of health-related careers in six Lehigh Valley health care facilities are available to college, graduate, and medical students. Five areas are suitable for medical students: emergency medicine, infection control, respiratory therapy, clinical surgery, and research surgery. Salary is $200/week. Deadline: March 20.

Roswell Park Cancer Institute—Summer Oncology Research Program

A structured 8-week summer program that gives you the opportunity to expand your horizons in the care and treatment of the cancer patient by participating in state-of-the-art clinical research. Dates are set; contact institute for specifics. Stipend is $250/week. Deadline is February 15. Contact: Arthur M. Michalek, PhD, Roswell Park Cancer Institute, Carlton and Elm Streets, Buffalo, NY 14263. Phone: (585) 845-2300. E-mail: *michalek@sc3102.med.buf falo.edu*. Web site: *www.roswellpark.org*

University of Texas M. D. Anderson Cancer Center—Medical Student Summer Research Program in Biomedical Sciences

The purpose of this 10-week program is to provide participants with firsthand biomedical research experience in the basic or clinical sciences. Student projects are submitted by faculty mentors at the Cancer Center and will reflect ongoing research efforts in the institution's clinics and laboratories. Students will actively participate in both the technical aspects of their project as well as interpretation of experimental data. Stipend is $2,500 for the summer. Deadline is in late February. Contact: Michael Ahearn, PhD, Summer Research Program for Medical Students, University of Texas M. D. Anderson Cancer Center, 1515 Holcombe Boulevard, Box 240, Houston, TX 77030. Phone: (713) 745-1205. E-mail: *mahearn@notes.mdacc.tmc.edu*

NEUROSURGERY AND NEUROLOGY

The American Association of Neurological Surgeons (*www.neurosurgery.org*) does not have a student membership or any specific awards for medical students, but their Web site is informative and worth checking out for those interested in the field.

American Association of Neurology (AAN)

Student Interest Group in Neurology (SIGN) brings together medical students who are interested in exploring the practice of neurology. The American Academy of Neurology (AAN) supports each SIGN chapter along with the neurology department or dean's office at each member's institution. Benefits of SIGN membership include free AAN membership. Firsthand experience:

- Shadow a neurologist.
- Be matched with a mentor.
- Meet professors.
- Meet neurologists in private practice.
- Meet attendings.
- Meet residents.

AAN Medical Student Essay Awards

These awards seek to stimulate interest in the field of neurology as an exciting and challenging profession by offering highly competitive awards for the best essay. Four awards are offered in the following categories:

- G. Milton Shy Award in Clinical Neurology
- Saul R. Korey Award in Experimental Neurology
- Roland P. MacKay Award in Historical Aspects
- Extended Neuroscience Award

Recipients are expected to give a poster presentation based on the selected manuscript at the AAN 55th Annual Meeting. Recipient will receive:

- Certificate of recognition
- $350 prize (Shy, Korey, and MacKay)
- $1,000 prize (Extended Neuroscience)
- Complimentary registration for Annual Meeting
- One-year complimentary subscription to *Neurology* journal
- Reimbursement for Annual Meeting travel, lodging, and meal expenses (up to 2 days)
- Recognition at Awards Luncheon at Annual Meeting

Contact Melissa Meath at *mmeath@aan.com* for more information.

AAN Medical Student Prize for Excellence in Neurology

Awarded annually to a graduating medical student who exemplifies outstanding scientific achievement and clinical acumen in neurology or neuroscience, and outstanding personal qualities of integrity, compassion, and leadership. A Certificate of Recognition and a check for $200 will be presented on behalf of the AAN during the graduation or awards ceremony at each institution. The names of the awardees will be listed in *AANews* and on the AAN Web site. Press releases will be sent to local newspapers. All application material must be received by March 15, 2003. Submit material to: Medical Student Prize for Excellence in Neurology, Gloria Barnard, American Academy of Neurology, 1080 Montreal Avenue, St. Paul, MN 55116. For additional information, contact Gloria Barnard at *gbarnard@aan.com*. Phone: (651) 695-2733. Fax: (651) 695-2791.

Michael S. Pessin Stroke Leadership Prize

This award recognizes emerging neurologists who have a strong interest in, and have demonstrated a passion for, learning and expanding the field of stroke research. Applicants should have an active involvement in providing patients with the highest quality of compassionate care. This award is intended to stimulate and reward individuals who demonstrate a passion for stroke in the developmental stages of their careers. Recipient will receive:

- Certificate of recognition and $1,500 prize
- Complimentary registration for 55th Annual Meeting
- Recognition at 2003 Awards Luncheon at 55th Annual Meeting

Contact DeAnn Mbuve at *dmbuve@aan.com* for more information.

AAN 2003 Aventis Minority Scholars Award

The 2003 Aventis Minority Scholars Award is funded by Aventis Pharmaceuticals and was established to increase diversity among neurologists. It provides up to eight scholarships for medical students meeting eligibility requirements. Award recipients will receive:

- $2,000 stipend
- Complimentary registration for the AAN Annual Meeting
- Educational program fees at junior member rates for the AAN Annual Meeting

All application materials must be received by November 1, 2002. Mail all applications and materials to: Aventis Pharmaceuticals Minority Scholarship, American Academy of Neurology, Education & Research Foundation, 1080 Montreal Avenue, St. Paul, MN 55116.

Medical Student Summer Research Scholarship

Sponsored by the AAN's Undergraduate Education Subcommittee, the Medical Student Summer Research Scholarship program offers members of the AAN's Student Interest Group in Neurology (SIGN) program a summer stipend of $3,000 to conduct a project either in an institutional, clinical, or laboratory setting where there are ongoing programs of research, service, or training, or in a private practice. Only applicants from schools with established SIGN chapters are eligible to apply. The scholarship program was established to stimulate individuals to pursue careers in neurology in either research or practice settings.

The AAN will award up to 20 scholarships to first- or second-year medical students who have a supporting preceptor and a project with clearly defined goals. The project is to be conducted through a U.S. or Canadian institution of the student's choice and jointly designed by the student and sponsoring institution. More than one student from an institution may apply, but only one student will be selected from an institution.

For application forms and guidelines or SIGN chapter registration materials, contact Gloria Barnard at *gbarnard@aan.com*.

Medical Student Scholarships to the Annual Meeting

The AAN and the Association of University Professors of Neurology (AUPN) are working together to stimulate medical students' interest in neurology programs and are jointly offering a scholarship to fund medical students' attendance at the AAN Annual Meeting. Through a grant from Aventis Pharmaceuticals, twenty $500 scholarships are available to SIGN chapter presidents or a designated SIGN representative nominated by their Program Director or SIGN Faculty Contact.

Scholarships are awarded on a first-come, first-served basis, based on the following criteria:

- Student must be from a registered SIGN chapter and serve as either the SIGN chapter president or a designated representative.
- Department chair will provide a supplemental grant to the student so that all expenses can be covered.
- Student must attend the SIGN meeting at the Annual Meeting in order to receive the scholarship. The award will be mailed to the student after the Annual Meeting.

For additional information, contact Gloria Barnard at *gbarnard@aan.com*.

American College of Neuropsychopharmacology—Pharmacia & Upjohn, Inc.—Minority Summer Fellow Program

This grant is made available to promote and enhance the interest of minority graduate students and residents in careers in psychopharmacology and the neurosciences. The grant provides support for one student to carry out a research project for 6 to 8 weeks in the summer. Stipend is $6,000 and covers room and board and transportation and funds to attend the Annual Meeting to present a poster covering the summer project. Deadline is April 1. Contact: Huda Akil, PhD, Mental Health Research Institute, 205 Zina Pitcher Place, University of Michigan, Ann Arbor, MI 48109. E-mail: *acnp@ctrvax.vander bilt.edu*. Web site: *www.acnp.org*

OPHTHALMOLOGY

National Society to Prevent Blindness Fight for Sight Fellowships

Student summer fellowships $500/month for 3-month maximum. Deadline: March 1. For more information, contact: Fight for Sight, Research Division, Prevent Blindness America, 500 East Remington Road, Schaumburg, IL 60173. Web site: *www.preventblindness.org*

University of California at Davis Ophthalmology Summer Fellowship

Summer fellowships in basic science research in ophthalmology available for first-, second-, or third-year medical students. Stipend is $1,500. Deadline: December. Web site: *www.ucdmc.ucdavis.edu*

ORTHOPEDICS

Hospital for Joint Diseases (NY) Summer Externships in Orthopedic Research

For 2 to 3 summer months. $500/month. Contact: Hospital for Joint Diseases, 301 East 17th Street, New York, NY 10003.

Harvard Pinkney Summer Scholar Program in Orthopaedics

The purpose of this award is to allow the recipient to pursue some scholarly activity in either clinical or basic orthopaedic science at the Massachusetts General Hospital for 2 months during the summer. The student may be in any year of medical school. The award is $1,000. Deadline: March 15. Contact: Henry J. Mankin, MD, Massachusetts General Hospital, Department of Orthopaedic Surgery, Gray Building, Room 606, 55 Fruit Street, Boston, MA 02114-2696. Phone: (617) 724-3700. E-mail: *mankinh@medex.mgh.harvard.edu*

UROLOGY

American Foundation for Urological Disease & American Urological Association Medical Student Summer Fellowship

Outstanding medical students who wish to work on an introductory research fellowship in an established urology laboratory in the summer immediately prior to or during medical school. An accredited medical research institution/department must sponsor the candidate by guaranteeing adequate support, including responsibility for the adequacy of the environment for research and development. Deadline for application is February 1. A salary stipend of $2,000 is paid directly to the scholar by AFUD. The stipend will be payable for 2 months (July 15 and August 15) at $1,000 per month.

For more information, contact: Kym Liddick, Manager, Research Scholar Program, 1128 N. Charles Street, Baltimore, MD 21201. Phone: (410) 468-1812. Fax: (410) 468-1808. E-mail: *kym@afud.org*

OTORHINOLARYNGOLOGY (ENT)

American Otological Society Medical Student Research Training Fellowships

The society's main interest is to study otosclerosis, Ménière's disease, and related disorders. Fellowship applications must be postmarked by January 31 of the year in which the grant is to begin. Grants run July to June. Information and material may be obtained from: Jeffrey P. Harris, MD, PhD, Research Fund of the American Otologic Society, Inc., Professor and Chairman, Department of Otolaryngology–Head and Neck Surgery, University of California, San Diego, 200 W. Arbor Drive, 8895, San Diego, CA 92103-8895. Phone: (619) 543-7896. Fax: (619) 543-5521. E-mail: *jpharris@ucsd.edu*. Inquiries about the program go to: *mseva@ucsd.edu*.

So, you want to be a surgeon? Check out . . . *www.facs.org/residencysearch* for an online medical student's guide to finding and matching with the best possible surgical residency.

Index

Pages followed by f indicate figure; those followed by t indicate table.